MASTER TECHNIQUES IN ORTHOPAEDIC SURGERY

Editor-in-Chief
Bernard F. Morrey, M.D.

Founding Editor
Roby C. Thompson Jr, M.D.

Volume Editors

Surgical Exposures
Bernard F. Morrey, M.D.
Matthew C. Morrey, M.D.

The Hand
James Strickland, M.D.
Thomas Graham, M.D.

The Wrist
Richard H. Gelberman, M.D.

The Elbow
Bernard F. Morrey, M.D.

The Shoulder
Edward V. Craig, M.D.

The Spine
David S. Bradford, M.D.
Thomas L. Zdeblick, M.D.

The Hip
Robert L. Barrack, M.D.

Reconstructive Knee Surgery
Douglas W. Jackson, M.D.

Knee Arthroplasty
Paul Lotke, M.D.
Jess H. Lonner, M.D.

The Foot & Ankle
Harold B. Kitaoka, M.D.

Fractures
Donald A. Wiss, M.D.

Pediatrics
Vernon T. Tolo, M.D.
David L. Skaggs, M.D.

Soft Tissue Surgery
Steven L. Moran, M.D.
William P. Cooney III, M.D.

Sports Medicine
Freddie H. Fu, M.D.

Orthopaedic Oncology and Complex Reconstruction
Franklin H. Sim, M.D.
Peter F.M. Choong, M.D.
Kristy L. Weber, M.D.

Master Techniques in Orthopaedic Surgery

Orthopaedic Oncology and Complex Reconstruction

Editors

Franklin H. Sim, M.D.
Professor
Department of Orthopaedic Oncology and Orthopaedic Surgery
Mayo Clinic
Rochester, Minnesota

Peter F.M. Choong, M.D., M.B.B.S.
Sir Hugh Devine Chair of Surgery
Head, Department of Surgery
University of Melbourne
St. Vincent's Hospital
Chair, Sarcoma Service
Peter MacCallum Cancer Centre
Director of Orthopaedics
St. Vincent's Hospital
Melbourne, Victoria, Australia

Kristy L. Weber, M.D.
Professor
Departments of Orthopaedics and Oncology
Johns Hopkins School of Medicine
Baltimore, Maryland

 Wolters Kluwer | Lippincott Williams & Wilkins
Health

Philadelphia • Baltimore • New York • London
Buenos Aires • Hong Kong • Sydney • Tokyo

Acquisitions Editor: Robert Hurley
Product Manager: Elise M. Paxson
Production Manager: Bridgett Dougherty
Senior Manufacturing Manager: Benjamin Rivera
Marketing Manager: Lisa Lawrence
Design Coordinator: Doug Smock
Production Service: SPi Global

Printed in China

Library of Congress Cataloging-in-Publication Data
Orthopaedic oncology and complex reconstruction / editors, Franklin H. Sim, Peter F.M. Choong, Kristy L. Weber. — 1st ed.
    p. ; cm. — (Master techniques in orthopaedic surgery)
  Includes bibliographical references.
  ISBN 978-1-60831-043-2 (hardback)
 1. Bones—Cancer. 2. Bones—Surgery. 3. Orthopedic surgery. I. Sim, Franklin H.
(Franklin Hindson), 1940- II. Choong, Peter F. M. III. Weber, Kristy L. IV. Series: Master techniques in orthopaedic surgery.
  [DNLM: 1. Bone Neoplasms—surgery. 2. Orthopedic Procedures—methods. 3. Reconstructive Surgical Procedures—methods. 4. Soft Tissue Neoplasms—surgery. WE 258]
  RC280.B6O78 2011
  616.99'471—dc23

                                       2011014512

To purchase additional copies of this book, call our customer service department at (800) 638-3030 or fax orders to (301) 223-2320. International customers should call (301) 223-2300.

Visit Lippincott Williams & Wilkins on the Internet: at LWW.com. Lippincott Williams & Wilkins customer service representatives are available from 8:30 am to 6 pm, EST.

                             10 9 8 7 6 5 4 3 2 1

This book on complex reconstructions is dedicated to the "reconstructive team" including surgeons, bioengineers, materials scientists and manufacturers who have devoted their energy, expertise and commitment to restoring function in our brave cancer patients with limb salvage, as well as those with bone loss associated with trauma or failed arthroplasties. Multiple disciplines working together have improved the outcome for our inspiring patients.

Contributors

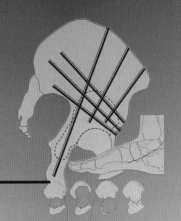

Luis A. Aponte-Tinao, M.D.
Orthopaedic Oncology Service
Institute of Orthopedics "Carlos E. Ottolenghi"
Italian Hospital of Buenos Aires
Buenos Aires, Argentina

Miguel A. Ayerza, M.D., Ph.D.
Associate Professor
Department of Orthopaedics
University of Buenos Aires
Chief
Orthopaedic Oncology Section
Italian hospital of Buenos Aires
Buenos Aires, Argentina

George C. Babis, M.D.
First Department of Orthopaedics
Athens University Medical School
Athens, Greece

Christopher P. Beauchaump, M.D.
Chair, Surgical Committee
Associate Professor
Mayo Graduate School of Medicine
Mayo Clinic
Scottsdale, Arizona

Peter F. M. Choong, M.B.B.S., M.D., F.R.A.C.S, F.A.Orth.A.
Sir Hugh Devine Professor of Surgery and Head
Department of Surgery
University of Melbourne
Director of Orthopaedics
Department of Orthopaedics
St. Vincent's Hospital Melbourne
Fitzroy, Victoria, Australia

Timothy A. Damron, M.D.
Vice-chair and David G. Murray Professor of Orthopedics
SUNY Upstate Department of Orthopedic Surgery
SUNY Upstate Medical University
Upstate Bone and Joint Center
East Syracuse, New York
Attending Orthopedic Surgeon
SUNY Upstate Department of Orthopedic Surgery
SUNY Upstate University Hospital
Syracuse, New York

Peter A. J. de Leeuw, M.D.
Academic Medical Center
Department of Orthopaedic Surgery
University of Amsterdam
Amsterdam, The Netherlands

Martin Dominkus, M.D.
Associate Professor
Department of Orthopaedics
Medical University of Vienna
Vienna, Austria

Costantino Errani, M.D., Ph.D.
Department of Orthopaedic Service
University of Bologna
Research Fellow
Department of Orthopaedic Service
Istituto Ortopedico Rizzoli
Bologna, Italy

Nicola Fabbri, M.D.
Associate Professor of Orthopaedic Surgery and Attending
    Surgeon
Department of Musculoskeletal Oncology
Istituto Ortopedico Rizzoli
Bologna, Italy

German L. Farfalli
Orthopaedic Surgeon
Department of Surgery
Italian Hospital of Buenos Aires
Buenos Aires, Argentina

David Jacofsky, M.D.
Chairman
The Center for Orthopaedic Research and Education
Phoenix, Arizona

Fazel A. Khan, M.D.
Resident
Department of Orthopaedic Surgery
Mayo Clinic
Rochester, Minnesota

Rainer Kotz, M.D.
Medical University of Vienna Department of Orthopaedic
  Surgery
Vienna General Hospital
Vienna, Austria

Andreas F. Mavrogenis, M.D.
Orthopaedic Surgeon
Holargos, Athens, Greece

Mario Mercuri, M.D.
Associate Professor
Department of Orthopaedic Service
University of Bologna
Chief
Department of Orthopaedic Service
Istituto Ortopedico Rizzoli
Bologna, Italy

Bernard F. Morrey, M.D.
Professor in Orthopaedics
Mayo Clinic College of Medicine
Emeritus Consultant of Orthopaedic Surgery
Department of Orthopaedic Surgery
Mayo Clinic
Rochester, Minnesota

S. M. Javad Mortazavi, M.D.
Associate Professor
Department of Orthopaedic Surgery
Tehran University of Medical Sciences
Director of Education
Department of Orthopaedic Surgery
Imam University Hospital
Tehran, Iran

D. Luis Muscolo, M.D.
Professor
Department of Orthopaedic Surgery
University of Buenos Aires
Honorary Chief

Orthopaedic Department
Italian Hospital of Buenos Aires
Buenos Aires, Argentina

Mary I. O'Connor, M.D.
Associate Professor
Chair
Department of Orthopedic Surgery
Mayo Clinic
Jacksonville, Florida

Panayiotis J. Papagelopoulos, M.D., D.Sc.
Professor
Department of Orthopaedics
Athens University Medical School
Amarousio, Athens, Greece
Chairman
Department of Orthopaedics
Attikon University General Hospital
Haidari, Athens, Greece

Javad Parvizi, M.D.
Professor
Department of Orthopaedic Surgery
Thomas Jefferson University Hospital
Vice Chairman Research
Department of Orthopaedic Surgery
Rothman Institute
Philadelphia, Pennsylvania

Mikel L. Reilingh, M.D.
Academic Medical Center
Department of Orthopaedic Surgery
University of Amsterdam
Amsterdam, The Netherlands

Peter S. Rose, M.D.
Assistant Professor
Department of Orthopedic Surgery
Mayo Clinic
Rochester, Minnesota

Vasileios I. Sakellariou, M.D.
Department of Orthopaedics
Attikon University Hospital
Athens, Greece

Joaquin Sanchez-Sotelo, M.D., Ph.D.
Associate Professor
Department of Orthopedic Surgery
Mayo Graduate Medical School
Consultant
Orthopedic Surgery
Mayo Clinic
Rochester, Minnesota

Adam J. Schwartz
Instructor

Senior Associate Consultant
Department of Orthopedic Surgery
Mayo Clinic Arizona
Phoenix, Arizona

Franklin H. Sim, M.D.
Professor
Department of Orthopaedic Oncology and Orthopaedic
    Surgery
Mayo Clinic
Rochester, Minnesota

Bryan D. Springer, M.D.
Attending Orthopedic Surgeon
Ortho Carolina Hip and Knee Center
Charlotte, North Carolina

Roger M. Tillman, F.R.C.S., F.R.C.S., Orth.
Consultant Orthopaedic Surgeon
Royal Orthopaedic Hospital
Senior Lecturer
University of Birmingham
Birmingham, United Kingdom

Norman S. Turner III, M.D.
Assistant Professor
Consultant
Department of Orthopedic Surgery
Mayo Clinic
Rochester, Minnesota

Timothy J. van de Leur, M.D.
Department of Orthopaedics
Fort Wayne Orthopaedics
Fort Wayne, Indiana

C. Niek van Dijk, M.D., Ph.D.
Academic Medical Center
Department of Orthopaedic Surgery
University of Amsterdam
Amsterdam, The Netherlands

Maayke N. van Sterkenburg, M.D.
Academic Medical Center
Department of Orthopaedic Surgery
University of Amsterdam
Amsterdam, The Netherlands

Kristy L. Weber, M.D.
Professor
Department of Orthopaedic Surgery and Oncology
John Hopkin's University School of Medicine
John Hopkin's Hospital
Baltimore, Maryland

Michael J. Yaszemski, M.D., Ph.D.
Krehbiel Family Endowed Professor of Orthopedic Surgery
    and Biomedical Engineering
Mayo Clinic College of Medicine
Chair, Division of Spine Surgery
Department of Orthopedic Surgery
Mayo Clinic
Director, Tissue Engineering and Biomaterials Laboratory
Departments of Orthopedic Surgery and of Physiology and
    Biomedical Engineering
Mayo Clinic College of Medicine
Rochester, Minnesota

Series Preface

Since its inception in 1994, the *Master Techniques in Orthopaedic Surgery* series has become the gold standard for both physicians in training and experienced surgeons. Its exceptional success may be traced to the leadership of the original series editor, Roby Thompson, whose clarity of thought and focused vision sought "to provide direct, detailed access to techniques preferred by orthopaedic surgeons who are recognized by their colleagues as 'masters' in their specialty," as he stated in his series preface. It is personally very rewarding to hear testimonials from both residents and practicing orthopaedic surgeons on the value of these volumes to their training and practice.

A key element of the success of the series is its format. The effectiveness of the format is reflected by the fact that it is now being replicated by others. An essential feature is the standardized presentation of information replete with tips and pearls shared by experts with years of experience.

Abundant color photographs and drawings guide the reader through the procedures step-by-step.

The second key to the success of the *Master Techniques* series rests in the reputation and experience of our volume editors. The editors are truly dedicated "masters" with a commitment to share their rich experience through these texts. We feel a great debt of gratitude to them and a real responsibility to maintain and enhance the reputation of the *Master Techniques* series that has developed over the years. We are proud of the progress made in formulating the third edition volumes and are particularly pleased with the expanded content of this series. Six new volumes will soon be available covering topics that are exciting and relevant to a broad cross section of our profession. While we are in the process of carefully expanding *Master Techniques* topics and editors, we are committed to the now-classic format.

The first of the new volumes is *Relevant Surgical Exposures,* which I have had the honor of editing. The second new volume is *Essential Procedures in Pediatrics*. Subsequent new topics to be introduced are *Soft Tissue Reconstruction, Management of Peripheral Nerve Dysfunction, Advanced Reconstructive Techniques in the Joint, Sports Medicine,* and *Orthopaedic Oncology and Complex Reconstruction*. The full library thus will consist of 16 useful and relevant titles.

I am pleased to have accepted the position of series editor, feeling so strongly about the value of this series to educate the orthopaedic surgeon in the full array of expert surgical procedures. The true worth of this endeavor will continue to be measured by the ever-increasing success and critical acceptance of the series. I remain indebted to Dr. Thompson for his inaugural vision and leadership, as well as to the *Master Techniques* volume editors and numerous contributors who have been true to the series style and vision. As I indicated in the preface to the second edition of *The Hip* volume, the words of William Mayo are especially relevant to characterize the ultimate goal of this endeavor: "The best interest of the patient is the only interest to be considered." We are confident that the information in the expanded *Master Techniques* offers the surgeon an opportunity to realize the patient-centric view of our surgical practice.

Bernard F. Morrey, M.D.

Preface

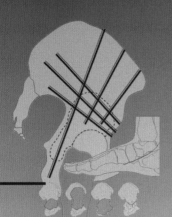

With the introduction of principles related to surgical margins, W. F. Enneking opened the door to modern management of musculoskeletal tumors. The success of surgery when combined with chemotherapy and radiation therapy reinforced the need for more innovative ways of resection and reconstruction in order to preserve the limb rather than amputate it. The greater sophistication of patient knowledge and expectation has also driven growth in the repertoire of surgical interventions, which, in turn, has leveraged advances in reconstructive surgery for nonneoplastic disease.

This text has been assembled to describe state-of-the-art techniques employed in musculoskeletal tumor surgery with a focus on the indications, contraindications, and requirements for such surgery. Special attention has been given to highlighting key points and focusing surgeons' understanding by the use of bullet points where appropriate. This has prepared the foundation for in-depth descriptions of the surgical techniques by recognized leaders in the field. Inclusion of reviews of the available literature and "pearls and pitfalls" from the experts round off this comprehensive approach to reconstruction of the pelvis and extremities after oncologic and nononcologic surgery.

The chapters are written by experts with an international reputation for reconstructive tumor surgery, who serve in institutions regarded as major global centers for bone and soft tissue tumor management. Thus, the contributions represent extensive experiences in an area of care recognized as rare and highly specialized. The chapters have been assembled to provide both depth and breadth and aim to be instructive in the preparation and execution of surgery.

This text is meant as a reference for those training or practicing in the field of musculoskeletal oncology and as a valuable resource for any department or library where surgery pertinent to this area of cancer care is practiced. It is our hope that the information contained within this text will help surgeons maximize the potential for limb-sparing surgery and bring greater benefit to patients afflicted with musculoskeletal tumors.

Franklin H. Sim, M.D.
Peter F. M. Choong, M.D., M.B.B.S.
Kristy L. Weber, M.D.

Contents

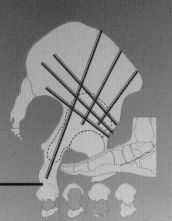

SECTION FIVE: ANKLE

PART II   Upper Extremity   283

SECTION SIX: SHOULDER

SECTION SEVEN: ELBOW AND WRIST

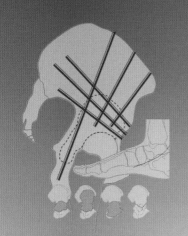

Part ONE

Lower Extremity

1 General Considerations

Peter F. M. Choong

Reconstructions of defects in the bony pelvis are some of the most complex challenges in surgery. The approach to such surgery is heavily influenced by the etiology of the pelvic defect, the anatomy of the pelvis, the reconstructive techniques used, and the acute physiologic disturbance experienced by the patient. The morbidity of pelvic reconstruction is high and pelvic reconstruction should be practiced in a team setting with adequate technical, physical, and expert resources available.

STRATEGIC APPROACH TO PELVIC RECONSTRUCTION

The complexity of pelvic reconstruction mandates a strategic approach to surgery.

- A clear understanding of the cause of the pelvic defect is fundamental to its management. For example, recognizing the differences in primary or secondary tumor behavior will determine the approach to resection and the subsequent residual defect. Similarly, an appreciation of the causes of acetabular prosthetic failure will lead to the appropriate choice of reconstruction.
- Thorough imaging allowing careful scrutiny of the anatomy is mandatory. Recognizing the extent of the pelvic defect helps to identify what reconstructive technique may be required.
- Classification systems that define the potential defect are important for determining the approach and reconstructive options.
- Understanding the anatomy of the pelvis allows anticipation of danger zones that may be encountered or avoided.
- Careful selection of the surgical approach is important for visualising the region of interest and for achieving adequate access for each step of the procedure. This will be determined by the location of the tumor or, in the case of acetabular revision, the nature of prosthetic failure. The surgical approach will determine how the patient is positioned and draped.

• Pelvic surgery is frequently prolonged and complicated by heavy blood loss. Managing the physiologic upset during the procedure is an important consideration and requires a close working relationship with the anesthetic team.

ETIOLOGY OF PELVIC DEFECTS

The two commonest causes for pelvic defects include resection of pelvic tumors and periacetabular prosthetic complications. While the etiologies and implications of these two problems may differ substantially, the same methodical and meticulous approach must be employed in executing the surgical plan. In some cases, very similar surgical techniques are required to address the bone defect.

Primary Tumors

The pelvis is a common site (10%) for the development of primary tumors. The commonest primary pelvic tumors include chondrosarcoma, Ewing sarcoma, and osteosarcoma (1). Primary malignancies may be treated with curative intent. If systemic spread has occurred, then the prime aim of pelvic surgery is the local control of disease. The principle of tumor resection is to achieve a wide surgical margin for clearance, which is defined as at least 2 cm of clear bone in the line of the bone and a cuff of normal tissue, which is a named anatomic layer such as muscle, or fascia that is parallel to the cortex of the bone (2). Surgery may be combined with neoadjuvant chemotherapy or radiotherapy. The extent of the wide margins will determine the amount of bone loss and the subsequent reconstruction. Furthermore, inclusion of soft tissue as part of the margin may add to the complexity by extending the dead space and compromising safe wound closure.

Secondary Tumors

Bone metastases occur in almost 60% of carcinomas (3). The pelvis is one of the most common sites for metastases with breast, lung, prostate, kidney, and thyroid carcinoma being the primary sources (3). With the exception of renal carcinoma, most metastatic bone tumors are permeative, poorly circumscribed, sclerotic, lytic or mixed, and not associated with a large soft tissue component. In contrast, renal carcinoma metastases are characterized by large cannon-ball–like lesions which are profoundly lytic and associated with a large soft tissue component and hypervascularity.

Unlike primary bone malignancies which are solitary and are treatable by wide surgical margins, metastatic disease is conventionally treated with bone-conserving procedures such as curettage or the removal of only macroscopically affected tissue. This is because true solitary metastases are uncommon with the high likelihood that there are micrometastatic lesions within the same bone at the time of diagnosis. In light of this, bone metastasis should be regarded as a locally progressive disease with the expectation that despite surgical intervention, recurrence of disease will occur. Periprosthetic recurrence of tumor may rapidly lead to failure of the device; therefore, reconstructions should aim for maximum durability in the setting of ongoing bone loss and a shortened patient survival. For example, the entire length of tubular and flat bones should be spanned when considering internal fixation to avoid fracture through unprotected bone distal to a fixation device. The judicious use of cement as filler or to supplement fixation should be encouraged rather than relying solely on individual screws which are easily loosened by tumor progression. Cemented prosthetic fixation is preferred when considering hip arthroplasty for the same reason.

Primary pelvic tumors are characterized by late presentation. The capacious volume of the pelvis or the abundant fat and muscle around the pelvic girdle frequently masks the presence and development of pelvic tumors until they have reached enormous sizes. Soft tissue sarcomas are frequently painless as compared to bone malignancies which often cause painful symptoms. These later symptoms, however, are often vague and can be misinterpreted as musculoskeletal injury or as pain referred from the lumbar spine. Symptoms from intrapelvic soft tissue tumors are often from their compressive effect on adjacent viscera.

The frequently large tumor size can make dissection difficult by distorting normal anatomy, and displacing viscera and major neurovascular structures from their known course (Fig. 1.1A). Large primary pelvic tumors which necessitate wide resection margins may be complicated by the need to protect vital neurovascular structures that lie within the resection margin. For example, the lumbosacral nerve trunk, which passes downwards and laterally in front of the sacral alar toward the sciatic notch, can be compressed by tumors arising from the sacrum and sacroiliac joint or may be vulnerable to injury when the resection margin passes through the sacral alar for a large iliac sarcoma (Fig. 1.1B). Tumors that overhang the sciatic notch may obscure the passage of the sciatic nerve and the branches of the internal iliac vessels as they traverse the notch, making them vulnerable to injury. Tumors of the anterior pelvis may compress the bladder, or obstruct the superficial femoral artery and vein or the femoral nerve as these structures course across the superior pubic ramus. Structures which are held to the pelvis by fascia such as the lumbosacral nerve trunk or the femoral vessels and nerve are particularly vulnerable to tumor compression or iatrogenic trauma.

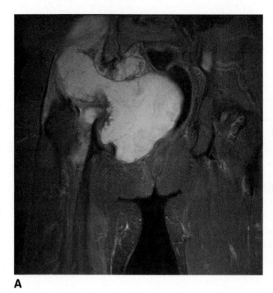

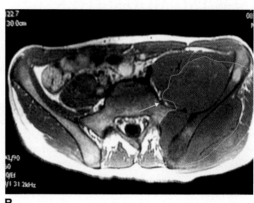

A   **B**

FIGURE 1.1

A: Thirty-eight-year-old woman with large intrapelvic chondrosarcoma that is compressing the bladder and also the contents of the sciatic notch as it emerges through the sciatic notch into the buttock. **B:** Eighteen-year-old man with Ewing sarcoma of the left sacroiliac joint with extension into the ilium and sacrum. Note the large soft tissue component of the tumor (*dotted white line*) and the lumbosacral trunk being compressed by the intrapelvic extent of the soft tissue component (*white arrow*).

Periacetabular Prosthetic Complications

Periacetabular prosthetic complications requiring revision represent some of the most challenging surgeries in orthopaedics (Fig. 1.2). With an increase in the numbers of joint replacements worldwide and the legacy of early generation components and implantation techniques, the requirement for complex acetabular revisions is certain to rise. The same meticulous approach to managing pelvic tumors may be applied to acetabular prosthetic complications.

Reconstructing acetabular defects after removal of acetabular prostheses is influenced by the quality of the residual bone, which is often poor. Frequently, the defects are cavitatory or segmental and are caused by osteolysis, the abrasion of a mobile acetabular component, and the damage caused by removal of the implant (4–6). What bone remains is commonly sclerotic with a paucity of good trabecular bone for interdigitation of cement or a reliable surface on which to support a cementless prosthesis. Central acetabular protrusion in bone softening conditions such as osteoporosis, osteomalacia, chronic steroid use, or Paget disease add to the difficulty that arthroplasty surgeons face. If acetabular loosening is accompanied by sepsis, then additional soft tissue debridement is required and surgery to reconstruct the pelvis may require a staged approach. What is sometimes also observed is the presence of significant and occasionally multiple, large serpiginous evaginations of the hip capsule containing darkly discolored pultaceous material. The latter is the by-product of metallic, polyethylene, and/or cement interface wear. The impact of this residue on newly revised bearing surfaces is unclear, but its total removal with excision of the granulomatous lining of the capsule should be undertaken. Backside acetabular wear is becoming a well-recognized cause of damage to the periacetabular bone and large

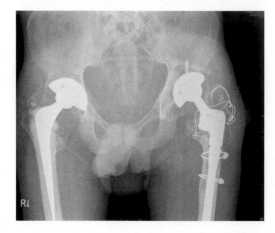

FIGURE 1.2

Thirty-six-year-old man with chronic rheumatoid arthritis and hip replacements in situ. Left hip prosthesis has been revised on both the femoral and acetabular sides on two separate occasions. He now presents with symptoms requiring further revision surgery.

cystic cavities may develop. Early modular implants gave rise to the unexpected phenomenon of polyethylene wear (7–10), which is now being addressed by better materials and design (8,11–13). Large cysts need to be appropriately curetted and grafted as part of the operative procedure.

IMAGING MODALITIES

Regardless of whether reconstructive surgery is contemplated for tumor or revision arthroplasty surgery, appropriate and adequate imaging should always be available.

Plain Radiography

Biplane and Judet views of the pelvis give an adequate assessment of the position and the quality of the anterior and posterior walls of the acetabulum. Plain radiographs also give an assessment of the symmetry of the pelvis and allow creation of a template for the size and relative positioning of prostheses. Should pelvic allografts be required, plain radiographs allow size and anatomic matching to occur. Some tumors have characteristic radiographic features which assist in diagnosis, and preliminary screening of the pelvis with radiographs can be useful for indicating the potential sites of bone destruction from metastatic disease.

Nuclear Scintigraphy

This modality is particularly useful for metastatic screening. Identifying more than one lesion in a single bone may have an impact on the type of surgery to be performed when operating for metastatic disease. Large tumors are frequently associated with central necrosis. Nuclear scintigraphy is very helpful for identifying regions of viable tumor which may be targeted for biopsy (Fig. 1.3A–C). The extent of tracer avidity within bone may

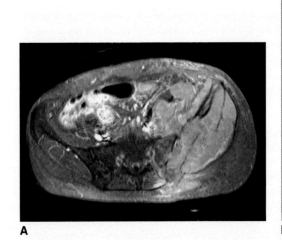

A

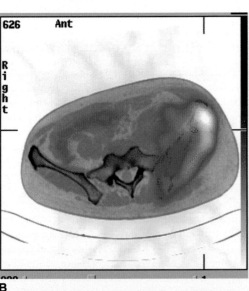

B

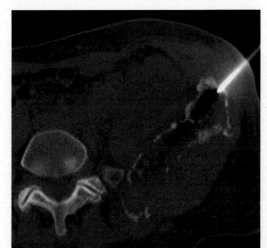

C

FIGURE 1.3

A: Sixty-three-year-old woman with iliac tumor and extensive intra- and extrapelvic soft tissue component. **B:** Co-registration of nuclear scintigraphy with computed tomographic scan identifies area of intense metabolic activity along the iliac crest and the periphery of the tumor signifying viable tumor. The central portion of the tumor is metabolically inert, suggesting necrosis. **C:** Area of high metabolic activity is then targeted for CT-guided needle core biopsy.

also influence the size of the surgical margins when operating on primary tumors. In nonneoplastic conditions, tracer avidity may indicate areas of occult fracture, prosthetic loosening, or sepsis.

Computed Tomography

Multislice computed tomography (CT) is an excellent modality for assessing the integrity of cortical and trabecular bone. As the pelvis is a complex three-dimensional structure, CT scanning can provide excellent multiplanar views from which three-dimensional images may be constructed. Destructive or cystic lesions are easily defined using this technique. With appropriate attenuation of the CT images such as when employing bone windows, metal artifacts may be suppressed to permit an assessment of the bone cement or bone prosthetic interface. With more sophisticated computer software, whole prostheses within individual images may be suppressed to provide better visualization of periprosthetic bone.

Magnetic Resonance Imaging

Magnetic resonance imaging (MRI) provides unsurpassed soft tissue contrast. This modality is mandatory for assessing all primary tumors of the pelvis because it allows a very accurate display of all important vascular and neural structures, the relationship of the viscera to the tumor, and the intraosseous extent of tumor. Because of these characteristics, MRI is a fundamental staging tool for planning surgical margins.

Angiography

Angiography is important for determining the vascularity of pelvic tumors or the relationship of the vessels that are adjacent to the planned operative site. Certain histotypes such as renal carcinoma, thyroid carcinoma, and myeloma can give rise to very vascular lesions. Curettage of these metastases may lead to life-threatening hemorrhage. Nonmalignant lesions such as aneurysmal bone cysts may also be associated with a hypervascular lesion. In these and other cases, preoperative embolization may be advantageous in controlling intraoperative bleeding. Preoperative embolization should be considered within 36 hours before surgery to minimize the return of flow to the embolized lesion. Angiography may also be important in severe protrusion of an acetabular component where revision is considered. Damage to the medial acetabular wall during migration or removal of the acetabular prosthesis may compromise adjacent vascular structures when the prosthesis is extracted. Angiography may be performed via femoral artery cannulization. Alternately, newer noninterventional methods such as CT or MRI angiograms may be performed. Although the images are multislice reconstructions, they provide sufficient information to allow an assessment of the potential for vascular damage during surgery. Embolization, however, requires femoral artery puncture and deployment of radio-opaque coils or beads.

ANATOMIC CONSIDERATIONS

Review of the anatomy of the pelvis must be undertaken in a methodical manner to avoid unexpected laceration of vital neurovascular or visceral structures. The combination of CT and MRI scans provides an excellent opportunity to scrutinize the relationship of the tumor to vital structures. However, distortion of anatomy may occur in the setting of prominent tumors, previous surgery, or gross acetabular loosening and migration; so care must be exercised when dissecting around areas where the anatomy cannot be clearly defined. Review of the anatomy should be orderly, beginning from the posterior pelvic ring and passing forward to the pubic symphysis.

Sacrum and Sacroiliac Joint

Major neurovascular structures pass medial to the sacroiliac joint, which is a key anatomic landmark that is characterized by an obvious ridge on the inner wall of the posterior pelvis. The common iliac vessels pass anterior to the sacral alar as they move downward and forward. The lumbosacral (L5-S1) trunk is also well medial of the sacroiliac joint but approaches the joint at its most inferior extent (Fig. 1.4). This structure is closely applied to the inner table of the pelvic ring and is frequently invested with a thick fascia that may obscure it from view unless it is specifically sought. Sacral tumors that emerge from the anterior surface of the sacrum or sacral alar are liable to threaten the safety of these vessels and the lumbosacral trunk. An osteotomy lateral to the sacroiliac joint is unlikely to injure the sacral nerves, while osteotomies medial to the sacroiliac joint need to be performed under direct vision with special attention paid at the inferior end of the osteotomy where the lumbosacral trunk joins the other sacral nerve roots to form the sciatic nerve at the level of the sciatic notch (Fig. 1.5). The decision regarding placement of the osteotomy in relation to the sacroiliac joint will depend on the involvement of the sacroiliac joint by tumor which can easily be assessed by CT or MRI scans.

Sciatic Notch

The sciatic notch is the key to pelvic surgery because of the very important structures traversing this portal. The sciatic nerve emerges below the piriformis muscle within the notch with the inferior gluteal artery and vein lying next to it. The superior gluteal vessels emerge from the notch above the piriformis muscle and are closely

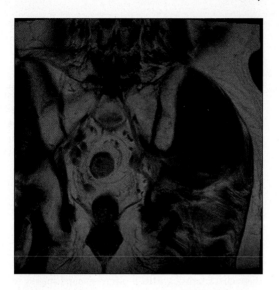

FIGURE 1.4

Coronal T1 magnetic resonance image of buttock tumor. Note the S1 nerve root and internal iliac vessels approaching the sciatic notch at the lower extent of the sacroiliac joint.

related to the top of the notch (Fig. 1.4). Occasionally, the superior gluteal vessels are fixed to the bone at this level by a posterior branch which may be avulsed during dissections at the notch. Avulsion of the superior gluteal vessels can be problematic as they retract into the pelvis. It is imperative that these vessels are sought and carefully dissected out and ligated under direct vision. The inferior gluteal vessels tend to follow the gluteus maximus muscle flap that is reflected downward and posteriorly after detachment from the iliac crest. The sciatic nerve may be held tightly in the sciatic notch if the pyriformis muscle is bulky, or tendonous. Dividing the sacrospinous ligament increases the space in the sciatic notch, which should allow greater freedom for dissection of the nerve and vessels. The sacrospinous ligament is a stout structure passing from the tip of the spinous process backwards towards the outer edge of the sacrum at its inferior extent. The internal pudendal nerve and vessels are located close to the tip of the spinous process; therefore, great care must be taken to avoid injury when dividing the ligament. A subperiosteal dissection of the ligament off the spinous process beginning at the base of the spinous process and working toward its tip may allow the tendon and the adjacent internal pudendal vessels and nerves to be swept off the spinous process without injury (Fig. 1.5). Ensuring that the sciatic nerve and the gluteal vasculature are released from attachment to the notch then permits a finger to be admitted into the pelvis via the sciatic notch. This is important to confirm that all structures are clear of the notch, allowing retractors to be inserted to protect these structures as osteotomies for iliac or periacetabular resections emerge at the notch. If the sciatic notch is filled by tumor, safe dissection of the nerve and vessels may not be possible. Under such circumstances, it may be wise to consider external hemipelvectomy rather than attempting limb-sparing surgery by dissecting free the neurovascular structures in the sciatic notch and accidentally breaching the tumor capsule in the process.

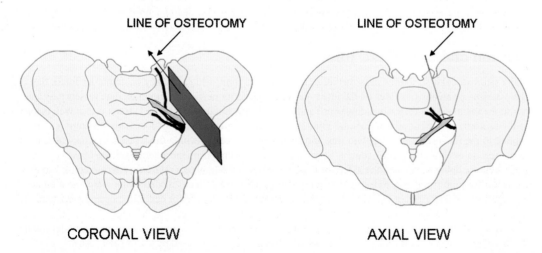

FIGURE 1.5

The proximity of the lumbosacral trunk to the sacroiliac joint places it in danger of injury when an osteotomy of the sacral alar is contemplated. The lumbosacral trunk has to be retracted (blue malleable retractor) and the osteotomy performed from within under direct vision (coronal and axial views).

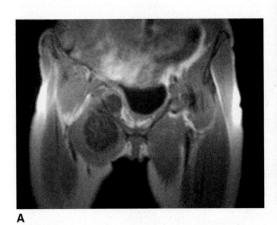
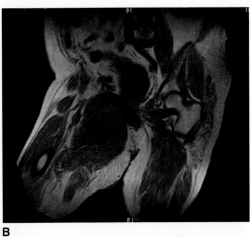

A   **B**

FIGURE 1.6

A: T1-weighted coronal magnetic resonance image of the pelvis demonstrating a pubic chondrosarcoma displacing but not invading the bladder. Note the well-preserved fat plane between tumor and bladder.
B: T1-weighted coronal magnetic resonance image of the pelvis demonstrating a pubic sarcoma invading the bladder neck. Note the loss of the fat plane between tumor and bladder and thickening of the bladder wall suggesting invasion.

Iliac Wing

The iliac wing is a dispensable bone. The iliacus and gluteal muscle provide an excellent margin when resecting iliac wing tumors. The main anatomic structure to be aware of is the femoral nerve, which emerges from between the psoas and iliacus muscles as it then courses under the iliacus fascia on top of the iliacus muscle before swinging forward to emerge lateral to the superficial femoral nerve at the midpoint of the inguinal ligament.

Hip Joint

Involvement of the hip joint will necessitate an extra-articular resection of the joint. Tumors that are associated with periacetabular or intracapsular fractures should be considered as having intracapsular contamination. Although a joint effusion may be sympathetic to periacetabular disease, this should be regarded with great suspicion for joint involvement. A conservative trochanteric osteotomy with attached gluteus medius should be performed where possible to preserve some stabilizing muscular function around the hip. The anterior capsule of the hip joint passes more distally than the posterior capsule and should not be accidentally breached when performing a subtrochanteric osteotomy in an extra-articular resection.

Anterior Pelvis

The anterior pelvis extends from the symphysis pubis to where the periacetabulum meets the pubic rami. The main structures at risk with tumors or dissection in this area include the superficial femoral vessels and femoral nerve as they pass over the pelvic brim to enter the femoral triangle where they are closely held to bone via the femoral fascia. This requires careful dissection for release. The pectineus muscle separates these structures from the superior pubic ramus. The obturator nerve and vessels are vulnerable with tumors arising from the obturator muscles or the superior and inferior pubic rami. Sacrifice of the obturator vessels is inconsequential. Division of the obturator nerve, however, will result in weakness of hip adduction. Behind the symphysis pubis lies the bladder neck and from here the urethra passes forward underneath the arch of the symphysis. This latter structure can be injured in dissections of this area, particularly when splitting the symphysis pubis. Invasion of the base of the bladder has to be identified prior to operations for tumors of the anterior pelvis as this will require planned bladder resection and reconstruction (Fig. 1.6A,B).

CLASSIFICATION OF PELVIC RESECTIONS AND ACETABULAR DEFECTS

Classifications of pelvic resection and nonneoplastic acetabular defects allow use of a common language when discussing the location of tumors or the nature of periacetabular deficiencies. Further, the use of a consensus classification permits comparisons between experiences derived from different institutions. A range of reconstructive options are now available depending on the site of the pelvic tumor or the type of periacetabular defect.

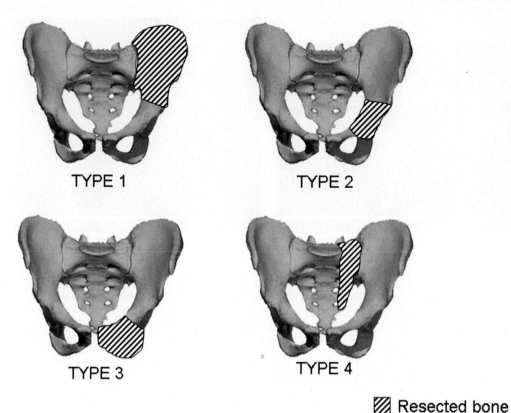

TYPE 1   TYPE 2

TYPE 3   TYPE 4

▨ Resected bone

FIGURE 1.7

Classification of pelvic resections. Type 1 involves the ilium, type 2 involves the periacetabulum, type 3 involves the pubic rami, and type 4 involves the sacral alar. Resections may also include combinations of types.

CLASSIFICATION OF PELVIC RESECTIONS

Resections of the pelvis are divided into internal hemipelvectomy (limb preserving) and external hemipelvectomy (amputation). Internal hemipelvectomy is characterized by the resection of part or the whole of a hemipelvis. There are four types of internal hemipelvectomy (14) (Fig. 1.7), including type 1 (ilium), type 2 (periacetabular), type 3 (pubic), and type 4 (sacral alar). Each type may be extended to include adjacent areas, for example, type 1–4 (iliosacral), type 1–2 (ilio periacetabular), type 2–3 (pubo periacetabular). External hemipelvectomy was previously known as hindquarter amputation and is regarded as an extended hemipelvectomy when the sacral alar is included and is also referred to as a modified hemipelvectomy when part of the ilium remains.

CLASSIFICATION OF PERIACETABULAR DEFECTS

There are a variety of classification systems for acetabular defects (4,6,15). These aim to define the various types of acetabular deficiencies and to guide reconstruction based on the extent of the defect. Conforming to a classification system allows better communication between treating surgeons.

ANESTHETIC CONSIDERATIONS

Anesthesia for pelvic surgery is challenging because of the extensive tissue trauma, the prolonged operative time, exposed bleeding bone, and, in the case of malignancy, the impact of neoadjuvant therapies. Postoperatively, patients face a number of major physiologic insults including ongoing blood and fluid loss, the effects of massive blood transfusion, ileus, and pain. Typically, postoperative pain is severe and multimodal anesthetic techniques are required to provide safe and effective analgesia. While much has been written about pelvic resection and reconstruction, little is reported about the anesthetic techniques (16) employed in the surgery for these patients.

In a well-planned surgery, preoperative anesthetic assessment begins sometime prior to the scheduled surgery date. Ideally, the patient is seen by the anesthetist, but patients from somewhere a great distance from the hospital may be contacted by telephone consultation.

While preoperative assessment includes a routine review of all systems, of particular importance is knowledge of location and pathology of the tumor and type and impact of preoperative adjuvant therapy. An understanding of the type, location, and size of tumor helps the anesthetist assess the possible extent of surgery required. For example, large tumors, requiring extensive resection with close proximity to vascular structures, will be more likely to have larger blood loss, greater tissue trauma, and need for intensive postoperative support than those which are smaller and in a more favorable surgical position. Tumors that are situated posteriorly in the pelvis more often involve complicated and prolonged dissection around the lumbosacral plexus. The internal iliac vessels are more likely to be troublesome when tumors are situated posteriorly in the pelvis. Equally, anterior pelvic tumors that require dissection near the bladder neck are challenging because of the great tendency for the perivesical venous plexus to bleed heavily or continuously. Osteotomies expose bleeding bone and can provide a sustained source of hemorrhage. In anticipation of major blood loss during surgery, the hospital blood transfusion service should be notified of the date of surgery and the amount of blood and blood components that may be required. In most hemipelvectomy cases an order for 20 units of packed red cells, 10 units of fresh frozen plasma, and 10 units of platelets should be made.

Preoperative chemotherapy or radiotherapy may have a deleterious effect on bone marrow function. Complete blood examinations are therefore required to ascertain if anemia, profound leucopenia, or thrombocytopenia exists. Consultation is made with the patient's oncologist to determine whether the hematological disturbances will correct themselves prior to surgery or whether further specific treatment is required. The hospital intensive care unit (ICU) is also notified at this stage of the date and type of surgery, as well as the possible duration of stay in the ICU, so that resources can be allocated in advance.

As with any prolonged surgery, careful attention needs to be given to prevention of peripheral nerve compression. The patient should be positioned in the lateral position with the side supports holding the upper body at the sternum and mid-thoracic region well clear of the flank and abdomen. This allows the patient's body, when the operating table is rolled laterally from left to right side, to move through an arc of 90 degrees, from −45 to +45 degrees. The benefit of this position to the surgeon is that the rolling maneuver allows both anterior and posterior parts of the pelvis to be accessed. The consequences for the patients are that the points of potential nerve compression change each time the patient is moved and there is a risk of breathing circuit disconnection or dislodgement. Checking by the anesthetist for areas at risk of compression neuropathy needs to be performed each time the patient is rolled from one side to the other. Although surgery to revise an acetabular component may require a fixed pelvis, the same precautions regarding pressure care must be applied.

The method used for postoperative analgesia will be dependent on the technique chosen for anesthesia. In our institution a combination of general and spinal anesthetic and a postoperative epidural catheter with a continuous infusion of ropivacaine 2 mg/mL with fentanyl 4 f.Lg/mL is preferred. The infusion is usually commenced in the ICU or recovery room once the patient has become hemodynamically stable. The infusion may be extended for up to 6 days. It is important that endotracheal intubation rather than laryngeal mask intubation is used because massive transfusion may cause subglottic and supraglottic edema which is more safely managed using an endotracheal tube rather than a laryngeal mask. In the postoperative period further bleeding can be expected, requiring transfusion of approximately another third of the amount given during surgery.

INCISION

The most extensile approach to the pelvis is the iliofemoral incision with an anterior limb that extends along the inguinal canal (Fig. 1.8). Beginning at the posterior inferior iliac spine, the incision passes along the length of the iliac crest before sweeping downward and forward from the anterior superior iliac spine to a point 2 inch anterior to the midpoint of the greater trochanter. From here the incision courses downward and posteriorly to cross the

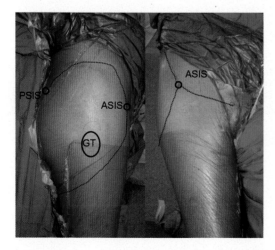

FIGURE 1.8

Key landmarks of the universal iliofemoral incision that creates the buttock flap, namely the posterior superior iliac spine, the anterior superior iliac spine, and the greater trochanter. An inguinal limb of the incision passes from the anterior superior iliac spine to the pubic tubercle and allows greater exposure of the anterior pelvis, bladder, and femoral neurovascular structures.

femur at the junction of its upper and middle thirds. The incision is then extended to the outer part of the buttock crease. When required, an anterior limb of the incision is created from the anterior superior iliac spine that passes forward along the inguinal ligament. The posterior-based gluteus maximus buttock flap so created exposes the proximal femur, the gluteus medius as it inserts into the greater trochanter and the sciatic nerve as it emerges from under the piriformis. The anterior inguinal incision allows dissection of the superficial femoral artery and vein as well as the femoral nerve, which lies laterally and deep to the course of the femoral artery.

Any biopsy should be performed in the line of this incision, thus allowing excision of the biopsy tract when formally creating the operative incision. Should there be a requirement to convert the resection to an external hemipelvectomy, then continuing the inferior limb of the incision around the buttock crease and emerging on the medial side of the thigh should allow completion of the amputation when the inferior incision joins with the medial end of the anterior inguinal incision.

If surgery for a revision hip replacement is being contemplated, incisions should be through previous operative scars. The extensile incision used in pelvic surgery may be adapted to meet the requirements of greater pelvic exposure should the need arise in arthroplasty surgery.

REFERENCES

1. Unni KK, ed. *Dahlin's Bone Tumors. General Aspects and Data on 11, 087 Cases.* 5th ed. Philadelphia, PA: Lippincott-Raven; 1996.
2. Choong P. Staging and surgical margins in musculoskeletal tumors. In: Bulstrode C, Buckwalter J, Carr A, et al., eds. *Oxford Textbook of Orthopaedics and Trauma.* Oxford, UK: Oxford University Press; 2002:110–120.
3. Janjan N. Bone metastases: approaches to management. *Semin Oncol.* 2001;28:28–34.
4. Paprosky WG, Burnett RS. Assessment and classification of bone stock deficiency in revision total hip arthroplasty. *Am J Orthop.* 2002;31:459–464.
5. Paprosky WG, Momberger NG. Preoperative recognition of acetabular defects: paths of reason. *Orthopedics.* 2000;23:959–960.
6. Bradford MS, Paprosky WG. Acetabular defect classification: a detailed radiographic approach. *Semin Arthroplasty.* 1995;6:76–85.
7. Barrack RL, Folgueras A, Munn B, et al. Pelvic lysis and polyethylene wear at 5–8 years in an uncemented total hip. *Clin Orthop Relat Res.* 1997;335:211–217.
8. Della Valle AG, Rana A, Furman B, et al. Backside wear is low in retrieved modern, modular, and nonmodular acetabular liners. *Clin Orthop Relat Res.* 2005;440:184–191.
9. Kurtz SM, Ochoa JA, White CV, et al. Backside nonconformity and locking restraints affect liner/shell load transfer mechanisms and relative motion in modular acetabular components for total hip replacement. *J Biomech.* 1998;31:431–437.
10. Yamaguchi M, Bauer TW, Hashimoto Y. Deformation of the acetabular polyethylene liner and the backside gap. *J Arthroplasty.* 1999;14:464–469.
11. Kligman M, Furman BD, Padgett DE, et al. Impingement contributes to backside wear and screw-metallic shell fretting in modular acetabular cups. *J Arthroplasty.* 2007;22:258–264.
12. Usrey MM, Noble PC, Rudner LJ, et al. Does neck/liner impingement increase wear of ultrahigh-molecular-weight polyethylene liners? *J Arthroplasty.* 2006;21:65–71.
13. Mayman DJ, Anderson JA, Su EP, et al. Wear data and clinical results for a compression molded monoblock elliptical acetabular component: 5- to 9-year data. *J Arthroplasty.* 2007;22:130–133.
14. Yuen A, Ek ET, Choong PF. Research: Is resection of tumours involving the pelvic ring justified? A review of 49 consecutive cases. *Int Semin Surg Oncol.* 2005;2:9.
15. D'Antonio JA, Capello WN, Borden LS, et al. Classification and management of acetabular abnormalities in total hip arthroplasty. *Clin Orthop Relat Res.* 1989;243:126–137.
16. Molnar R, Emery G, Choong PF. Anaesthesia for hemipelvectomy—a series of 49 cases. *Anaesth Intensive Care.* 35:536–543.

2 Iliofemoral Pseudoarthrosis and Arthrodesis

Nicola Fabbri, Mary I. O'Connor, Mario Mercuri, and Franklin H. Sim

The treatment and prognosis of musculoskeletal neoplasms have dramatically improved during the past three decades. However, the surgical management of malignant pelvic tumors remains a challenging problem from both oncological and functional standpoints. With respect to tumor control, a limb salvage procedure has been shown to be a reliable alternative to hemipelvectomy when an adequate surgical margin can be obtained or when an amputation does not provide a better margin (1–4). In general, if chances of tumor local control are the same, a limb sparing procedure is preferable because it usually is associated with superior function than hindquarter amputation and prosthetic fitting (5,6). In this setting, postoperative function depends upon tumor location, extent of resection, and whether pelvic stability, defined as the ability to withstand physiologic loading, is maintained or restored at the time of surgery (3). The best functional results are usually seen when pelvic stability is maintained, either by preservation or by surgical reconstruction of effective load transmission through femorosacral continuity (3,7).

A schematic approach to pelvic anatomy and classification in four regions (2,3) is helpful in order to visualize these concepts (Fig. 2.1). In resections involving the ischiopubic region (region III) or incomplete resections of the ilium (region I), the continuity between the femur and the ipsilateral sacrum is maintained along with an essentially normal weight-bearing capability. In these circumstances, bone reconstruction is usually not required and functional results are uniformly quite satisfactory (1–4). Management of a malignant tumor involving the acetabulum (region II) is in general a more complex surgical challenge for the following reasons:

TUMOR EXTENSION

Lesions are usually of larger size and often extending into region I and/or region III, requiring a wider exposure and a more extensive dissection.

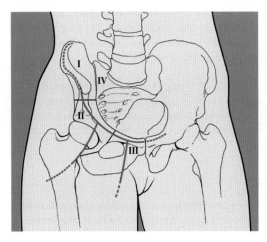

FIGURE 2.1

Classification of pelvis and sacrum anatomy in four regions. The red lines represent the utilitarian incision we routinely use for pelvic sarcomas.

PROXIMITY TO NEUROVASCULAR STRUCTURES AND VISCERA

Anteriorly, external iliac and femoral artery and vein and the femoral nerve have to be adequately exposed and mobilized in order to gain access to the inner portion of the pelvis and medial wall. Posteriorly, exposure of the greater sciatic notch and sciatic nerve is mandatory to approach supra- and retroacetabular areas. Depending upon medial soft tissue extension and region III involvement, considerable work may be necessary to dissect the retropubic space, including urethra, urinary bladder, and ipsilateral ureter.

PELVIC STABILITY AND RECONSTRUCTION

Resection of the acetabulum by definition causes femorosacral discontinuity and pelvic instability. In terms of function, creation of a flail hip remains a better option than hemipelvectomy but is often associated with considerable disability. Reconstruction should be therefore at least considered in these instances in order to restore stability and improve function.

INDICATIONS

Selection of the reconstructive technique is a very important step in the overall management and is based on careful evaluation of numerous factors related to

- Patient characteristics
- Tumor features
- Surgeon's experience and preference

The role of the above factors in the selection of optimal technique may be summarized as follows:

Patient Characteristics

Age, Functional Demands, and Expectations   Skeletal immaturity is relevant because of the patient's size and growth potential, usually discouraging the use of massive implants and suggesting a more biologic approach. Potential for recreational activities, type of employment, and required level of function, namely the capability to weight bear and sustain load, are important considerations at any age.

Overall Medical Condition and Relationship With Tumor Prognosis   Careful assessment of the general medical condition is important when facing a usually long and demanding procedure, sometimes associated with severe postoperative complications. Particularly, the presence of an immunocompromised status, as it occurs during multiagent chemotherapy, and other relatively common comorbidities, such as diabetes and obesity, has to be kept in mind because of the increased risk of infection.

Tumor Features

Diagnosis, Stage, and Prognosis   Important considerations related to the tumor are the need for chemotherapy and/or radiotherapy and the presence of distant metastasis. While previous radiation therapy dramatically increases the risk of wound problems and infection, delay in resuming chemotherapy because of postoperative complications may severely impact survival. In these instances, an effort should be made to minimize morbidity of surgery. Not uncommonly, a patient presenting with pelvic sarcoma and lung metastasis may still be a candidate for surgery. Particular attention should then be paid to minimize the risks of surgery, maximize the role of adjuvant medical management, and focus on quality of residual life.

Tumor Location, Type of Resection, and Extent of Surgery   Reconstructive technique may vary depending upon tumor extension and type of resection. Tumor involvement of zone I requiring partial or complete resection of the ilium and soft tissue involvement are important factors to consider. In fact, while iliac resection reduces the bone available for fixation, involvement and resection of the gluteus medius and/or superior gluteal nerve will cause loss of active abduction.

Surgeon's Experience and Preference

Level of training and personal experience of the surgeon also play a relevant role. Common sense is as important as technical skills in pelvic surgery and avoidance of possibly catastrophic complications may outweigh

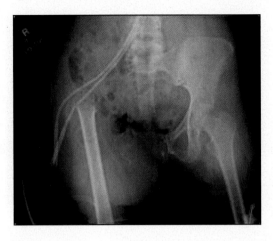

FIGURE 2.2

Example of flail limb after resection of the whole hemipelvis and proximal femur (P1,2,3,H1).

the potential functional benefit associated with a massive implant, such as a mobile hip and the absence of substantial limb shortening.

A detailed description of advantages and disadvantages pros of each technique is beyond the purpose of this chapter; however, a brief outline of the main inherent features is pertinent to the subject discussed.

Overview of Surgical Options

Various surgical options are available today following pelvic resection for a tumor involving the acetabulum. They can be schematically divided in three groups:

Flail Hip, Hip Transposition to Sacrum   Flail hip (Fig. 2.2) is at the opposite end of the concept of pelvic stability and has been historically associated with significant limb shortening and substantial disability (2,3,8,9). Recent literature has reported excellent results in a subgroup of young patients, emphasizing the role of careful soft tissue reconstruction and prolonged rehabilitation as key for success (10). Hip transposition to the sacroiliac joint has been also described following resection of the whole hemipelvis (11). According to the authors, a stable pseudoarthrosis between the sacrum and the femur is obtained using a polyethylene terephthalate mesh tube (Trevira; Implantcast, Buxtehude, Germany) to augment soft tissue reconstruction and create a neo-joint capsule (Fig. 2.3). Functional and quality of life assessment indicate superior outcome of this technique when compared to prosthetic replacement and amputation (11).

Iliofemoral Arthrodesis and Pseudoarthrosis, Ischiofemoral Arthrodesis and Pseudoarthrosis   Iliofemoral and ischiofemoral arthrodesis or pseudoarthrosis have been employed successfully for many years in limb salvage for malignant pelvic tumors (1–4). The basic principle of both techniques is to obtain continuity of the hip with residual pelvis, by either fusion or coaptation, improving pelvic stability and weight-bearing potential (Figs. 2.4 and 2.5). Stability of the construct and functional results are depending upon the amount of pelvic bone left after resection. Both options are associated with limb shortening,

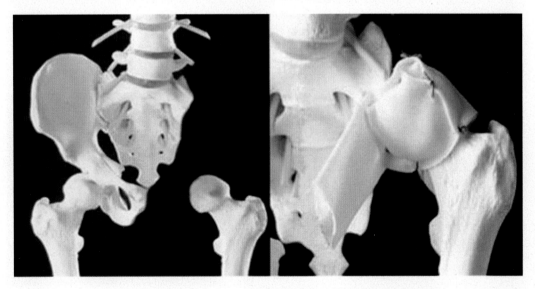

FIGURE 2.3

Hip transposition to the sacrum has been described following resection of the whole hemipelvis (11). A stable pseudoarthrosis between the sacrum and the femur is obtained using synthetic material. (Reprinted from Hoffmann C, Gosheger G, Gebert C, et al. Functional results and quality of life after treatment of pelvic sarcomas involving the acetabulum. *J Bone Joint Surg Am.* 2006;88:575–582.)

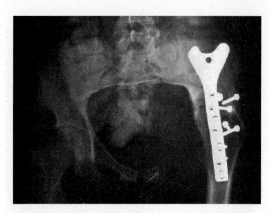

FIGURE 2.4
Iliofemoral arthrodesis following type II and III resection.

usually less severe in ischiofemoral techniques. Because intrinsically more stable, however, iliofemoral reconstructions have been predictably associated with better functional results than ischiofemoral reconstructions, which have lost popularity during the last 2 decades. Limb shortening, usually ranging 3.5 to 6 cm, may be easily compensated by a shoe lift without major impact on function (12).

Massive Implants (Pelvic Allograft or Allograft-Prosthetic Composite, Autoclaved or Irradiated Autograft, Pelvic Prosthesis, Saddle Prosthesis)   The use of massive implants to restore hip motion and more physiologic function has been also pursued with enthusiasm in many centers more recently (Figs. 2.6 to 2.8). However, while good function in this setting has been reported mainly for allograft-prosthetic composite and occasionally for pelvic prosthesis, an high incidence of severe complications including infection, graft fracture, hip instability, and need for secondary hindquarter amputation has been associated with all these techniques (13–19).

Indications for Iliofemoral Arthrodesis and Pseudoarthrosis

The ideal candidate for iliofemoral fusion, either arthrodesis or pseudoarthrosis, is a patient requiring a type II or type II and III pelvic resection in which the proximal osteotomy through the ilium is close to the acetabulum. Availability of most of the ilium minimizes limb length discrepancy and allows wider bone contact and solid fixation, enhancing either fusion in iliofemoral arthrodesis or hip stability when pseudoarthrosis is preferred (12). In arthrodesis, rigid fixation is usually achieved with a plate, while cable wires or heavy mersilene sutures are used for pseudoarthrosis (1,3,12).

Iliofemoral fusion is preferable for young and active patients because it provides stable and durable construct capable to withstand high-demand functional requirements. Iliofemoral pseudoarthrosis appears indicated for more sedentary and older patients. Although the construct is less stable than iliofemoral fusion, maintaining the ability to flex the hip seems to be appreciated by older patients with a more sedentary lifestyle (1,12). In addition, iliofemoral pseudoarthrosis is usually a shorter and technically less demanding procedure possibly associated with a lower complication rate than iliofemoral pseudoarthrosis, features particularly appealing in older patients. When the proximal osteotomy is above the neck of the ilium, the iliac wing becomes thin, and obtaining solid fixation and fusion may be very difficult because of reduced bone contact and inadequate screw fixation. In this instance, iliofemoral arthrodesis is less than ideal while pseudoarthrosis remains a viable option (1,12).

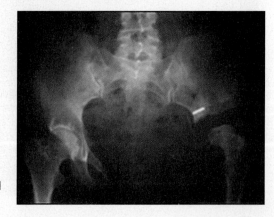

FIGURE 2.5
Iliofemoral pseudoarthrosis after type II and III resection.

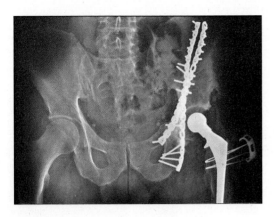

FIGURE 2.6
Example of allograft-prosthetic composite reconstruction.

CONTRAINDICATIONS

Extension of the tumor in zone I and inadequate iliac bone stock after the resection is the most important and common contraindication to iliofemoral arthrodesis. When the entire ilium is resected with the acetabulum, as it occurs in type I and II and type I to III resections, a different surgical strategy has to be considered to maximize function in the light of the overall clinical scenario. Flail limb, ischiofemoral arthrodesis or pseudo-arthrosis, or a massive hemipelvic implant may be selected based on the factors previously discussed.

The need to sacrifice the sciatic or femoral nerve because of tumor involvement is not per se a contraindication to limb salvage surgery in general nor to iliofemoral arthrodesis or pseudoarthrosis in particular. However, since the rationale for undertaking limb salvage surgery is providing superior function than external hemipelvectomy, a realistic evaluation of the postoperative function versus perioperative complications is crucial in this setting.

PREOPERATIVE PLANNING

Tumor control remains the first priority of surgery and correlates with achievement of adequate surgical margin (1–3,20–23). The minimum surgical margin required for tumor control is a wide margin, which implies en bloc removal of the tumor completely surrounded by normal tissue (24). The goal of preoperative planning is to ensure the best chances to obtain an adequate margin and a stable reconstruction minimizing the risk of complications.

Successful preoperative planning is in our opinion based on three main steps:

Physical Examination and Staging Studies Review

Thorough review of the regional anatomy and careful evaluation of good quality recent staging studies are mandatory. History and physical examination may provide important clues such as limb edema, urinary symptoms, sciatic or out of proportion regional pain, possibly suggesting deep venous thrombosis or involvement of adjacent visceral or neurologic structures. The presence of previous incisions for abdominal or pelvic procedures (e.g., hernia repair, caesarian section) should be noted and taken into account as potential problem because of scarring and sometimes interference with ideal incision line. Because of the need to excise the biopsy track en bloc with the tumor (24–26), evaluation of the biopsy site is also important. A poorly

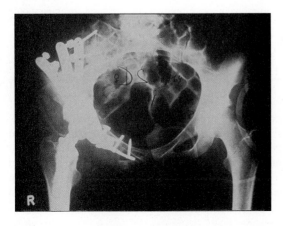

FIGURE 2.7
Pelvic prosthesis following periacetabular resection.

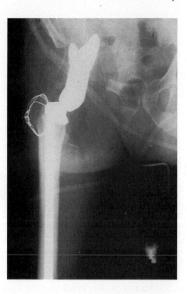

FIGURE 2.8

Use of saddle prosthesis after type II and III resection. The "saddle" is engaged in the residual ilium.

performed biopsy complicates surgical management, often requiring modification of the incision and surgical conduct in order to obtain an adequate margin (3,25,26). Plastic surgery counseling and assistance for evaluation of skin flaps viability and potential need for soft tissue reconstruction with regional or free flaps is mandatory for these patients. Staging studies review is crucial in order to assess bone and soft tissue extension, suggest the dissection planes and osteotomy levels, and anticipate potential problems and need for multidisciplinary involvement. Good quality standard radiography and magnetic resonance imaging (MRI) are golden standard but integration with computerized tomography (CT) scan may be very helpful, especially when dealing with bone forming or calcified tumors. Occasionally, further diagnostic studies such as angiography, angio-CT or urinary tract imaging modalities may be selectively considered to finalize the surgical plan.

Multidisciplinary Approach and Strategy

A multidisciplinary team approach including experienced urologist, neurosurgeon, plastic, general, and vascular surgeons is highly recommended and mandatory to maximize chances of success. The team should be familiar with the basic principles of musculoskeletal oncology and involved in the staging studies review and decision-making process in order to optimize overall surgical strategy and timing. Even when no visceral nor neurovascular involvement can be suspected on preoperative staging studies, team members should be available because of the risk for intraoperative complications.

Patient Preparation

Because of the magnitude of the procedure and the potential for significant blood loss and other relevant complications, pelvic surgery requires detailed review of the medical status. Lower bowel preparation and urinary catheter and ureteral stent(s) insertion should be done routinely. A urinary catheter maintains the bladder deflated and allows easier identification of the urethra when retropubic dissection is needed, as it occurs in tumors involving region III. Moreover, intraoperative methylene blue injection through the catheter may be very helpful in order to reveal bladder lacerations. Similarly, palpation of ureteral stent(s) is very useful intraoperatively, facilitates dissection in lesions presenting with significant intrapelvic mass, and allows easier repair in case of accidental lesion. Perioperative intravenous antibiotics are definitely recommended; due to potential for contamination from urinary and/or gastrointestinal tracts, Gram-negative bacteria coverage should be considered along with routine prophylaxis.

SURGICAL TECHNIQUE

Positioning and Draping

A loose lateral decubitus that allows moving the patient from an almost full supine position to an approximately 45-degree anterior tilt is usually preferred and achieved with well-padded supports over the sternum and thoracolumbar region. The lower chest, abdomen, pelvis, and ipsilateral lower limb are prepared and draped well past anterior and posterior midline, including umbilicus, pubic symphysis, median crest of the sacrum, and lower lumbar spinous processes. The genitalia and the anus are draped out of the field. The surgical field then extends from the rib cage to the ipsilateral toes. A mild compression bandage is applied over the lower limb to improve venous flow and minimize the risk of deep venous thrombosis.

Landmarks

Several bony landmarks can be identified not only to plan the incision but also as useful guide throughout the procedure:

- Anterior superior iliac spine (ASIS)
- Pubic tubercle and symphysis
- Iliac crest and tubercle
- Posterior superior iliac spine (PSIS)
- Ischial tuberosity
- Greater trochanter
- Femoral pulse/femoral head

The inguinal ligament runs from the *ASIS* to the *pubic tubercle*. The femoral artery enters the thigh under the inguinal ligament and the *femoral pulse*, corresponding to the *femoral head*, may be palpated approximately at the mid-inguinal point.

Surgical Incision

Different surgical incisions and techniques have been proposed for management of pelvic tumors (2,4,9,27,28).

We routinely prefer an extended approach combining basically an ilioinguinal with a modified iliofemoral incision; additionally, a descending vertical branch approximately perpendicular to the ilioinguinal incision may be associated in large lesions arising from the obturator ring to improve exposure of the anterior pelvic arch (27,28) (Fig. 2.1). The main ilioinguinal incision permits access to the all pelvis, the lateral femoral portion is always necessary to adequately visualize zone II, and the medial obturator extension further improves exposure of zone III (28). The ilioinguinal incision starts from the PSIS and follows the iliac crest and then the inguinal ligament toward the pubic symphysis. The lateral branch of the ilioinguinal incision starts approximately at the junction of the lateral and middle third of the inguinal ligament, runs distally, and curves toward the junction of the proximal with middle third of the lateral aspect of the thigh. When needed, the medial vertical branch of the incision usually begins in proximity of the symphysis and spans distally over the genitofemoral region (Fig. 2.1). This utilitarian approach allows intraoperative flexibility to accommodate different clinical situations with respect to tumor size and location (28). In fact, slight modification of the length and direction of each branch of the incision may improve the exposure. Sometimes, for management of tumors originating in zone III and extending to zone II (see case 1), the femoral and obturator branch may be comprised in a single incision extending over the anterior or anteromedial aspect of the proximal thigh. In addition, the need to remove the biopsy track en bloc with the tumor not uncommonly requires variation of the ideal incision.

In specific circumstances dictated by tumor location and extension, the exposure can be further improved by

- Extending the ilioinguinal incision across the symphysis
- Starting the femoral branch more medially and closer to the femoral vessels if significant vascular dissection may be anticipated
- Extending the vertical incision to the ischial tuberosity and eventually in the subnatal crease

Case 1—Iliofemoral Pseudoarthrosis

The case of a 57-year-old woman with a 6-year history of progressive pain and swelling of the left pubic region is shown. Staging studies reveal a large radiolucent lesion arising from the anterior pelvic arch and extending to the acetabulum, with overall radiographic features (lobular architecture and intratumoral calcifications) quite suggestive for low-grade chondrosarcoma (Figs. 2.9 to 2.11). There is no evidence of distant metastasis. Histologic confirmation has been obtained elsewhere by incisional biopsy, and the patient then referred. The patient is morbidly obese, is on oral agents for type II diabetes mellitus, and has a rather sedentary lifestyle. Preference in this setting is given to an intra-articular resection of pelvic zone II and III, and reconstruction by iliofemoral pseudoarthrosis, associated with a lower incidence of surgical complications and an acceptable function for this patient's lifestyle.

A long ilioinguinal incision incorporating the biopsy track and extending anteromedially over the proximal thigh is selected to provide adequate exposure (Fig. 2.12). After dissection through subcutaneous fat, the ilioinguinal fascia (aponeurosis of the external oblique muscle) is exposed, divided in line with its fibers and the spermatic cord (male) or round ligament (female) then identified and retracted. While care must be taken to protect the spermatic cord, the round ligament can actually be sacrificed without consequences. The internal oblique and transverse abdominis muscles are then released from the iliac crest and divided distally, where they form the posterior wall of the inguinal canal, gaining access to the abdominal cavity and visualizing the extraperitoneal fat. The inguinal ligament, rectus abdominis, and pyramidalis muscles are released off the pubis at adequate distance from the tumor, exposing the superior border of the symphysis. By blunt finger dissection, the retropubic prevesical space (space of Retzius) is entered and developed exposing the posterior wall of

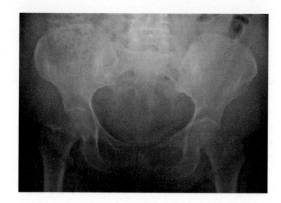

FIGURE 2.9

Case 1. Standard AP view of the pelvis showing a radiolucent destructive lesion containing mineralization, involving zone II and III on the left side.

FIGURE 2.10

Coronal MRI T1 **(A)** and proton density fat saturated **(B)** sequences revealing the extent of periacetabular involvement and need for a type II and III resection.

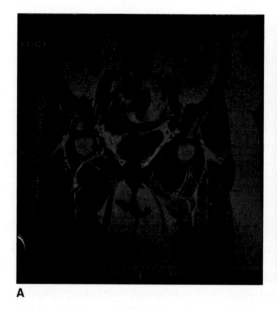

A

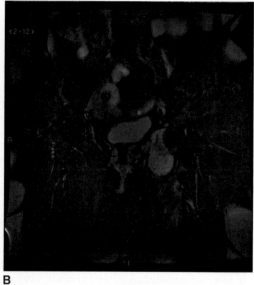

B

FIGURE 2.11

Axial MRI T2 fat-saturated sequence **(A)** and CT scan **(B)**, demonstrating soft tissue extension and intratumoral calcifications, overall rather suggestive for low-grade chondrosarcoma.

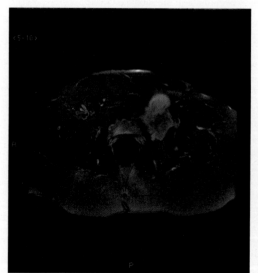

A

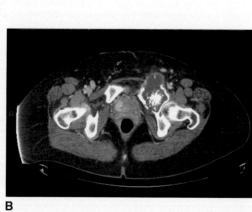

B

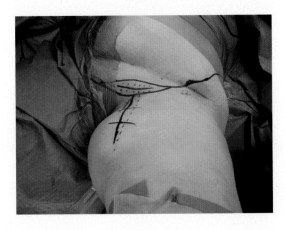

FIGURE 2.12

The utilitarian ilioinguinal incision, incorporating the biopsy track and extending anteriorly to improve zone III exposure.

the symphysis. The bladder is gently retracted backward, the urethra is identified, and the inferior pubic arch can then be palpated. During this phase, attention should be paid to the retropubic venous plexus, a potential source of significant bleeding. Once developed, the retropubic space is maintained by packing with one or more large sponges, for hemostasis and as intraoperative landmark. The pubic region at this point is prepared for osteotomy through the symphysis, using either an osteotome or a Gigli saw. Regardless of the technique, attention should be paid to protect the urethra and the retropubic venous plexus (Fig. 2.13). With the hip slightly flexed, abducted, and externally rotated, dissection through the vertical incision is carried out and adductors and gracilis muscles are divided at appropriate distance from the tumor. Laterally, the sartorius, tensor fasciae latae, and direct head of rectus femoris are released off the anterior superior and anterior inferior iliac spine, improving exposure of the hip and femoral vessels. The femoral sheath is then identified and dissected after ligation and division of a few branches to the abdominal wall, including deep circumflex iliac and inferior epigastric vessels (Fig. 2.14). The iliopsoas is laterally retracted and the femoral vessels further mobilized and elevated from the osteomuscular plane. Use of a broad rubber band is helpful during this phase. Lateral retraction of the iliopsoas and femoral nerve and elevation of the femoral vessels permit at this point division of pectineus, obturator externus, and quadratus, exposing the entire obturator ring (Fig. 2.15). The obturator vessels and nerve are tied and divided. The gluteus maximus is released off the iliac crest as necessary, and maintaining the hip flexed and externally rotated, circumferential capsulotomy, visualization of the femoral head, and section of the round ligament are performed. The supra-acetabular region of the ilium is then approached from the inner and outer aspects of the pelvis in order to expose the greater sciatic notch. The gluteus medius and minimus are released from the gluteal surface of the iliac wing, while the iliacus is mobilized from the iliac fossa. Care must be taken to maintain adequate soft tissue coverage around the tumor. Once exposed the notch, the sciatic nerve is identified and protected with either a sponge or Homann retractors (Fig. 2.16). Osteotomy through the supra-acetabular region is then performed at the desired level using either a Gigli saw or an oscillating saw. The hip is now dislocated and the specimen is mobilized to visualize remaining soft tissue insertions. Applying gentle traction, the residual external rotators (obturator internus, superior and inferior gemellus muscles, quadratus femoris) are divided from the femur, while hamstrings are released off the ischial tuberosity, carefully avoiding the sciatic nerve. By externally rotating the specimen, the urogenital diaphragm is divided from the inner aspect of the ischium, entering the ischiorectal fossa. Particularly in males, bleeding may occur during this phase when dissecting the corpus cavernosum (crus of penis). The ischiorectal fossa may then be accessed and developed, the pelvic floor (levator ani muscle) visualized and divided along with the sacrospinous and sacrotuberous ligaments, and the specimen then removed (Fig. 2.17).

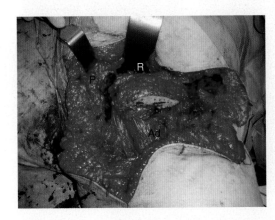

FIGURE 2.13

In zone III, the retropubic space has been developed, bladder and urethra protected, and osteotomy carried out through the pubic symphysis (P, pubic symphysis; R, retropubic space with a wet sponge for bladder protection; Ad, adductor muscles).

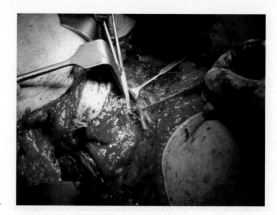

FIGURE 2.14

Dissection to mobilize the femoral vessels sheath.

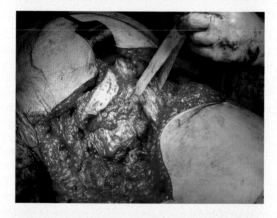

FIGURE 2.15

Exposure of the anterior pelvic arch and obturator ring. Femoral vessels are elevated and mobilized over a broad loop.

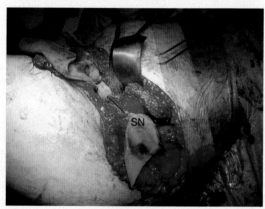

FIGURE 2.16

The supra-acetabular region and sciatic notch (SN) exposed. A green sponge fills the notch and protects the sciatic nerve in preparation of the supra-acetabular osteotomy (*black line*).

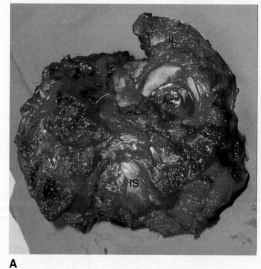

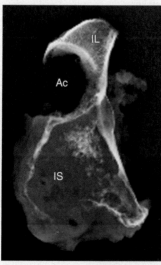

FIGURE 2.17

A: The resection specimen: acetabulum (Ac), ilium (IL), and ischium (IS) are indicated.
B: Radiograph of a coronal cross section of the specimen showing the same anatomic regions.

A   B

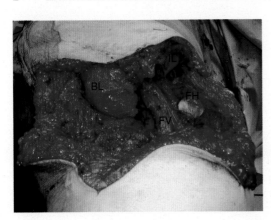

FIGURE 2.18

The pelvic defect after tumor removal. The bladder (BL), femoral vessels (FV), femoral head (FH), and remaining ilium (IL) are indicated.

The reconstructive phase of the procedure, aiming to restore a stable femoropelvic continuity, is then started (Fig. 2.18). The thicker portion of the iliac stump is shaped in a concave fashion to approximately match the femoral head size in order to create a neo-acetabular cavity for the pseudoarthrosis (Fig. 2.19). Holes are drilled through the ilium and the femoral head to allow the passage of either cable wires or heavy mersilene sutures (Fig. 2.20). The articular cartilage is left intact and usually three holes are drilled through the femoral head, approximately with the same orientation as the holes in the iliac wing. Care must be taken during this phase to avoid drilling injury to surrounding anatomic structures such as vessels and viscera. Three heavy gauge wires are then passed through the ilium and femoral head to form three parallel loops that are sequentially tightened on the outer aspect of the pelvis, as desired to secure fixation (Fig. 2.21). In our opinion, the fixation should maintain the pseudoarthrosis stable in neutral abduction and allow about 45 degrees of hip flexion. Careful hemostasis and frequent irrigation are recommended throughout the procedure. Routine wound closure in layers over suction drains is then undertaken. Special attention is paid to accurate soft tissue reconstruction, closing the abdominal wall with the gluteal and femoral muscles. Maintaining slight flexion of the hip may be helpful to approximate and repair the inguinal ligament and conjoined tendon with the gluteal and femoral fascia (Fig. 2.22). In case of soft tissue loss due to tumor resection or suboptimal quality of the closure, the repair may be augmented with either synthetic (soft polypropylene mesh) or biologic (dermal or fascial allograft) material in order to prevent herniations. After routine skin closure and wound dressing, the limb is placed slightly flexed and abducted in a foam-rubber brace to prevent rotational stresses, and then postoperative radiographs are obtained (Fig. 2.23). Limb shortening of the operated side is about 2.5 cm.

Case 2—Iliofemoral Arthrodesis

A 16-year-old girl with known Ewing's sarcoma of the anterior pelvic arch is now discussed. She has undergone induction multiagent chemotherapy with remarkable tumor response and is evaluated for local treatment. Restaging of the disease confirms resectability by an intra-articular type II-III resection (Fig. 2.24).

This is a young active patient with high functional requirements and expectations. The reconstruction of choice is therefore iliofemoral arthrodesis, providing a stable and durable construct associated with acceptable complication rate and functional result superior to pseudoarthrosis.

The same utilitarian incision is used for pelvic approach and dissection. When planning iliofemoral arthrodesis, however, osteotomy of the greater trochanter improves exposure of the hip, facilitates optimal plating fixation, and enhances healing potential by reinsertion of the trochanter and abductors over the fusion site.

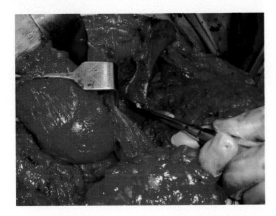

FIGURE 2.19

The residual ilium is shaped in a concave fashion using a curette or high-speed burr.

FIGURE 2.20

Holes are drilled in the ilium **(A)** and femoral head **(B)** to pass either cable wires or heavy sutures.

A   **B**

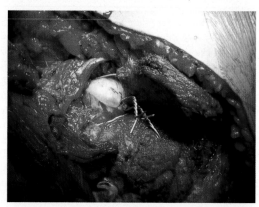

FIGURE 2.21

The wires are tightened on the outer aspect of the pelvis.

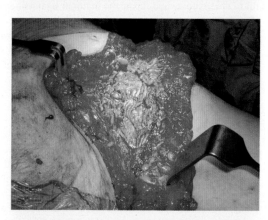

FIGURE 2.22

Meticulous closure of the abdominal wall.

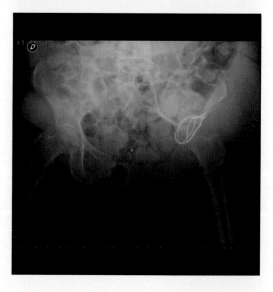

FIGURE 2.23

Postoperative radiograph showing satisfactory bone contact and minimal shortening.

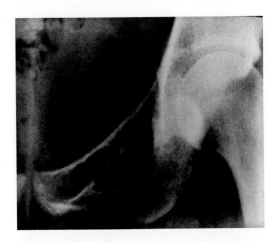

FIGURE 2.24
Ewing's sarcoma of the pubis extending to the acetabulum.

After tumor removal, the top portion of the femoral head is carved appropriately to fit over the remaining ilium and maximize bone contact and stability (Fig. 2.25). Care must be taken to check the overall alignment and rotation of the limb before fixation. Ideal position for hip fusion is neutral abduction, about 15 to 20 degrees of flexion and slight external rotation equal to the opposite side. The proximal femur is then approximate to the ilium and plate fixation is applied posterolaterally, spanning from the ilium to the diaphysis (Fig. 2.26). Locking nuts may be used to enhance fixation on the inner aspect of the pelvis (Fig. 2.27). Autogenous bone grafts from the iliac crest may be added and the greater trochanter with abductors is then reinserted over the fusion site, maximizing the healing potential (Fig. 2.28). Excellent bone contact and solid fixation are obtained, and shortening of the operated limb at the end of the procedure is 4.5 cm. (Fig. 2.29).

Pearls and Pitfalls

- The surgeon should not be afraid of extending the incision in case of inadequate exposure. While a slightly longer incision in this setting is not associated with increased risk of infection, excessive traction on wound flaps, prolonged operative time, and suboptimal visualization easily associate with increased risks of wound complications and neurovascular or visceral injury.
- Opening the femoral vessels sheath and extensively dissecting artery and vein expose to the risk of vascular injury and postoperative lymphatic drainage. The latter may be a serious problem, constantly associated with delayed wound healing and frequently with secondary infection.
- Excessive traction of the femoral vessels, especially in older patients, may cause intraoperative venous and/ or arterial thrombosis, with obvious catastrophic consequences. Care should be taken to use wide loops and avoid excessive and prolonged traction of neurovascular structures.
- Regular irrigation and maintaining wound flaps adequately wet is helpful in reducing wound complications. Before closure, wound flap inspection and excision of skin and subcutaneous areas of questionable viability enhance chances of healing.

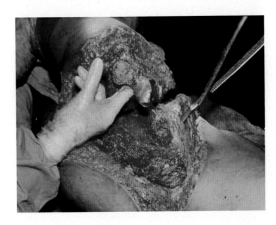

FIGURE 2.25
The femoral head is carved to fit over the remaining ilium for optimal stability.

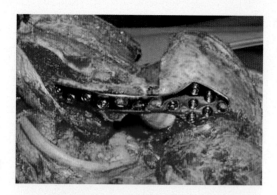

FIGURE 2.26

Plate fixation spans from the ilium to the femoral diaphysis.

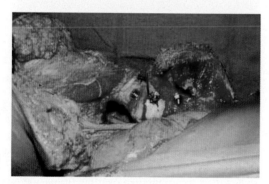

FIGURE 2.27

Plate is applied posteriorly and fixation is enhanced by locking nuts on the inner aspect of the pelvis. (Reprinted from Fuchs B, O'Connor MI, Kaufman KR, et al. Iliofemoral arthrodesis and pseudarthrosis: a long-term functional outcome evaluation. *Clin Orthop Relat Res.* 2002;397:29–35.)

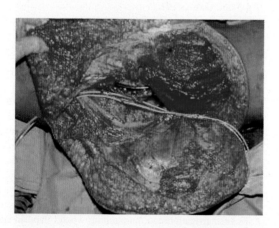

FIGURE 2.28

Posterior view after reinsertion of the trochanter before closure.

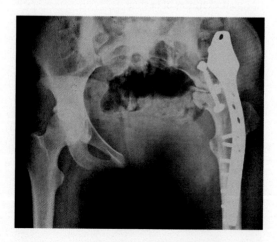

FIGURE 2.29

Postoperative radiograph shows solid fixation and moderate shortening.

- Significant blood transfusion and fluid administration are frequently necessary throughout the procedure. Dilution of preoperative antibiotics may increase the risk of infection, and additional intraoperative antibiotics administration should be always considered.

POSTOPERATIVE MANAGEMENT

The wound is closely monitored during the early postoperative phase, and prompt attention should be paid to any evidence of wound slough, sieroma/hematoma, or frank infection. Aggressive operative management by thorough irrigation and debridement is usually recommended. Early removal of urinary catheter and drains is encouraged. Intravenous antibiotics are usually given for a few days postoperatively and discontinued only after drain removal. Even if controversial, wide-spectrum oral antibiotics are then generally recommended for 4 to 6 weeks to prevent early hematogenous colonization of the operative site.

The immobilization regimen of the hip varies according to the type of reconstruction. For pseudoarthrosis, we prefer a hip-spica cast for 1 month, followed by hip brace for 2 months. The hip flexion hinge is maintained locked for the first 3 to 4 weeks, and then progressive motion and weight bearing as tolerated is allowed during the third month. Since heavy patients poorly tolerate hip-spica cast, hip brace in a locked position of the hip may be preferable in this setting. A more conservative regimen is indicated for iliofemoral arthrodesis, with hip-spica cast maintained for 2 months followed by hip brace for additional 2 to 3 months. Partial progressive weight bearing is started after radiographic evidence of at least initial fusion, usually at 4 to 6 months from surgery. The use of short hip-spica cast or knee hinged brace is encouraged whenever possible to prevent knee stiffness. Prophylactic anticoagulation therapy consisting of either low molecular weight heparin or warfarin is usually maintained until the patient is at least partially weight bearing and is possibly modified based on overall risk of thromboembolic events.

COMPLICATIONS

Limb salvage surgery for pelvic sarcomas is associated with considerable morbidity and significant complications. Incidence of complications correlates with the extent of resection, complexity of the reconstruction, and patient-related factors, such as underlying medical conditions or need for adjuvant chemotherapy and/or radiotherapy. The reported risk of complications is uniformly high and varies from 30% to more than 50%, with infection being the most common and probably most difficult to prevent (1,3,8,14,15,17,18,23). A meta-analysis combining all the reported data during a decade has shown an overall complication rate of 33% (23% wound related) and a perioperative mortality close to 0% (29).

Interpretation of retrospective data is obviously limited, among the other variables, by the fact that different type of reconstruction may be inherently related with different incidence and severity of complications. However, the general risk of complications when dealing with periacetabular sarcomas requiring a type II or a type II-III resection can be reasonably summarized as follows:

- Wound healing problems (20% to 40%)
- Deep infection (12% to 40%)
- Local recurrence (13% to 24%)
- Nerve palsy (5% to 15%)
- Visceral injury (5% to 10%)
- Vascular injury (3% to 5%)
- *DVT and PE (10% to 30%)*
- Perioperative mortality (1% to 3%)

The use of custom pelvic prostheses and saddle prosthesis has been associated in large series with high incidence of infection ranging from 22% to 60% (14,15,17,18). Additional risk of implant-related mechanical complications, including hip dislocation, implant migration, or loosening, has been also reported as ranging from 20% to 37% (14,15,17,18). Similarly, up to 100% infection rate and 29% risk of early dislocation have been reported with allograft or allograft-prosthetic composite (16,17,19).

Iliofemoral pseudoarthrosis and arthrodesis compare favorably with these data because they are associated with milder complications. In fact, besides infection rate of 23% (3), a nonunion rate of 14% has been reported as a main long-term complication for iliofemoral arthrodesis (12). Loss of fusion translates into pseudoarthrosis, leaving a situation still functional, even though at a lower level (12).

RESULTS

Oncologic Outcome

Tumor stage, surgical margin, and local recurrence correlate with prognosis of pelvic sarcomas. Achievement of a wide margin is reported in 50% to 70% of cases. Overall local recurrence rate ranges 15% to 35% and increases to more than 50% when associated with inadequate margins in high-grade sarcomas (1–3,20–23,30–35).

According to reported series, the overall disease-free survival ranges as follows:

- 5-year survival low-grade tumor: 77% to 88% (1,3,20,23,35)
- 5-year survival high-grade tumors: 25% to 55% (1,3,20,23,35)
- 10-year survival chondrosarcoma: 54% to 69% (22,32)
- 5-year survival high-grade osteosarcoma: 22% to 41% (21,30,31,33,34)

Functional Outcome

Middle- to long-term functional results of iliofemoral arthrodesis and pseudoarthrosis are now available (12). In a large and homogeneous series, the functional outcome was evaluated using the Musculoskeletal Tumor Society and the Toronto Extremity Salvage scores at mean follow-up of 97 months (range from 14 to 226 months). Success rate in obtaining radiographic fusion of iliofemoral arthrodesis was 86%. The overall Toronto Extremity Salvage and Musculoskeletal Tumor Society scores for arthrodesis and pseudoarthrosis were 64% and 48%, respectively. The functional outcome of patients with a primary solid fusion was significantly better than patients with pseudoarthrosis (Toronto Extremity Salvage Score, 76%; Musculoskeletal Tumor Society Score, 71% versus Toronto Extremity Salvage Score, 52%; Musculoskeletal Tumor Society Score, 25%). In patients with pseudoarthrosis, there was no difference whether this was obtained with the primary procedure or as the end result of a failed attempt to fusion and subsequent hardware removal (12). These data confirm earlier reports of satisfactory and durable functional results (1–4).

Iliofemoral arthrodesis and pseudoarthrosis remain a valuable reconstructive option for management of pelvic tumors. Current data show that both functional outcome and incidence of complications compare favorably with other reconstructive techniques.

REFERENCES

1. Campanacci M, Capanna R. Pelvic resections: the Rizzoli Institute experience. *Orthop Clin North Am.* 1991;22:65–86.
2. Enneking WF, Dunham WK. Resection and reconstruction for primary neoplasms involving the innominate bone. *J Bone Joint Surg Am.* 1978;60:731–746.
3. O'Connor MI, Sim FH. Salvage of the limb in the treatment of malignant pelvic tumors. *J Bone and Joint Surg Am.* 1989;71:481–494.
4. Steel HH. Partial or complete resection of the hemipelvis. An alternative to hindquarter amputation for periacetabular chondrosarcoma of the pelvis. *J Bone Joint Surg Am.* 1978;60:719–730.
5. Davis AM, Wright JG, Williams JI, et al. Development of a measure of physical function for patients with bone and soft tissue sarcoma. *Life Res.* 1996;5:508–516.
6. Enneking WF, Dunham W, Gebhardt MC, et al. A system for the functional evaluation of reconstructive procedures after surgical treatment of tumors of the musculoskeletal system. *Clin Orthop Relat Res.* 1993;286:241–246.
7. Gerrand CH, Bell RS, Griffin AM, et al. Instability after major tumor resection: prevention and treatment. *Orthop Clin North Am.* 2001;32:697–710.
8. Apffelstaedt JP, Driscoll DL, Karakousis CP. Partial and complete internal hemipelvectomy: complications and long term follow-up. *J Am Coll Surg.* 1995;181:43–48.
9. Karakousis CP, Emrich LJ, Driscoll DL. Variants of hemipelvectomy and their complications. *Am J Surg.* 1989;158:404–408.
10. Schwartz AJ, Kiatisevi P, Eilber FC, et al. The friedman-eilber resection arthroplasty of the pelvis. *Clin Orthop Relat Res.* 2009;467:2825–2830.
11. Hoffmann C, Gosheger G, Gebert C, et al. Functional results and quality of life after treatment of pelvic sarcomas involving the acetabulum. *J Bone Joint Surg Am.* 2006;88:575–582.
12. Fuchs B. O'Connor MI, Kaufman KR, et al. Iliofemoral arthrodesis and pseudarthrosis: a long-term functional outcome evaluation. *Clin Orthop Relat Res.* 2002;397:29–35.
13. Aboulafia AJ, Buch R, Mathews J, et al. Reconstruction using the saddle prosthesis following excision of primary and metastatic periacetabular tumors. *Clin Orthop Relat Res.* 1995;314:203–213.
14. Abudu A, Grimer RJ, Cannon SR, et al. Reconstruction of the hemipelvis after the excision of malignant tumors. Complications and functional outcome of prostheses. *J Bone Joint Surg Br.* 1997;79(5):773–779.
15. Aljassir F, Beadel GP, Turcotte RE, et al. Outcome after pelvic sarcoma resection reconstructed with saddle prosthesis. *Clin Orthop Relat Res.* 2005;438:36–41.
16. Bell RS, Davis AM, Wunder JS, et al. Allograft reconstruction of the acetabulum after resection of stage-IIB sarcoma. Intermediate-term results. *J Bone Joint Surg Am.* 1997;79:1663–1674.
17. Hillmann A, Hoffmann C, Gosheger G, et al. Tumors of the pelvis: complications after reconstruction. *Arch Orthop Trauma Surg.* 2003;123:340–344.
18. Renard AJ, Veth RP, Schreuder HV, et al. The saddle prosthesis in pelvic primary and secondary musculoskeletal tumors: functional results at several postoperative intervals. *Arch Orthop Trauma Surg.* 2000;120:188–194.
19. Yoshida Y, Osaka S, Mankin HJ. Hemipelvic allograft reconstruction after periacetabular bone tumor resection. *J Orthop Sci.* 2000;5:198–204.
20. Han I, Lee YM, Cho HS, et al. Outcome after surgical treatment of pelvic sarcomas. *Clin Orthop Surg.* 2010;2:160–166.
21. Kawai A, Huvos AG, Meyers PA, et al. Osteosarcoma of the Pelvis. *Clin Orthop Relat Res.* 348:196–207.

22. Pring ME, Weber KL, Unni KK, et al. Chondrosarcoma of the pelvis. A review of sixty-four cases. *J Bone Joint Surg Am.* 2001;83:1630–1642.

23. Windhager R, Karner J, Kutschera HP, et al. Limb Salvage in Periacetabular Sarcomas. Review of 21 Consecutive Cases. *Clin Orthop Relat Res.* 1996;331:265–276.

24. Enneking WF, Spanier SS, Goodman MA. A system for the surgical staging of musculoskeletal sarcoma. *Clin Orthop Relat Res.* 1980;153:106–120.

25. Mankin HJ, Lange TA, Spanier SS. The hazards of biopsy in patients with malignant primary bone and soft-tissue tumors. *J Bone and Joint Surg Am.* 1982;64:1121–1127.

26. Mankin HJ, Mankin CJ, Simon MA. The hazards of the biopsy, revisited. *J Bone and Joint Surg Am.* 1982;78:656–662.

27. Campanacci M, Langlais F. Les resections du bassin pour tumeurs. *Encycl Méd Chirs* (Editions Scientifiques et Médicales Elsevier SAS, Paris). *Techniques Chirurgicales - Orthopédie-Traumatologie.* 1992;1–7:44–505.

28. Fabbri N, Mercuri M, Campanacci M. Resection of ischiopubic tumours (pelvic region 3). (Editions Scientifiques et Médicales Elsevier SAS, Paris). *Techniques Chirurgicales - Orthopédie-Traumatologie.* 2001;55-470-D-10:5.

29. Conrad EU III, Springfield D, Peabody T D. Pelvis. In: Simon MA, Springfield DS, ed. *Surgery for Bone and Soft-Tissue Tumors.* Philadelphia, PA: Lippincott-Raven Publishers; 1998.

30. Fuchs B, Hoekzema N, Larson DR, et al. Osteosarcoma of the pelvis: outcome analysis of surgical treatment. *Clin Orthop Relat Res.* 2009;467:510–518.

31. Grimer RJ, Carter SR, Tillman RM, et al. Osteosarcoma of the pelvis. *J Bone Joint Surg Br.* 1999;81:796–802.

32. Ozaki T, Hillmann A, Lindner N, et al. Chondrosarcoma of the pelvis. *Clin Orthop Relat Res.* 1997;337:226–239.

33. Ozaki T, Flege S, Kevric M, et al. Osteosarcoma of the pelvis: experience of the Cooperative Osteosarcoma Study Group. *J Clin Oncol.* 2003;21:334–41.

34. Saab R, Bhaskar NR, Rodriguez-Galindo C, et al. Osteosarcoma of the pelvis in children and young adults: the St. Jude Children's Research Hospital Experience. *Cancer.* 2005;103:1468–1475.

35. Shin K, Rougraff BT, Simon MA. Oncologic outcomes of primary bone sarcomas of the pelvis. *Clin Orthop Relat Res.* 1994;304:207–217.

3 Allograft Prosthetic Composites in the Pelvis

Peter F. M. Choong

Primary tumors of the pelvis account for almost 15% of all primary malignant bone tumors and present a considerable management challenge. Their location frequently involves the acetabulum and surgery to this part has significant implications for mobility and independence. Pelvic tumors often present late and may be quite substantial at the time of diagnosis, which adds to the difficulty of surgery and also has a negative influence on survival. The three most common sarcomas are chondrosarcoma, osteosarcoma, and Ewing sarcoma and the roles of adjuvant therapy in each case and their respective impacts differ widely. Surgery, however, is the mainstay of treatment and in the past, transpelvic or hindquarter amputation was traditionally performed for all resectable tumors. For the majority of these tumors, advances in the efficacy of chemotherapy have led to a profound improvement in survival and with greater sophistication of imaging modalities, the possibilities for limb-sparing surgery have increased. Indeed, the expectations of patients have now also increased in light of the increased success of limb-sparing surgery in general and pelvic surgery specifically.

Resections of the bony pelvis with oncologic margins almost always lead to large segmental defects in the pelvic ring with pelvic discontinuity. This is particularly important if resections include the acetabulum because the hip joint has a pivotal role in weight transmission, limb function, and mobility. In recognition of the importance of the acetabulum and the poor function that follows resection without periacetabular reconstruction, a wide variety of techniques has been developed to maintain the function of the hip joint and these include biologic reconstructions with allograft or autograft bone, prosthetic reconstructions including pelvic and saddle prostheses, and combinations of biologic and prosthetic reconstructions such as allograft prosthetic composites.

Allograft reconstructions have a number of advantages, including a readily available source, the ability to be size matched, a shape that can be customized to fit the defect created by tumor resection, biologic union with host bone, which may arguably provide better stability than the fixation of a prosthetic pelvic device, and reestablishment of acetabular anatomy, which in turn allows hip arthroplasty with conventional joint prostheses. The acetabular defect may be segmental or total and may include part of the ilium, ischium, or pubis (Fig. 3.1).

INDICATIONS

- Wide resection with allograft pelvic reconstruction and prosthetic joint replacement is indicated when a primary tumor involves the periacetabulum (Fig. 3.2). Extension of the tumor into the hip joint should not prevent this type of reconstruction.
- The extent of encroachment into the ilium or pubic rami should raise concerns if this spread is large because the quality of support provided to the allograft and fixation to ilium and pubic rami gets poorer the further away from the periacetabulum the osteotomy is made.

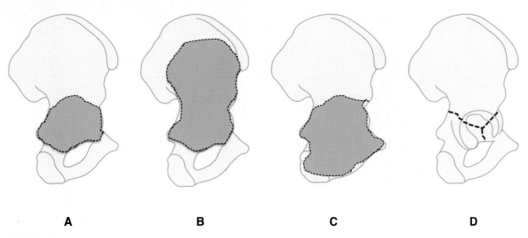

FIGURE 3.1

Allograft prosthetic composite may be considered when pelvic resection is confined to **(A)** the acetabulum or if acetabular resection extends into the **(B)** ilium or **(C)** ischium. Acetabular resection may also be **(D)** segmental.

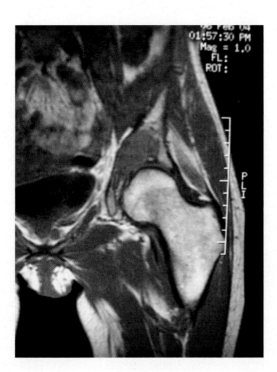

FIGURE 3.2

T1-weighted coronal MRI of the left hip joint demonstrating a chondrosarcoma involving the dome and medial wall of the acetabulum.

CONTRAINDICATIONS

- Patients undergoing chemotherapy are at high risk of developing secondary infections from their immunosuppression and neutropenia. The use of large segmental allografts during a prolonged surgical procedure also brings with it its own risk of infection. Performing allograft surgery in the presence of pre-existing sepsis in immunocompromised patients raises the certainty of infection to unacceptable levels and pre-existing sepsis should be regarded as an absolute contraindication to allograft transplantation.
- True solitary metatases are rare. Often they represent the first presentation of what is usually widespread disease. Therefore, the role of wide resection and allograft reconstruction for a putative solitary metastasis may be questionable. If systemic metastasis is evident, the risk of surgery may outweigh the benefits in a patient with only a limited survival chance.
- Some tumors are associated with a large soft tissue component (Fig. 3.3). This may render safe dissection around the major neurovascular structures or viscera impossible without violation of the tumor boundaries and contamination of these structures. In this scenario, hindquarter amputation may be a safer option than

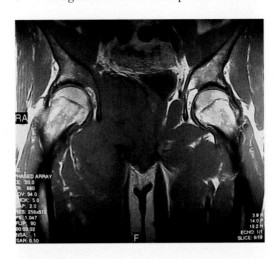

FIGURE 3.3

T1-weighted coronal MRI of the pelvis demonstrating an extensive soft tissue extension of a periacetabular Ewing sarcoma. Note displacement of the bladder.

limb-sparing surgery. If periacetabular resection is also associated with sciatic or femoral nerve sacrifice, not only does the patient face a dysfunctional lower limb but the stability of the reconstructed hip joint may also be jeopardized. In this scenario, limb-sparing surgery is contraindicated.

- If tumor resection requires sacrifice of the whole hemipelvis, only the sacrum will be left to provide a wide surface against which to seat a pelvic allograft. Attempts at achieving union with the contralateral pubis have been disappointing and with only the sacrum and the contralateral pubis for attachment, the allograft pelvis is left unsupported over a wide expanse. This predisposes the allograft to fracture and early failure.
- Major pelvic resections and management of subsequent complications require a team approach for successful completion. Skilled surgical staff, intensive care facilities, an experienced anesthetic team, ready access to a blood bank, and excellent ward facilities are mandatory when undertaking major pelvic resections and reconstructions. Absence of any elements of the above will require careful consideration prior to embarking on such complex surgery.

PREOPERATIVE PREPARATION

Staging Investigations

Staging investigations should be performed at the time of diagnosis as part of the patient workup and after neoadjuvant chemo- or radiotherapy to assess the response to treatment immediately prior to surgery. The surgical margins are calculated based upon the imaging performed immediately before surgery except in cases where there has been a poor response to neoadjuvant treatment. In the latter situation, surgical margins should be based on the studies obtained at the time of initial diagnosis.

Plain Radiographs

Plain radiographs should be obtained to allow rough planning and sizing of allograft material (Fig. 3.4). Further, it is important to preoperatively create a template of prostheses and preselect of a range of pelvic reconstruction plates that will be required to span and support the graft.

Bone Scan

Technetium methyl-diphosphonate bone scans should be obtained to identify the presence of any osseous metastases.

Computed Tomography

Computed tomography (CT) of the lungs is mandatory prior to surgery. Evidence of pulmonary metastases is a contraindication to major pelvic resection or reconstruction. CT is an excellent modality for delineating cortical or trabecular destruction (Fig. 3.5). Further, periosteal new bone formation is best detected using this modality and this will be critical in planning margins. The availability of three-dimensional reconstructed images may assist in planning the type and shape of allograft reconstruction to be employed.

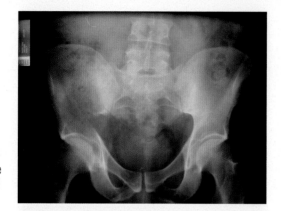

FIGURE 3.4

Plain radiograph of the pelvis demonstrating a malignant fibrous histrocytoma (MFH) of bone affecting the right periacetabulum. Full size radiographs are useful for accurate size matching of allograft material.

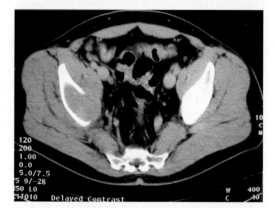

FIGURE 3.5

CT scans are excellent modalities for defining the degree of bone destruction in the pelvis. Not only does it clearly show defects in cortical and trabecular bone, replacement of the intramedullary bone by tumor is well demonstrated by the density of tissue that is higher than marrow fat.

Magnetic Resonance Imaging

Magnetic resonance imaging (MRI) provides unsurpassed soft tissue contrast and this characteristic should be exploited when deciding upon the appropriate soft tissue margins. This is particularly relevant when the soft tissue component of tumors lie adjacent to major neurovascular structures such as the lumbosacral trunk, the internal iliac vessels, the sciatic nerve, and gluteal vessels in the greater sciatic notch. Involvement of the hip joint may also be suspected by the presence of a joint effusion or changes in the signal characteristics of the hip joint fat pad or ligamentum teres. MRI is also an excellent modality for assessing the intraosseous extension of tumor which has implications for the planning of surgical margins (Fig. 3.6).

Functional Nuclear Imaging

Positron emission tomography and thallium scanning are two nuclear medical techniques that reflect the metabolic activity of tumors. They are ideal for assessing the most metabolically active part of the tumor for targeted biopsy as well as for assessing the response of tumors to neoadjuvant therapy. Poorly responsive tumors should be excised with far wider margins than those that are applied for good responding tumors.

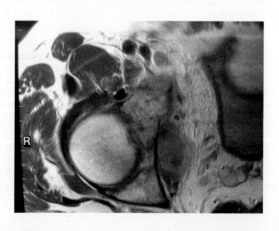

FIGURE 3.6

MRI scans of the pelvis are extremely valuable for determining the intra- and extraosseous soft tissue extent of tumor which is critical for planning surgical margins.

Blood Cross-Matching

Pelvic resections may be associated with considerable blood loss and this should be anticipated prior to the commencement of surgery. Cross-matching of blood should be performed early to identify the presence of any particular antibodies in the recipient that may make high-volume transfusion during surgery hazardous. Initial blood cross-matching demands should include 15 units of packed cells, 10 units of fresh frozen plasma, and 10 units of platelets. Further blood requirements may be determined on intraoperative testing of the patient's hemoglobin.

Preoperative Optimisation

Most patients on chemotherapy will experience a fall in peripheral blood products as a consequence of marrow suppression. The level of suppression is dependent on the health status of the patient, the type of cytotoxic drugs employed, and their dose and intensity of delivery. Advice should be sought from the treating chemotherapists as to what would constitute a safe minimum level of red cells, neutrophils, and platelets for surgery to be undertaken. In some circumstances, GM-CSF may be used to stimulate bone marrow activity. It is important to ensure that the patient has good renal function prior to surgery. The extensive blood loss and potential for intraoperative hypotension in the setting of preoperative chemotherapy may lead to renal failure. Some chemotherapeutic agents, for example doxorubicin, may also have a cardiotoxic effect. It is important that the state of the cardiac function is established prior to surgery so that appropriate intraoperative monitoring and care may be provided by the anesthetic team. Close collaboration with internal medicine physicians is required to optimize the preparation of the patient for surgery.

Informed Consent

It is critical that patients and their carers understand the full extent and sequelae of surgery. Information about the material risk must be furnished to patients to guide their acceptance or refusal of the complications and hardship of a failed reconstruction. If patients have understood the real risk of complications they may elect to accept hindquarter amputation or a flail hip in place of allograft reconstruction. Further, they need to understand the need for prolonged recumbency or rehabilitation to ensure safe healing and return of function to the operated limb. Finally, patients also need to understand the impact that surgery and the subsequent prolonged recovery phase will have on the quality of their lives over the ensuring 1 to 2 years. This is important because the risk of local or systemic recurrence of disease within the first 2 years is great and the patients will need to balance what limited time they may have after surgery with the incursion that postoperative convalescence and complications may have on that time.

TECHNIQUE

Patient Position and Draping

The patient is placed in a "floppy" lateral position with loosely applied supports resting against the thoracic spine and sternum. This allows the patient to be flopped forward to provide better visualization of the back of the pelvis or flopped backward to allow better visualization of the front of the pelvis. An axillary support is used to elevate the contralateral chest wall off the downside arm to avoid prolonged axillary and brachial neurovascular compression. The ipsilateral arm is excluded from the operative field under the drapes but is supported by a thoracic armrest to allow it to move with the body when the body is rolled from side to side as well as to reduce the weight of the arm against the chest wall that may cause axillary and brachial neurovascular compression. A protective plastic drape may be applied to shut out the upper body and the contralateral limb, ensuring that the margins of this drape cover the genital and perineal areas to avoid pooling of caustic or alcoholic antiseptic wash that may collect on the operating table or in skin creases and cause chemical skin burns or intraoperative fires sparked by electrocautery. The abdomen is draped free to allow access to the entire abdominal field. The ipsilateral limb is draped free to allow manipulation during surgery and preparation of the proximal femur for joint replacement. Access to the pubic symphysis is important to determine the correct position of the anterior pelvic osteotomy and also to protect the bladder and the bladder neck. Padding under pressure points such as the downside ankle, knee, and trochanter is important to avoid pressure necrosis of skin.

Anesthetic Considerations

Central venous and arterial access is vital for monitoring blood volume and pressure intraoperatively. The former also provides a reliable access for fluid resuscitation and drug delivery. Other intravenous lines are also inserted according to anesthetic preference. All patients are usually subjected to endotracheal intubation and volatile agent anesthesia and then ventilated during surgery. In some institutions, regional anesthesia is combined with general anesthesia. This achieves two purposes, namely, a reduction in the depth of general anesthesia during surgery because of the presence of regional anesthesia and the ability to continue regional anesthesia postoperatively, which may help to reduce the requirement of intravenous narcotic analgesia.

Urinary Catheterization

In the case of large pelvic tumors, the decision may be made to insert ureteric catheters prior to the commencement of surgery to assist in the identification of these structures during dissection. These are usually placed endoscopically and secured to a bladder catheter which is inserted at the same time for intra- and postoperative urine volume measurements.

Prophylactic Antibiotic

The risk of infection is high because of the immunosuppression, prolonged surgery, extensive soft tissue trauma, and the implantation of foreign biologic and synthetic material. Combination antibiotic therapy to cover staphylococcal and Gram-negative organisms is recommended. Vancomycin and ceftriaxone in combination provide adequate coverage and may be continued safely postoperatively. These should be given preoperatively and allowed to circulate prior to the commencement of surgery. Vancomycin should be given slowly over 30 minutes to avoid a vascular reaction sometimes referred to as "red man" syndrome.

Incision

A curved iliofemoral incision begins at the posterior superior iliac spine and follows the course of the iliac crest to the anterior superior iliac spine. It then passes distally a few inches in front of the greater trochanter before sweeping slightly distally and posteriorly a hand span distal to the center of the greater trochanter (Fig. 3.7A). The skin incision is carried down to and through the deep fascia. This creates a posteriorly based gluteal flap. Tumors that are covered by the gluteus medius muscle spare the gluteus maximus muscle which carries the blood supply to the overlying skin through the inferior gluteal vessels. If required, a second incision can be created that passes from the anterior superior iliac spine forward to the pubic tubercle (Fig. 3.7B). Should a second

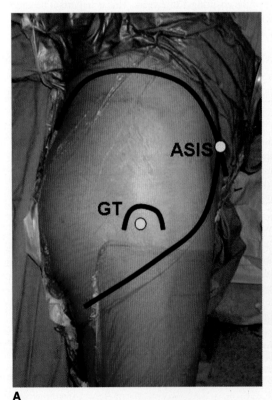
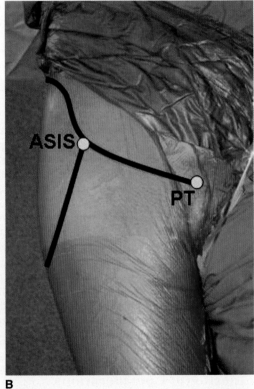

A   **B**

FIGURE 3.7

With the patient in the floppy lateral position, the incision used for pelvic resection includes **(A)** iliofemoral and **(B)** inguinal limbs. Key landmarks include the anterior superior iliac spine (ASIS), the greater trochanter (GT) and the pubic tubercle (PT).

incision be required, a triradiate incision is created, which gives an extensile approach to the hemipelvis. The anterior limb of the triradiate incision is created to provide better access to the vital neurovascular structures as they cross the inguinal ligament. A disadvantage of the triradiate incision is the potential for skin ischemia at the junction of the three limbs of the skin incision.

Exposure of the Posterior Pelvis

The deep fascia is incised along the iliac crest and continued to the anterior superior spine where the split between the sartorius muscle and the tensor fascia lata is found and incised. As the incision is carried inferiorly the gluteus maximus flap is reflected posteriorly. The gluteus maximus muscle is attached via a stout tendon to the outer border of the linea aspera below the greater trochanter. Division of the tendonous insertion of gluteus maximus allows the muscle to be reflected a considerable distance posteriorly to expose the posterior hip and pelvis, the sciatic nerve as it courses up to the sciatic notch, and the trochanteric attachments of the other glutei and short external rotators of the hip.

The sciatic nerve is followed up to the sciatic notch where it and the inferior gluteal vessels traverse the portal between the inner and outer pelvis. This space is quite confined and inadvertent injury to the vessels within the notch is possible if care is not taken. Increasing the dimensions of the sciatic notch allows much easier dissection, safer identification and tagging of the inferior gluteal vessels, and careful separation of the sciatic nerve from its adventitial attachments to the notch walls. Division of the sacrospinous and sacrotuberous ligaments allows a virtual dilation of the notch such that several fingers may be admitted into the true pelvis.

Division of the Sacrospinous Ligament

The anterior bony margin of the notch is followed distally to the point of the spine of the pelvis. The sacrospinous ligament is attached up to 1 cm or more along the spine from its tip. The internal pudendal nerve and vessels cross the sacrospinous ligament near the tip of the spine of the pelvis and these should be protected to avoid injuring the nerve, which may impact on bowel and bladder function, and rupturing the vessels which may cause troublesome bleeding. Once the nerve and vessels have been identified, the ligament attachment proximal to the tip of the spine is found, incised, and dissected subperiosteally off the spine. Release of this ligament increases the space of the sciatic notch and allows the pudendal nerve and vessels to drop back into the pelvis, thus moving away from danger.

Division of the Sacrotuberous Ligament

The sacrotuberous ligament is a strong falciform ligament that passes from the lower lateral border of the sacrum to the ischial tuberosity. Once the sacrospinous ligament is divided, the sacrotuberous ligament becomes obvious as a significant structure. This can be divided under direct vision between two Hohmann retractors. Releasing the sacrospinous and sacrotuberous ligaments is best done early. In periacetabular resections the sacrospinous ligament must be detached before that segment of the acetabulum can be extracted. If a type II/III resection is contemplated, then release of the sacrotuberous ligament is also required.

Exposure of the Inner Wall of the Pelvis

The external oblique muscle is incised with a coagulating diathermy along the line of the iliac crest and, if required, extended to its attachment along the inguinal ligament. The transversalis and internal oblique muscles are likewise incised. It is best to breach all three layers along the iliac crest whereupon two fingers may be admitted into the retroperitoneal space and pushing these fingers outward to tent the overlying abdominal musculature, the remaining part of the incision can be safely completed by cutting down on to the fingers. Extending the incision medial to the lateral border of the rectus abdominis needs to be done carefully to avoid injury to the inferior epigastric artery. Preservation of this structure should be attempted in case the rectus abdominus muscle that it supplies is required as a transposition flap to fill a groin defect.

Entry into the retroperitoneal space is signaled by the presence of a large amount of retroperitoneal fat. This can be pushed away to reveal the external iliac artery and vein. The vein is more medially and deeply placed in relation to the artery. Carefully following these vessels proximally will reveal the internal iliac vessels. Vessel loops should be applied at this stage to allow control of the vessels if required. The psoas major muscle lies along the brim that separates the greater and lesser pelvis. Dividing the psoas allows it to be retracted out of the way to provide much better exposure to the internal iliac vessels and the lumbosacral trunk as they pass toward the inner portal of the sciatic notch. Good exposure here is required to safely ligate and divide vessels and to avoid injury to the sciatic nerve. The vessels lie superficial to the lumbosacral trunk within the pelvis but emerge from beneath the sciatic nerve when viewed from the external side of the notch. A finger that is run up the external surface of the sciatic nerve toward the notch can be passed up into the notch to carefully dissect the nerve from its notch attachments without injuring the internal iliac branches as they lie deep to the nerve.

Superficial Femoral Vessels

The superficial femoral vessels are exposed by following the external iliac vessels to the inguinal ligament. The ligament is then freed from its attachment to the anterior superior iliac spine and retracted distally and forward. The vessels are held quite firmly by an investing fascia to the underlying pectineus muscle over the superior pubic ramus. They need to be carefully freed and then retracted with vessel loops that are passed around them.

Femoral Nerve

The femoral nerve is easily found in the crease between the iliacus and psoas muscles. This can be followed distally by incising the iliacus fascia, which lies over it, before being carefully lifted free and a nerve loop passed around it. The nerve can be followed all the way to the inguinal ligament which it penetrates to enter the upper part of the femoral triangle where it lies lateral to the superficial femoral artery.

Bladder

If a more medial osteotomy of the pubic rami is required, the bladder can be swept to the opposite side and protected with a pack and retractor. The bladder neck area needs to be carefully protected as the urethra is held under the superior arch of the pubis by a fascia that may cause injury to the urethra if too much traction is applied to the bladder. The area directly behind the symphysis needs to be cleared down to the symphyseal arch. The back of the symphysis is recognized by a small midline crest which is encountered when a finger is run along the inner surface of the superior pubic ramus toward the other side.

Hip Dislocation or Excision

Intra-articular resection of the hip implies resection of the pelvis after dislocation of the hip, while extra-articular resection implies resection of the pelvis including the hip without opening the hip joint. For intra-articular resections, the abductors are preserved by trochanteric osteotomy. The hip is internally rotated in flexion and the short external rotators put on tension and divided at their femoral attachments. The hip is then externally rotated in extension and the pectineus and the obturator externus muscles divided from their attachment to the femoral neck. The psoas tendon may be divided at its attachment into the lesser trochanter. The posterior capsule is then incised and the capsulotomy continued around the femoral head to finally release the femoral head from its acetabular attachment.

For an extra-articular resection, the short external rotators are kept intact. The pectineus and obturator externus muscle may also be kept intact depending on the extent of the pubic or ischial osteotomies. The femur is transacted immediately below the lesser trochanter. If the loss of femoral length is to be minimized, an oblique osteotomy may be used just distal to the line of the capsular attachment of the hip along the intertrochanteric line.

Pelvic Osteotomy

The pelvic osteotomies for a periacetabular resection pass through the superior pubic ramus, the inferior pubic ramus or ischial tuberosity, and through the ilium beginning at the sciatic notch and emerging at the iliac crest or the anterior inferior iliac spine depending on the margins of the resection. If possible, a forward tongue of iliac crest and bone should be preserved to help support the allograft. The iliac crest is a strong strip of bone that acts as an I-beam for the pelvis and is a useful strut against which to attach the allograft.

Attachment of the Allograft

The allograft should be securely fixed to the host bone with compression screws that pass through the acetabulum into the ilium and, if possible, also into the ischium or superior pubic ramus. The construct is then further supported by spanning pelvic reconstruction plates which add strength to the allograft (Fig. 3.8). If a tongue of iliac crest is preserved, screws may be directed from the allograft through the iliac crest or vice versa. All attempts should be made to size match the pelvis and information such as the gender and height, and plain radiograph of the pelvis should be provided to the relevant bone bank when acquiring allograft bone.

Hip Arthroplasty

The simplest hip arthroplasty is a bipolar arthroplasty. The large head size provides added stability. If a standard hip arthroplasty is performed, it is best to use a cemented cup which provides immediate acetabular fixation.

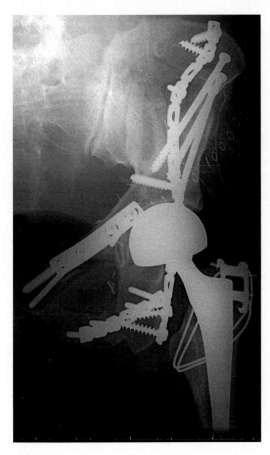

FIGURE 3.8

Allograft reconstruction after a type II periacetabular resection. Note the bipolar prosthesis for increased hip stability and large fragment interfragmentary screws and spanning plates to support the allograft.

Cementless cups do not capitalize on any ingrowth and the interference fit may cause allograft bone to fracture on impaction if the cup is oversized.

Stability of the hip is an issue. Preserving and reattaching the abductors where possible is of great value. Reconstructing a hip capsule by the use of polypropylene mesh has also been found to be useful. Occasionally, directional instability may be encountered. This can be improved by placement of allograft/autograft extensions around the rim of the acetabulum. A captured liner may also provide additional joint stability. Lengthening the limb may provide sufficient soft tissue tension to maintain the limb in position. Care must be taken to avoid overlengthening of the limb which is easy to do once a hip is disarticulated and the periacetabular soft tissue divided.

POSTOPERATIVE MANAGEMENT

The postoperative management must be clearly planned with the aim of minimizing complications, promoting healing of soft tissue, and protecting union of allograft to host bone.

Bed Rest

Patients should be confined to bed for the first 10 days to 2 weeks. The purpose of this is to allow the soft tissue trauma of the incision and the soft tissue reconstructions to settle and for the patient to recover from the injury and pain of surgery. Skin edge necrosis should be identified early and operative debridement and resuture undertaken.

Blood Loss

Up to 30% of the intraoperative volume of blood loss may also be lost in the drainage tubes in the first 24 hours after surgery. Close attention should be paid to hemoglobin levels to ensure that postoperative anemia does not become severe. There may be a heavy requirement for blood transfusions and postoperative coagulopathy may occur as a consequence. This should be treated with adequate fresh frozen plasma and platelet replacement as required. A soft spica constructed from Velband and crepe bandaging may be helpful for reducing hematoma formation, as well as for obliterating dead space in the upper thigh. Drainage tubes should be removed when flow rates are at a minimum (<10 mL/h for 4 consecutive hours).

Thromboprophylaxis

The use of low molecular heparin has become popular as prophylaxis against deep vein thrombosis. This may be combined with anti-thrombotic stockings and calf or foot compression devices. Ankle and foot exercises should be encouraged to promote venous circulation. The commencement of chemical thromboprophylaxis will be dependent on blood coagulation profiles and bleeding times.

Antibiotic Therapy

The selection of antibiotic therapy will be institution specific. However, specific agents to cover Gram-positive and Gram-negative cocci should be employed. We prefer vancomycin and ceftriaxone as the combination of choice. This is maintained for 10 days and then ceased. An oral cephalosporin is then administered for 3 months as this is the period of greatest susceptibility for infection.

Pressure Care

With prolonged bed rest, pressure care becomes important. Decubitus ulcers may be a source of hematogenous infection and should be avoided. Ripple or silicon mattresses should be utilized where possible. The operated leg frequently rolls outward and the motor power to the limb is insufficient to change its position. This predisposes the limb to heel and lateral malleolar pressure ulcers. Adequate precautions must be taken to avoid this.

Weight Bearing

Weight bearing should be avoided for up to 12 weeks to promote union. After 12 weeks, a program of graduated weight bearing may be instituted according to the surgeon's preference and by signs of union as seen on plain radiographs or CT scans. Once the patient begins to be mobile, a hip brace should be constructed to ensure stability of the hip and to prevent excursion of the joint to ranges that may predispose to dislocation. For example, a removal hip brace may be set to maintain the hip in 30 degrees of abduction with a range of flexion from 0 to 90 degrees.

COMPLICATIONS

Hemorrhage

Heavy intraoperative hemorrhage is a high risk with pelvic resections. Bleeding may be arterial or venous and also from the osteotomy surfaces. Certain areas are prone to bleeding; and these include the sciatic notch, the branches of the internal iliac vessels as they approach the sciatic notch, the venous plexus around the base of the bladder, and the obturator vessels as they emerge through obturator externus. The time of maximum bleeding seems to occur after the bone cuts and with extraction of the resected specimen from the pelvis. At this time, the bleeding from the osteotomy surfaces is poorly controlled and vessels which remain attached to the resected segment may be avulsed from their main branches. The internal iliac system is the most vulnerable during this part of the dissection. Techniques to minimize bleeding include blunt or finger dissection, use of argon beam diathermy, which is particularly good for bleeding surfaces of bone and also at the bladder neck, and early control of the main branches of the internal iliac before dissection into the pelvis.

Infection

Infection is a high risk of pelvic surgery and is further increased by the implantation of avascular biologic material such as allograft. All precautions should be taken to minimize infection which may be devastating. While patients have active sepsis, their chemotherapy must be curtailed and this may impact on the success of treatment. Active sepsis usually means removal of the allograft and conversion to a flail hip. If acute infection can be controlled by operative debridement and lavage, long-term antibiotic therapy is usually required to suppress ongoing infection.

Nerve Injury

Injury to the sciatic and femoral nerves is common with pelvic resections. This usually occurs from traction during exposure of the operative field or when the attempts are made to extract the resected segment from the pelvis. The latter is usually accompanied by rotation of the specimen as the final soft tissue attachments are divided. Injury of the sciatic nerve often occurs at the notch where it may be caught between the osteotomy surfaces, or traction is applied against the lumbosacral plexus which is firmly held to the inner surface of the pelvis by a thick fascia. Femoral nerve injury usually occurs with the dissection and retraction of the nerve as it crosses over the superior pubic ramus. Here it is often in the way of dissection and may be accidentally retracted with some force when one tries to free the femoral artery and vein. Nerve injury should be avoided at all cost because of the instability it may cause to the lower limb and the hip joint.

Dislocation

Dislocation of the hip joint is a common complication of acetabular reconstructions, whether by prostheses or allografts. The inclusion of the hip capsule with the operative specimen and the division of the short muscles of the hip predispose the hip to dislocation. Malposition of the allograft with subsequent seating of the acetabulum in an exaggerated anteverted, retroverted, or vertical inclination will exacerbate the tendency to dislocate. Size matching the pelvis affords the best opportunity of reconstructing the defect in an anatomical fashion.

RESULTS

Survivability

Periacetabular allografts for reconstructing the acetabulum now have an established place in oncologic and nononcologic surgery (1–15). A comparison between type 2 and type 1/2 or 1/2/3 resections for sarcoma reports that extending the resection beyond purely periacetabular is a much larger resection, and hence reconstruction is associated with a higher failure rate (1). The good survival rates of grafts that are utilized purely for revision hip arthroplasty and which are confined to the acetabulum support the notion that the smaller the allograft, the higher the success rate (9,11,12). The reason for the better results in smaller grafts is most likely attributable to the greater support that can be applied to smaller grafts.

Function

Good function depends on the stability of the reconstruction and the availability of the relevant motors to drive function about the hip joint. Given reconstructions that preserve good abductor, flexor, and extensor power about the hip, satisfactory function has been reported (1,3,5,6,8,16). Some have reported better function in patients 20 years old or younger as compared to older patients (3). In comparison to resections of other parts of the bony pelvis and despite the types of reconstructions utilized, resections that involve the acetabulum appear to have a greater negative impact on function and patient acceptance than those that do not include the acetabulum (17).

Complications

Allograft reconstructions are associated with significant complications (3,5,9,16). This is not surprising considering the extent and the duration of the surgery. The main complications include infection (1,3,11,15,16), nonunion (3), nerve injuries, and dislocation (11,12,15).

Use of Reinforcement Rings

The structural integrity of acetabular allografts depends on their ability to unite at the osteotomy sites and to tolerate the loading of the graft with weight bearing. Considerable work in hip revision surgery has confirmed the predictable nature in which bulk allografts will unite and be incorporated by host bone (9,18–21). While some reports following sarcoma resection show that good graft survival can occur and also directly support a cemented cup (11), roof-reinforcement rings have been shown to aid mechanical support and fixation and also have been shown to improve the performance of bulk acetabular allografts (4,22). Where possible, the allograft should be supported by rigid internal fixation, and adequate protection from load bearing must be provided to facilitate union at the osteotomy site (4,9,22,23).

REFERENCES

1. Beadel GP, McLaughlin CE, Wunder JS, et al. Outcome in two groups of patients with allograft-prosthetic reconstruction of pelvic tumor defects. *Clin Orthop Relat Res*. 2005;438:30–35.
2. Chen CH, Shih CH. Acetabular allograft reconstruction in total hip arthroplasty: preliminary report with clinical, roentgenographic and scintigraphic analyses. *J Formos Med Assoc*. 1994;93:781–787.
3. Delloye C, Banse X, Brichard B, et al. Pelvic reconstruction with a structural pelvic allograft after resection of a malignant bone tumor. *J Bone Joint Surg Am*. 2007;89:579–587.
4. Garbuz D, Morsi E, Gross AE. Revision of the acetabular component of a total hip arthroplasty with a massive structural allograft: study with a minimum five-year follow-up. *J Bone Joint Surg Am*. 1996;78:693–697.
5. Guest CB, Bell RS, Davis A, et al. Allograft-implant composite reconstruction following periacetabular sarcoma resection. *J Arthroplasty*. 1990;5(suppl):S25–S34.
6. Gul R, Jeer PJ, Oakeshott RD. Twenty-year survival of a cementless revision hip arthroplasty using a press-fit bulk acetabular allograft for pelvic discontinuity: a case report. *J Orthop Surg (Hong Kong)*. 2008;16:111–113.

7. Kumta SM, Kew J, Fu LK, et al. Massive diaphyseal and pelvic bone allograft for skeletal reconstruction. *Transplant Proc.* 1998;30:3776.

8. Mnaymneh W, Malinin T, Mnaymneh LG, et al. Pelvic allograft: a case report with a follow-up evaluation of 5.5 years. *Clin Orthop Relat Res.* 1990;255:128–132.

9. Paprosky WG, Martin EL. Structural acetabular allograft in revision total hip arthroplasty. *Am J Orthop.* 2002;31:481–484.

10. Parrish FF. Total and partial half joint resection followed by allograft replacement in neoplasms involving ends of long bones. *Transplant Proc.* 1976;8:77–81.

11. Piriou P, Sagnet F, Norton MR, et al. Acetabular component revision with frozen massive structural pelvic allograft: average 5-year follow-up. *J Arthroplasty.* 2003;18:562–569.

12. Saleh KJ, Jaroszynski G, Woodgate I, et al. Revision total hip arthroplasty with the use of structural acetabular allograft and reconstruction ring: a case series with a 10-year average follow-up. *J Arthroplasty.* 2000;15:951–958.

13. Stiehl JB. Acetabular allograft reconstruction in total hip arthroplasty. Part II: surgical approach and aftercare. *Orthop Rev.* 1991;20:425–432.

14. Stiehl, J.B. Acetabular allograft reconstruction in total hip arthroplasty. Part I: current concepts in biomechanics. *Orthop Rev.* 1991;20:339–341.

15. Yoshida Y, Osaka S, Mankin HJ. Hemipelvic allograft reconstruction after periacetabular bone tumor resection. *J Orthop Sci.* 2000;5:198–204.

16. Cheng MT, et al. Periacetabular giant cell tumor treated with intralesional excision and allograft reconstruction. *J Chin Med Assoc.* 2004;67:537–541.

17. Yuen A, Ek ET, Choong PF. Research: Is resection of tumours involving the pelvic ring justified? A review of 49 consecutive cases. *Int Semin Surg Oncol.* 2005;2:9.

18. Alexeeff M, Mahomed N, Morsi E, et al. Structural allograft in two-stage revisions for failed septic hip arthroplasty. *J Bone Joint Surg Br.* 1996;78B:213–216.

19. Hooten JP, Engh CA, Heekin RD, et al. Structural bulk allografts in acetabular reconstruction—Analysis of two grafts retrieved at post-mortem. *J Bone Joint Surg Br.* 1996;78B:270–275.

20. Oakeshott RD, Morgan DAF, Zukor DJ, et al. Revision total hip-arthroplasty with osseous allograft reconstruction—a clinical and roentgenographic analysis. *Clin Orthop Relat Res.*, 1987;225:37–61.

21. Stiehl JB, Saluja R, Diener T. Reconstruction of major column defects and pelvic discontinuity in revision total hip arthroplasty. *J Arthroplasty.* 2000;15:849–857.

22. Gross AE. Revision arthroplasty of the acetabulum with restoration of bone stock. *Clin Orthop Relat Res.* 1999:198–207.

23. Paprosky WG, Sekundiak TD. Total acetabular allografts. *J Bone Joint Surgery-Am.* 1999;81A:280–291.

4 Pelvic Prosthesis

Martin Dominkus and Rainer Kotz

Surgical reconstruction after pelvic resections remains a highly demanding procedure. More efficient chemotherapy in primary malignant bone tumors and a high percentage of long-term survivors have inspired greater interest in the development of pelvic reconstruction methods that permit limb salvage resections. The reconstructive procedures that are associated with pelvic reconstructions may be biological, endoprosthetic, or a combination of the two, and include pelvic allograft, saddle prosthesis, allograft prosthetic composites, and pelvic prosthesis reconstructions. This chapter gives an overview of the history, development, and state of the art of pelvic reconstruction with pelvic prostheses.

PREOPERATIVE PLANNING

Independent of the reconstruction method, accurate preoperative imaging of the intraosseous and extraosseous tumor extent is obligatory. This includes

- Computerised tomography (CT) scans, which provide the best information for detection of cortical lesions and offer the basic data for three-dimensional (3D) reconstruction (Fig. 4.1).
- MRI scans, which is ideal for demonstrating the intraosseous tumor extent, soft tissue involvement, and joint involvement (Fig. 4.2).
- Intravenous pyelography, which highlights the anatomical position of the ureter. Preoperative insertion of a ureteric catheter may prevent intraoperative damage.
- Arteriography or venography, which demonstrates the position and potential involvement of the iliac or femoral vessels. Recent generation MR angiographic techniques permit noninvasive assessment of the arterio and venous systems.
- Scintigraphy or whole body magnetic resonance imaging (MRI), which can diagnose or exclude metastatic disease (Fig. 4.3).
- The insertion of a vena cava filter, which can prevent fatal intraoperative or postoperative thromboembolism.

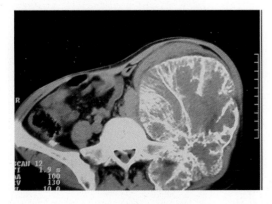

FIGURE 4.1

CT scan of a huge chondrosarcoma of the left ilium.

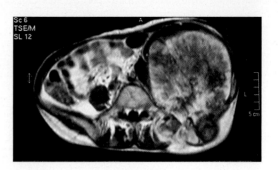

FIGURE 4.2

MRI scan of the same patient, showing soft tissue involvement and the anatomical position of the pelvic organs.

PREOPERATIVE CONSIDERATIONS

The patient should be in a good health condition with normal blood values before the operation. Sufficient amounts of blood products (packed cells, platelets, fresh frozen plasma) should be crossmatched and available, and a rapid blood warming-transfusion system should be available.

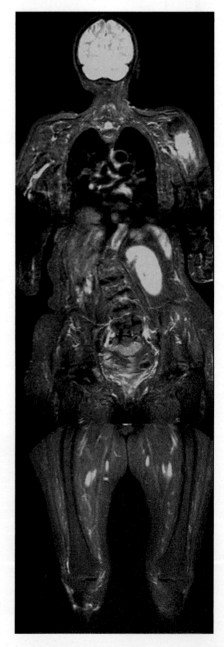

FIGURE 4.3

Whole body MRI.

OPERATIVE CONSIDERATIONS

- Newer computerized techniques that employ coregistration of CT and MRI images facilitate intraoperative computer navigation techniques for tumor resection and exact planning of the bone resection lines (Fig. 4.4).
- Depending on the type of endoprosthetic reconstruction additional preoperative planning has to be done. Most of the custom-made prostheses are designed via a 3D pelvic model, produced from the original CT data (Fig. 4.5A–F).
- More recently a virtual reality planning and simulation of endoprosthetic reconstruction of the pelvis has been reported (1). Using this technique, three-dimensional models are generated and manipulated in real time during the simulation of the pelvic operation. Cutting planes can be positioned in the 3D scene. The resected bone model is then used to determine the shape and geometry of the endoprosthesis. This technique prevents the time-consuming step of production of a solid pelvic model but the preoperative modeling of the prosthesis's size and position is critical for planning the intraoperative bone resection (Fig. 4.6A–D). An example of preoperative 3D visualization and determination of the bone resection, followed by computer aided design (CAD) designing and production of the prosthesis from the preoperative dataset and the exact intraoperative navigation of the appropriate bone resection, reporting a case of a patient with a metastatic destruction of the left acetabulum from a rectal carcinoma, was reported (2).

DISCUSSION

The first attempts of endoprostheses to reconstruct resected pelvic bone and to restore the pelvic ring can be found in the early 1970s. Scales and Rodney (*personal communication*) implanted a temporary spacer of acrylic cement and designed a steel prosthesis in the shape of the resected iliac bone. In a second surgery, they implanted the prosthesis by fixation with pins and cement. Unfortunately, the prosthesis had to be removed a few months later due to infection.

In 1974, Schöllner and Ruck (3) published the first case, in which resection of a chondrosarcoma in a 53-year-old truck driver was followed by implantation of a pelvic prosthesis during the same surgery. The extent of the planned resection was determined from x-rays of the patient. Next, a cast model was produced

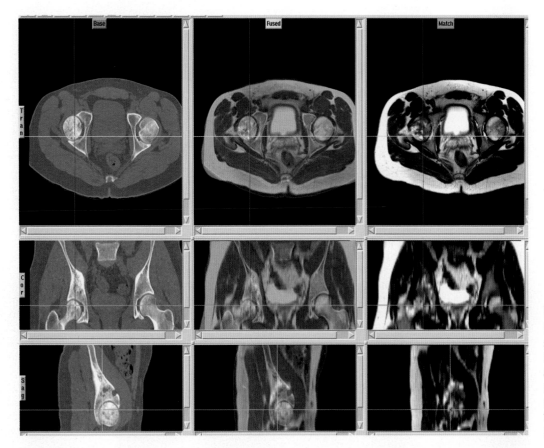

FIGURE 4.4

Digital fusion of the CT scan (**left row**) and the MRI data (**right row**) to a combined image (**mid row**) in a patient with an osteosarcoma of the right femoral head and right periacetabular region.

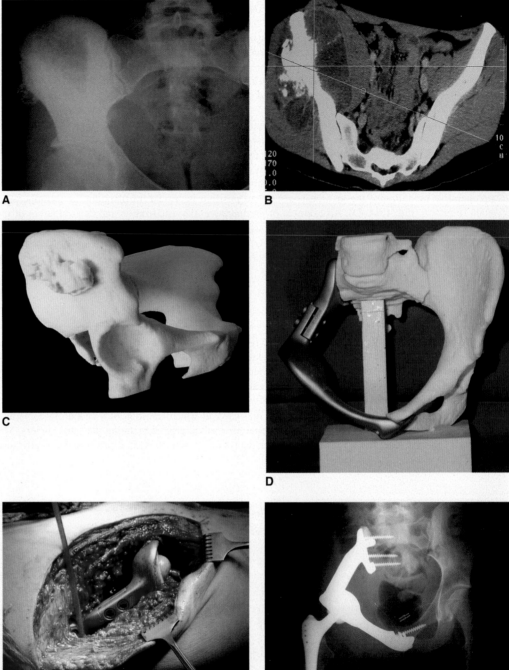

FIGURE 4.5

A: Plain x-ray of an osteosarcoma of the right iliac bone. Diffuse osteosclerosis of the iliac wing, periosteal destruction, and a lateral soft tissue extension can be seen. **B:** The CT scan confirms the bony destruction and demonstrates its extraosseous extent. Moreover, the medial dislodging of the musculus iliacus by the tumor mass is obvious. **C:** Pelvic model from the CT data set. **D:** Complete resection of the hemipelvis was chosen as an adequate oncologic treatment. According to the defined resection, a custom-made pelvic prosthesis was designed. **E:** Intraoperative view of assembling the prosthesis. **F:** Postoperative x-ray.

from a pelvic skeleton, which was similar in size to that of the patient. On this pelvic model, the resection lines were determined and a custom-made pelvic prosthesis was machined from steel. The tumor was removed by a Type II wide resection (4) and the prosthesis was implanted in the same procedure. The prosthesis was fixed to the remaining part of the ilium, ischium, and pubic bone by flanges and screws. The femoral part of the hip joint was reconstructed with a conventional Charnley-Mueller prosthesis. Five weeks after surgery the patient left the hospital, mobilized with partial weight-bearing, and at follow-up examination, the prosthesis was still in place without any signs of dislocation, loosening or infection, and the patient was able to walk with one cane and drive his car.

Johnson treated two patients after internal periacetabular resection with a reconstruction of the pelvic ring by cement reinforced Küntscher rods and Kirschner wires (5). One patient, who had adequate resection of a chondrosarcoma, was reported to be well and able to walk without a cane 5 years postoperatively, and the other patient, who had an inadequate resection of a high-grade chondrosarcoma, died after 2 years but was also able to walk with a cane.

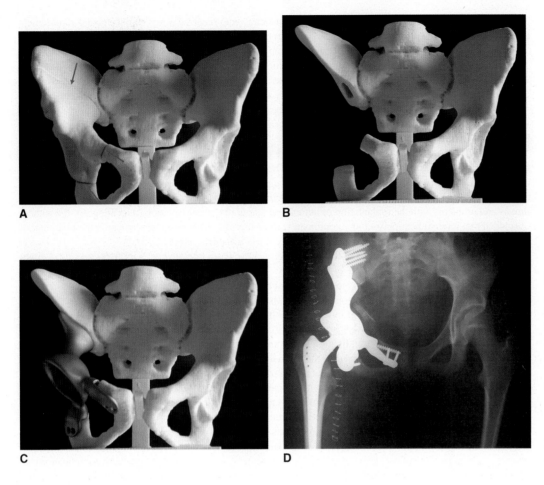

FIGURE 4.6
A: Precise preoperative planning of the pelvic osteotomies. **B:** The pelvic model after the simulated resection. This model is the basis for the custom-made prosthesis. **C:** The prosthesis with exact fit to the model. **D:** The postoperative x-ray after exact resection according to the planning.

Since that time attempts have been made to improve the accuracy of pelvic prosthesis production and design. Better imaging techniques now allow precise preoperative planning and 3D CT data help to obtain an exact model of the patients' pelvis.

Gradinger reported on 25 patients with internal hemipelvectomy and endoprosthetic reconstruction for primary bone tumors in 17 and metastases in 8 patients. Also in his series the first prostheses were custom-manufactured from plain x-rays. Intraoperatively, they were difficult to adopt and the anatomical orientation of the acetabulum was imprecise. Prostheses made from polyacetal could be adopted intraoperatively more easily, but still the orientation was insufficient. Since the use of CT and the possibility of computer-aided design of pelvic models, Gradinger developed a new custom-made, anatomically adoptable prosthesis. The anchorage into the remaining iliac bone was mainly provided by an intramedullary stem with additional plates and flanges with screw holes to also enable screw fixation. To reduce lateral shear forces, the pelvic ring was closed with a semidynamic connection mimicking the symphysis function. Twenty of these prostheses were used in his series and he reported a reduction of complications, for example, dislocation, reduction in operation time, and infection (6).

In a review of our own series, Windhager et al. reported on 21 consecutive cases who underwent limb salvaging surgery for periacetabular sarcomas between 1972 and 1990. In cases with preoperative conventional imaging techniques only 50% of the resection could achieve wide margins, whereas 100% wide margins were documented after 3D imaging. In nine of these patients, a custom-made endoprostheses (Howmedica) was used after defining the resection on a real-size model produced using computer-assisted reconstruction of CT sections. The functional outcome was best after reconstruction with a custom-made prosthesis, only satisfactory after saddle prosthesis and poor, when allografts or when no reconstruction was performed (7). A new ventral and dorsal approach was used in most of the patients, which offered the advantage of good exposition of the ischium and the lateral part of the sacrum.

Guo et al. (8) published a new design of a modular hemipelvic endoprosthesis to reconstruct periacetabular bone defect. Other than using custom-made prostheses, which needed a planning and production phase of some weeks, the use of a modular prosthesis provided immediate intraoperative prosthetic fitting to the given anatomical situation. The system consisted of an iliac fixation component with a variable length bush and a plate for screw fixation to the ilium, an acetabular component, and a pubic connection plate. All of the components were made of titanium. In 28 patients operated between 2001 and 2005, the complication rate after a mean follow-up of 30 months was 39%, mainly infection, wound necrosis, hip dislocation, and two patients with pubic connection breakage. About 7 patients could walk without supports; 21 patients needed at least one cane or crutch.

Falkinstein et al. (9) reported on the results of 21 patients, who received a new periacetabular replacement prosthesis (Stryker-Howmedica, Rutherford, New Jersey) between 2000 and 2006. The prosthetic design allowed the remaining ilium to support a horizontal acetabular component secured with internal fixation and bone cement. The pelvic ring is not closed. Compared to the conventional saddle prosthesis, this design offered an improved load distribution. About 10 were alive and 11 died after a mean follow-up of 20.5 months. The most common complication was deep infection in six patients, local recurrence in four, and dislocation in two patients.

Wirbel et al. (10) reported on 39 patients, most of them reconstructed with a polyacetal resin replacement, 8 with a custom-made vitallium prosthesis, and 2 had a saddle prosthesis. About 13 of the 19 surviving patients had good or excellent results. Six had a dislocation.

Bruns et al. (11) described long-term results on 15 patients with internal hemipelvectomy and endoprosthetic pelvic replacement over a period of 15 years. The six surviving patients, who had been implanted with custom-made pelvic prostheses (Link), had only a medium score of functional outcome, but a high subjective acceptance. Compared with even lower functional outcome of alternative surgical procedures such as pseudarthrosis and problems with the replantation of autoclaved autografts or implantation of an allograft, the authors concluded that internal hemipelvectomy combined with endoprosthetic pelvic replacement is the treatment of choice for acetabular lesion, provided a complete resection is feasible.

More recently, Tunn et al. (12) reviewed their 24 consecutive cases operated between 1994 and 2004. Eight patients survived the follow-up period of 98 months. The most common complications included infection (41.7%), femoral or sciatic nerve paralysis (33%), local recurrence (20.8%), and loosening of the endoprosthesis (16.7%). In three patients secondary external hemipelvectomy had to be performed due to infection. Five patients still had their endoprosthesis at follow-up, the function was good in two and fair in three. The authors had a high loosening and screw breakage rate in their prostheses used until 2000 (Stryker-Howmedica) and tried to close the pelvic ring by a rigid fixation of the prostheses. Since the year 2000, another endoprosthetic design has been used, which is only fixed to the ilium and does not close the pelvic ring (MUTARS, Implant cast). The reason for changing the endoprosthetic fixation concept was the idea that a rigid closure of the pelvic ring that does not allow micromotion as in a symphysis will lead to screw breakage and loosening.

The outcome of limb salvage pelvic procedures in children and adolescents using different types of reconstruction showed the best results for biologic reconstruction in children below 10 years of age. Older children or adolescents were mainly treated with endoprostheses or allograft and prosthesis composites, which showed a significantly higher complication rate (2.5) of reoperations per patient, compared to the group of patients with other reconstructions or without reconstruction (13). Hillmann et al. (14) found the same high complication rate of endoprosthetic reconstruction in their series of 110 primary pelvic tumor resections between 1982 and 1996. In contrast to Hillmanns finding, Zeifang et al. (15) reported a lower complication rate in 11 of 42 patients with endoprosthetic reconstruction of the pelvis compared to 18 patients with biological reconstruction.

In a most recent study on 776 patients with endoprosthetic reconstruction of the appendicular skeleton and pelvis, Jeys at al. (16) described a 10-year implant survival rate of pelvic prostheses of 59.9 %. However, their analysis did not include the type of implant or the type of pelvic fixation.

The main differences between the available pelvic prostheses are

- Modularity: Up to now, most of the implants require a preoperative acquisition of the anatomical shape via a solid pelvic model obtained from CT data of the patient, or via computer assisted planning, which leads to a time-consuming custom-made implant production. Only a few systems are routinely available and provide the possibility of intraoperative adaption according to the bone defect after tumor resection.
- The fixation of the prosthesis to the remaining bone and the feature of anatomically reconstructing the pelvic ring: Most of the implant designs aim to anatomically reconstruct the pelvic ring and the hip rotation center to provide a maximum of function. However, these implants are usually large and produce a significant soft tissue defect, which facilitates haematoma formation and infection. Rigid fixation to the contralateral pubic bone, which does not mimic the dynamic properties of the symphysis and does not allow micromotion during gait, often fails by screw breakage, dislocation, and loosening of the implant (Fig. 4.7). Other prosthetic

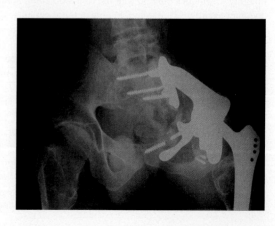

FIGURE 4.7

Loosening of a custom-made prosthesis reconstructing the entire hemipelvis in a male patient with multiple osteochondromas and a chondrosarcoma in the left ilium. Lateral force transmission led to failure and breakage of all screws with consecutive implant loosening.

TABLE 4–1 Complications After Custom-made Pelvic Prostheses After a Mean Follow-up of 163 Months (99 to 248 Months)

Complication	Number of Revisions	%
Infection	21	75
Wound healing disturbance	20	71
Prosthetic loosening	16	57
Hematoma	11	39
Dislocation	9	32
Thrombosis	5	18
Nerve palsy	2	7
Intraoperative exitus letalis	1	3
Local recurrence	1	3

designs are only fixed to the iliac bone and do not close the pelvic ring. These implants are smaller, and therefore soft tissue filling of the pelvic defect is easier, which may prevent the high rates of infection. However, these implants need at least a remaining part of the ilium and cannot be used in total internal hemipelvectomy.

In our own series of 28 patients, custom-made pelvic prostheses were implanted between March 1988 and May 2000. The mean age of these 17 female and 11 male patients was 33.6 years, ranging between 12 and 62 years. About 12 patients died after a mean of 26 months after surgery (1 to 64 months). The 16 patients who are still alive after a mean of 163 months have a follow-up period between 99 and 248 months. All of them had primary malignant bone tumors; chondrosarcoma was the most frequent tumor (11 patients), Ewing sarcomas and osteosarcomas were equally frequent (8 patients each), and 1 patient had a haemangiopericytoma. The main site for tumor was the ilium in 22 patients. Four patients had their tumors located in the proximal femur, but had to be treated by extra-articular hip joint resection, and two patients had their tumors in the pubic bone resulting in a periacetabular resection. Detailed results of some of these patients were published in 1996 by Windhager et al. (7). Later Schwameis et al. (13) found a complication and reoperation rate of 2.5 per patient after endoprosthetic reconstruction compared to 0.8 reoperations after no reconstruction or some other type of reconstruction. The most recent data of all our patients in the long-term follow-up showed that 3 out of 28 patients had no complication (10.7%). Nine patients had no revision (32%). The remaining patients had a total of 86 complications including one intraoperative death and one hemipelvectomy for local recurrence (Table 4.1). Summing up, the revision rate after long-term follow-up was 3.1 per patient. Infection, wound healing disturbances, and prosthetic loosening were the most frequent complication requiring revision. In some patients, additional periprosthetic bone bridging during the primary procedure or as a salvage procedure during revision was performed to allow a secondary closure of the pelvic ring, thereby reducing the shear forces to the prostheses (Fig. 4.8). In one patient, a spontaneous ankylosis of the hip joint from periarticular ossifications occurred (Fig. 4.9A–E).

Due to this high complication rate the concept of pelvic reconstruction was changed, and since the year 2000 we use a pedestal cup (Schoellner-cup, Zimmer) (Fig. 4.10A,B), originally designed for severe acetabular revision (17), in pelvic resections Enneking type (partly) I, II, and III. Complete resections of the iliac bone (resection Type I) were reconstructed biologically, and complete internal hemipelvectomies or resections, which also involved the lateral mass of the sacrum, were reconstructed by a hip transposition plasty (18).

Our results of the pedestal cup include 39 patients after tumor resection and 45 patients after revision of conventional hip prostheses. The 39 patients after tumor resection were 21 female and 18 male patients with a

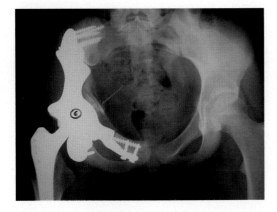

FIGURE 4.8

Complete osseous bridging and closure of the pelvic ring 3 years after primary surgery and bone grafting around the prosthetic body.

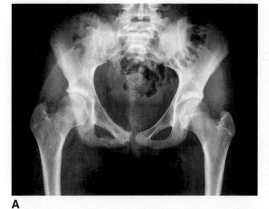

A

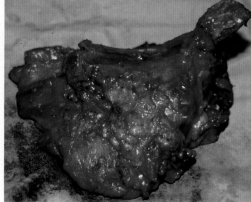

B

FIGURE 4.9

A: Plain x-ray of a 13-year-old girl with an Ewing sarcoma of the right pubic bone. **B:** The resected specimen after wide resection Enneking Types II and III. **C:** Radiograph 6 months postoperatively shows the implant in situ, but periarticular ossification had developed, leading to an ancylosis of the hip joint. **D:** Eleven months postoperative x-ray shows loosening and screw breakage at the symphysis anchorage. Clinically, a transvaginal fistel could be seen. **E:** During revision the pubic arm of the prosthesis was cut and removed intraoperatively using a Midas Rex device with diamond cutting blades. The prosthesis remained in situ and the fistel healed after a further two revisions with soft tissue coverage using an omentum majus flap and a gracilis flap, respectively.

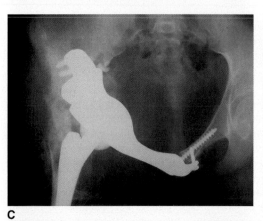

C

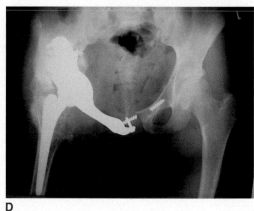

D

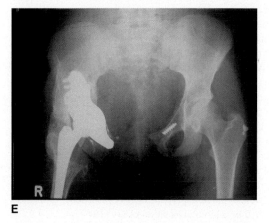

E

FIGURE 4.10

A: The design of the pedestal cup. Due to its asymmetric cup, the inclination angle can be adjusted at implantation by turning the cup around its axis. **B:** Typical orientation of the pedestal cup during implantation.

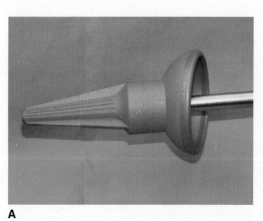

A

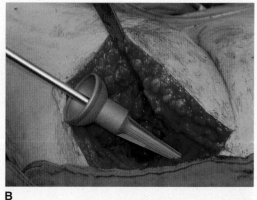

B

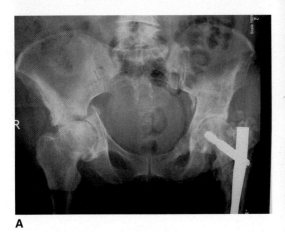

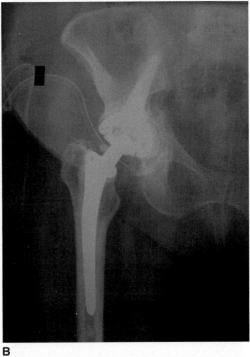

FIGURE 4.11
A: Pathologic supra-acetabular fracture and disrupture of the pelvic ring in a patient with breast cancer metastasis. **B:** Palliative reconstruction with cemented total hip arthroplasty using the pedestal cup.

mean age of 52 years (15.9 to 82.9 years). In this group of patients, a high number of implantations were carried out after periacetabular destruction due to bone metastases (17 patients) (Fig. 4.11). This explains the higher mean age in this group. Primary malignant tumors were treated in 18 patients. Two patients had acetabular destruction after tumor simulating diseases (histiocytosis X, pigmented villonodular synovitis [Fig. 4.12]), and one patient had a fibrous dysplasia and one a plasmocytoma.

Thirty-two patients received the pedestal cup in the primary procedure, and in seven patients it was implanted as a salvage procedure; two after custom-made pelvic prostheses failed (Fig. 4.13A–C) and five after other reconstruction techniques failed (Table 4.2).

Complications that required surgical revision occurred in 13 patients (33%): 5 dislocations (13%), 4 haematoma/necrosis (10%), 3 infections requiring prosthesis explantation (7%)—1 one-stage revision, 1 prosthesis explantation without further reconstruction and, 1 hip disarticulation—and 1 intraoperative fracture of the iliac bone leading to a consecutive implant loosening and exchanging of prosthesis (2%). Thus, 0.3 revisions were

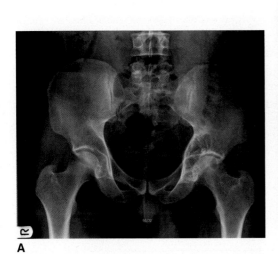

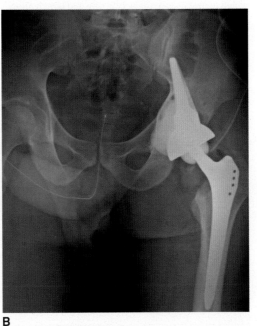

FIGURE 4.12
A: A rare case of a severe acetabular destruction in a 30-year-old male patient suffering from villonodular synovitis. **B:** The disrupted pelvic ring after complete curettage was reconstructed with the pedestal cup and a conventional femoral stem.

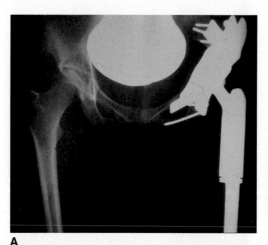

A

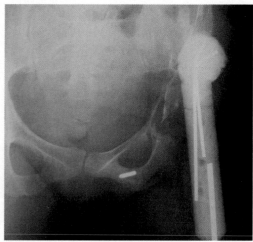

B

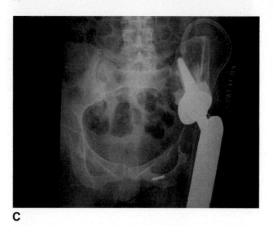

C

FIGURE 4.13

A: Reconstruction of a periacetabular osteo-sarcoma with a custom-made pelvic prosthesis and a proximal femur tumor endoprostheses. **B:** Explantation of the prosthesis after a late infection and implantation of a temporary cement spacer. **C:** Implantation of a pedestal cup in a second-stage procedure after healing of the infection.

necessary in the group of patients with pedestal cup. Dislocation was the most frequent complication in the beginning. However, since the routine use of an additional polyester band creating an artificial joint capsule, the dislocation rate has declined considerably (19) (Fig. 4.14A,B).

In conclusion, most of the procedures described above using pelvic prostheses to reconstruct the pelvic ring seem to fail mechanically. Micromotion through the sacroiliac joint and load transmission to a small and weak bone anchorage area lead to implant or screw fatigue failure in most cases. The concept of using implants, which do not restore the pelvic ring and which allow a more axial load transmission through their bony anchorage, may be one of the crucial factors in reducing loosening and implant failure. Moreover, these smaller implants allow a better soft tissue reconstruction and reduce the dead space within the pelvis after resection, leading to a lower incidence of haematoma, necrosis, and infection.

TABLE 4–2   Comparison of Complications Between Custom-Made Pelvic Prostheses and the Pedestal Cup

Complication	Custom-Made Prostheses		Pedestal Cup	
	Number of Revisions	%	Number of Revisions	%
Infection	21	75	3	7
Wound healing disturbance	20	71	1	2
Prosthetic loosening	16	57	1	2
Hematoma	11	39	3	7
Dislocation	9	32	5	13
Thrombosis	5	18	0	0
Nerve palsy	2	7	0	0
Intraoperative exitus letalis	1	3	0	0
Local recurrence	1	3	0	0

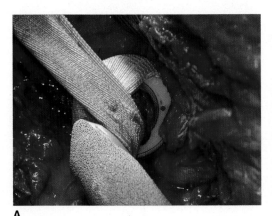

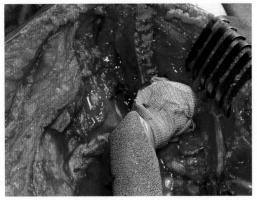

A   **B**

FIGURE 4.14

A: The polyester band is fixed with nonresorbable sutures around the pedestal cup and then around the femoral neck (anticlockwise on the right hip and clockwise on the left hip—this tightens the artificial capsule in outward rotation). **B:** After tightening in inward rotation of the leg, the artificial joint capsule is closed around the hip joint.

REFERENCES

1. Handels H, Ehrhardt J, Plötz W, et al. Simulation of hip operations and design of custom-made endoprostheses using virtual reality techniques. *Methods Inf Med.* 2001;40(2):74–77.
2. Wong KC, Kumta SM, Chiu KH, et al. Computer assisted pelvic tumour resection and reconstruction with a custom-made prosthesis using an innovative adaptation and its validation. *Comput Aid Surg.* 2007;12(4):225–232.
3. Schöllner D, Ruck W. Proceedings: pelvic prosthesis—an alternative to hemipelvectomy in tumor patients. *Z Orthop Ihre Grenzgeb.* 1974;112(4):968–970.
4. Enneking WF, Spanier SS, Goodman MA. A system for the surgical staging of musculoskeletal sarcoma. *Clin Orthop Relat Res.* 1980;153:106–120.
5. Johnson JT. Reconstruction of the pelvic ring following tumor resection. *J Bone Joint Surg Am.* 1978;60(6):747–751.
6. Gradinger R, Rechl H, Ascherl R, et al. Partial endoprosthetic reconstruction of the pelvis in malignant tumors. *Orthopade.* 1993;22(3):167–173.
7. Windhager R, Karner J, Kutschera HP, et al. Limb salvage in periacetabular sarcomas, review of 21 consecutive cases. *Clin Orthop Rel Res.* 1996;331:265–276.
8. Guo W, Li D, Tang X, et al. Reconstruction with modular hemipelvic prostheses for periacetabular tumor. *Clin Orthop Rel Res.* 2007;46:180–181.
9. Falkinstein Y, Ahlmann ER, Menendez LR. Reconstruction of type II pelvic resection with a new peri-acetabular reconstruction endoprosthesis. *J Bone Joint Surg Br.* 2008;90(3):371–376.
10. Wirbel RJ, Schulte M, Maier B, et al. Megaprosthetic replacement of the pelvis: function in 17 cases. *Acta Orthop Scand.* 1999;70(4): 348–352.
11. Bruns J, Luessenhop SL, Dahmen G Sr. Internal hemipelvectomy and endoprosthetic pelvic replacement: long-term follow-up results. *Arch Orthop Trauma Surg.* 1997;116(1–2):27–31.
12. Tunn PU, Fehlberg S, Andreou D, et al. Endoprosthesis in the operative treatment of bone tumours of the pelvis. *Z Orthop Unfall.* 2007;145(6):753–759.
13. Schwameis E, Dominkus M, Krepler P, et al. Reconstruction of the pelvis after tumour resection in children and adolescents. *Clin Orthop Relat Res.* 2002;402:220–235.
14. Hillmann A, Hoffmann C, Gosheger G, et al. Tumours of the pelvis: complications after reconstruction. *Arch Orthop Trauma Surg.* 2003;123(7): 340–344.
15. Zeifang F, Buchner M, Zahlten-Hinguranage A, et al. Complications following operative treatment of primary malignant bone tumours in the pelvis. *Eur J Surg Oncol.* 2004;30:893–899.
16. Jeys LM, Kulkarni A, Grimer RJ, et al. Endoprosthetic reconstruction for the treatment of musculoskeletal tumours of the appendicular skeleton and pelvis. *J Bone Joint Surg Am.* 2008;90(6):1265–1271.
17. Schoellner C, Schoellner D. Die Sockelpfannenoperation bei acetabulären Defekten nach Hüftpfannenlockerung. Ein progress report. *Z Orthop.* 2000;138:215–221.
18. Winkelmann W. A new surgical method in malignant tumors of the ilium. *Z Orthop.* 1988;126(6):671–674.
19. Dominkus M, Sabeti M, Kotz R. Functional tendon repair in orthopedic tumor surgery. *Orthopade.* 2005;34(6): 556–559.

5 Saddle Prosthesis

Kristy L. Weber

Saddle prosthesis reconstruction of a large acetabular/pelvic defect is a rare procedure with limited indications and substantial morbidity. This construct was originally designed for reconstruction in patients with large acetabular bony defects after total hip replacement with or without infection (Fig. 5.1). The most common current scenario is a patient with a primary or metastatic bone tumor located in the periacetabular region. Occasionally, it is still used in cases of massive bone loss after trauma or hip dysplasia or as a salvage procedure after failed hip reconstructive surgery. Resection types for pelvic tumors have been classified according to anatomic location (1). There are alternative reconstructive options after a Type 2 periacetabular resection that include a custom pelvic endoprosthesis, allograft-prosthetic composite hip reconstruction, iliofemoral arthrodesis or pseudarthrosis, ischiofemoral arthrodesis or pseudarthrosis, and flail hip. The benefits of a saddle prosthesis include stable limb reconstruction for early weight bearing, equal leg lengths, acceptable function, and relative ease of prosthesis placement compared to arthrodeses or allograft-prosthetic composites.

INDICATIONS

- Periacetabular (Type 2 or Type 2/3) resection of a primary or metastatic bone tumor (Fig. 5.2)
- Salvage procedure after multiple hip revision surgeries with periacetabular bone loss
- Periacetabular bone loss secondary to trauma
- Periacetabular bone loss due to severe hip dysplasia

CONTRAINDICATIONS

- Active pelvic infection within the operative field
- Lack of substantial remaining ilium. The saddle prosthesis requires a stable, thick area of medial ilium for attachment to the pelvis; otherwise, there is a risk of iliac wing fracture through the thinner (lateral, superior) bone.
- Lack of functional abductor muscles puts the patient at higher risk of dislocation.
- Severe osteoporosis predisposes the ilium to fracture during weight bearing.
- Patients receiving intensive chemotherapy may be at higher risk of infection.
- Compromise of the lumbosacral plexus *or* femoral neurovascular bundle by tumor in addition to involvement of the acetabulum/hip joint is generally an indication for an external hemipelvectomy (hindquarter amputation).
- No viable rectus abdominus musculature to fill the dead space if the iliopsoas or gluteal muscles are resected. This is a relative contraindication as free tissue transfer or local tissue rearrangement can also be used.
- Extensive medical comorbidities that preclude a prolonged surgical procedure or predict a lifespan <3 months

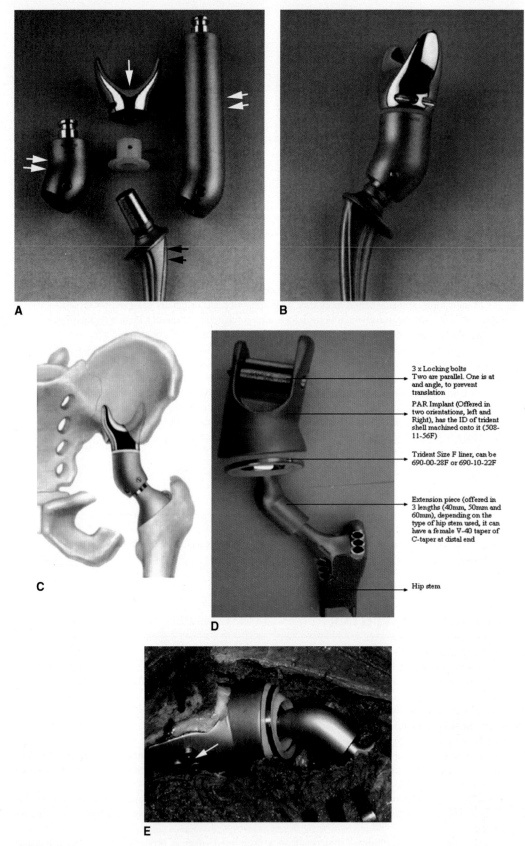

FIGURE 5.1

Examples of the saddle type prosthesis from two different manufacturers. **A:** Link saddle prosthesis disassembled showing the saddle component (*white arrow*), two sizes of body component (two *white arrows*), polyethylene component (*black arrow*), and femoral stem (two *black arrows*). **B:** Assembled Link prosthesis. **C:** Model of Link saddle prosthesis pelvic reconstruction. **D:** Stryker PAR pelvic implant. **E:** Stryker prosthesis implanted in the pelvis. Note the locking bolts (*arrow*) and cement holding the PAR component to the ilium.
(D and E Courtesy Lawrence Menendez, Los Angeles).

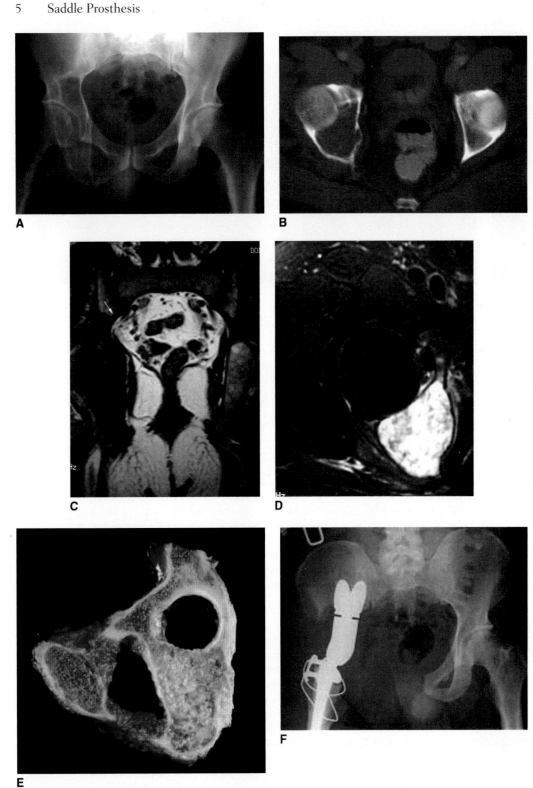

FIGURE 5.2

A: A pelvis radiograph showing a grade 2 chondrosarcoma of the right acetabulum in a 44-year-old man.
B: CT scan shows an osteolytic lesion in the posterior acetabulum with intralesional calcifications.
C: Coronal T1-weighted MRI shows the proximal extent of the tumor at the lower edge of the sacroiliac joint
(*arrow*). **D:** Axial T2-weighted, fat-saturated MRI revealing an expansile lesion in the posterior acetabulum.
E: Gross specimen after a Type 2/3 pelvic resection. **F and G:** Postoperative pelvis and AP right hip radiographs showing the Link saddle prosthesis in good position. Note the trochanteric osteotomy fixed with a
trochanteric claw and cables.

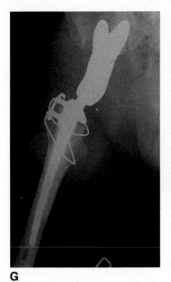
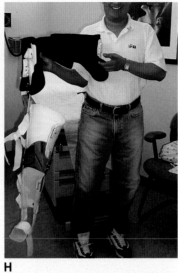
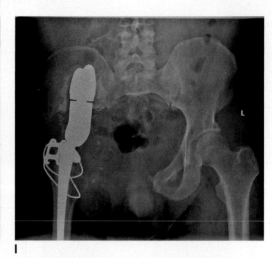

G   H   I

FIGURE 5.2 (*Continued*)

H: Six weeks postoperatively the patient is fully weight bearing out of the hip abduction brace. His iliopsoas and hip abductor muscles were maintained. **I:** AP pelvis radiograph 8 years postoperatively showing stable position of the saddle prosthesis with minimal bone formation around the saddle component. The patient walks with a very minimal limp and uses no assistive devices.

PREOPERATIVE PREPARATION

Patient Expectations

Pelvic resections are challenging procedures with potential complications. Patients should be adequately counseled on the risks for their particular situation. There are several different periacetabular reconstructive options, and the risks and benefits of each should be described so that the physician and patient can make the best decision to balance function with potential complications. After a saddle prosthesis reconstruction, patients are usually able to fully bear weight after the soft tissues have healed, and their leg lengths should be equal. However, they may have a permanent limp and require assistive devices to ambulate if the hip flexors or abductors are compromised from the tumor extension. The known risks of this reconstruction (dislocation, infection, fracture, neurologic compromise, etc.) should also be clearly outlined.

Workup

A detailed history and physical examination are performed preoperatively with attention to pain, tumor stage, expected lifespan, neurologic status, gait, lower extremity strength, presence of signs of infection, inguinal adenopathy, and location of prior incisions/biopsy tracts. Plain radiographs and cross-sectional imaging of the pelvis are necessary. An MRI scan is helpful in situations where an adequate tumor margin needs to be achieved, as this will show the marrow and soft tissue extent of the disease. In a case of traumatic bone loss or a failed hip arthroplasty, a CT scan can better outline the bony structures in the pelvis. Adequate medial iliac bone is required to allow a stable fit of the saddle portion of the prosthesis and avoid a postoperative iliac wing fracture. Staging studies to assess the presence of possible metastasis are performed to better assess the anticipated lifespan or likelihood of cure. Preoperative laboratory tests include a complete blood count, protime/prothrombin time, electrolytes, and a type and cross for blood products. For a highly vascular metastasis (renal, thyroid), preoperative embolization should be considered to decrease blood loss. A formal preoperative bowel prep is used to minimize the chances of infection if the bowel is perforated during surgery.

Surgical Team

For the resection, ensure the availability of appropriate surgical services. Depending on the extent of tumor, other services may include urology, gynecologic oncology, vascular surgery, general surgery, and plastic surgery. If a primary bone tumor such as chondrosarcoma, Ewing sarcoma, or osteosarcoma invades the bladder or vaginal wall, it is necessary to partially resect these structures en bloc with the tumor to achieve an adequate margin. Often there is a plane between tumor and bowel, which is carefully dissected by the orthopedic or general surgeon. The benefit of the plastic surgery team cannot be underestimated, as a saddle prosthesis reconstruction creates a large devascularized dead space with frequent loss of part or all of the iliopsoas muscle.

This becomes a potential area for accumulation of a hematoma and subsequent infection. An ipsilateral or contralateral rectus abdominus flap is often rotated into the wound at the end of the case if the inferior epigastric vessels are maintained.

Equipment

There are several companies that currently make a saddle type of prosthesis (Link, Hamburg, Germany [1979] and Stryker, Mahwah, New Jersey). As of early 2011, the Stryker PAR process remains in the 510(k) approval process at the FDA. Review the specific technique considerations. Template the femoral side and determine the likely gap after resection in order to select the correct length of the curved body (base) component. The femoral component is placed with methylmethacrylate. Heavy sutures will help secure the saddle component to the ilium. For surgeons who use computer navigation for pelvic resections, the specific equipment should be ordered. A ureteral stent is placed in the operating room by the urology team to protect one or both ureters during the resection. A formal abduction brace is often used postoperatively to prevent early dislocation and is ordered in advance so that it can be placed on the patient at the end of the case.

Anesthesia Considerations

Often a pelvic resection and reconstruction can require many hours in the operating room depending on the extent of the tumor. The anesthesia team should be aware of this in advance to plan for additional venous access, arterial lines, and blood products.

TECHNIQUE

Positioning

The patient is placed in a sloppy lateral position on a beanbag or other support after vascular access catheters, endotracheal tube, urinary catheter, and ureteral stent(s) are inserted. If there is a possibility of a rotational muscle flap, it is best to prepare and drape out the entire abdomen, leg, and the back to midline. Intravenous antibiotics are given and re-dosed throughout the procedure. If the dissection occurs around the bowel, additional antibiotic coverage may be warranted.

Resection

The resection technique depends on the specific location of the periacetabular tumor. An ilioinguinal or iliofemoral approach is used depending on the involvement of the anterior pelvis. For some resections, an additional "T" incision is made to raise the gluteus maximus as a posterior flap. In this case the anterior/inferior flap should be retracted with the origins of the sartorius and tensor fascia lata to maintain blood supply to this corner of the skin. Expose the retroperitoneal space with release of the abdominal muscles from the ilium. The inguinal ligament is transected carefully to preserve the underlying external iliac vessels. The spermatic cord is retracted medially. If the inferior epigastric vessels are maintained to the ipsilateral rectus abdominus, it can be used for a later rotational flap. If the superior pubic ramus requires exposure, the rectus abdominus muscle is released superiorly and the space of Retzius between the symphysis pubis and bladder is exposed. The femoral neurovascular bundle is elevated from the superior pubic ramus and freed distally to the profunda femoris artery to allow for adequate mobilization. If the anterior pelvis is part of the resection, the obturator vessels and nerve are ligated. If a medial portion of the superior and inferior pubic rami can be maintained, obturator neurovascular structures can potentially be saved. The adductor muscles are released from the symphysis, and eventually the hamstring muscles are released posteriorly from the ischium. If transection through the symphysis pubis is required, protect the urethra, which is just posterior to this area. The urinary catheter is usually palpable within the urethra. A Gigli saw is helpful for this cut. The external iliac vessels are dissected as proximal as necessary in the pelvis to allow the appropriate cut through the ilium. The hypogastric vessels are identified and preserved if possible or ligated if necessary. Often, depending on the soft tissue extension of the tumor, the iliopsoas obstructs an adequate view for dissection within the pelvis and needs to be partially or fully resected while maintaining the femoral nerve. The patient will have improved function if some or all of the iliopsoas is maintained. Maintenance may also preclude the need for a rotational muscle flap. At this time it is usually possible to assess whether there is involvement of the bowel, bladder, prostate, or vagina and intraoperative consultations are called if necessary. As the dissection continues proximally it is important to protect the ureter. The L5 nerve root lies over the sacral ala, and the lumbosacral plexus travels through the greater sciatic notch and both should be protected. Some tumors require an iliac cut to be made through the lateral sacrum and then superior to a point where a transverse cut across the entire ilium is safely made.

If a posterior flap is raised, the gluteus maximus is maintained along the posterior ilium and may or may not need to be partially or totally released from the iliotibial band or femur. The sciatic nerve is identified and followed proximally to the sciatic notch. The gluteus medius is either released from the iliac crest and retracted distally or it is released via a trochanteric osteotomy and elevated proximal to the level of the iliac osteotomy. The sciatic nerve and surrounding vessels are protected in the greater sciatic notch, and the ischial spine is identified as the most inferior border of the sciatic notch. The sacrospinous ligament is released from the ischial spine after the pudendal vessels are ligated. The pudendal nerve can occasionally be maintained. Usually, the sacrotuberous ligament is released from the ischial tuberosity. The external rotators (piriformis and gemelli) are released from the femur and tagged. The iliac osteotomy is made once the soft tissues are cleared and protected within and outside the pelvis. The femoral neck cut is then made so that the hip joint can be maintained intact with the resection in case there is tumor extension into the acetabulum. After all the cuts are made, the remaining hamstrings and pelvic floor are released to remove the specimen. *For cases after traumatic bone loss or as a salvage after failed hip reconstruction, much of this technique is not necessary. A more limited resection is done after débridement of the fracture fragments or removal of a prior acetabular reconstruction. In these situations, more bone and soft tissues can be maintained such that there is usually no need for a rotational flap.* After a tumor resection, the operative team changes gowns, gloves, and instruments and adds or changes the upper drapes to maintain a clean field. The pelvic cavity is irrigated with warm saline using a pulse lavage system, and hemostasis is obtained. Bone wax is placed on bleeding bone edges and care is taken to prevent stretch on the pelvic neurovascular structures.

Reconstruction

This technique is based on placement of the Link saddle prosthesis. The Stryker PAR prosthesis involves several modifications to allow the pelvic portion of the prosthesis to be bolted to the ilium and supplemented with cement (see Fig. 5.1). The reader is encouraged to read the specific technique manual depending on the specific implant used.

It is important to assess the thickness of the remaining medial ilium as this is where the saddle component is placed. The leg is medialized, which helps decrease the dead space. Using a high speed burr, a deep groove is created in the ilium to articulate with the symmetrical, saddle-shaped end piece. The medial horn of the saddle lies within the pelvis and the lateral horn is outside the pelvis. The ilium groove needs to be deep enough to minimize the risk of dislocation of the component. Occasionally, the remaining anterior ilium (ASIS) will be too prominent after the leg is medialized. The author has occasionally taken the most prominent bony section off using a saw and fixed it as a lateral buttress adjacent to the pelvic portion of the prosthesis using long screws.

Once the ilium is prepared, attention is directed to the femur. If the femoral head was not taken as part of the pelvic resection specimen, a femoral neck cut is made followed by standard preparation of the femur. Broaches are used to open the canal in preparation for the trial femoral stems.

The resection length is restored using a trial prosthesis comprising the femoral stem, curved body (base) component, and saddle component. Between the body component and the saddle is a polyethylene bearing, which allows movement between these metal parts. The movements allowed by the saddle itself include flexion, extension, and rotation around a central axis. A small screw is placed through the base of the saddle (on the lateral side to be accessible if later revision is necessary) to prevent dislocation of these components (see Fig. 5.1). The length is restored using the appropriate modular body component to balance between enough tension to prevent dislocation and no undue stretch on the neurovascular structures (common lengths are 70 to 90 mm). After the trial reduction is complete, the real femoral stem is cemented into the canal. After the cement hardens, the body and saddle components are assembled and placed in the medial ilium groove. Drill holes are placed in the adjacent ilium with heavy suture wrapped around the saddle component and through the bone to add stability during the closure and early postoperative period. Four additional set screws are added through the body component to fix it to the underlying Morse taper. The wound is reirrigated and inspected to assess the need for a muscle flap. Deep drains are placed exiting near the incision, and a layered closure is performed. The gluteus medius is either reattached to the ilium using drill holes or reattached distally using a trochanteric claw and cables. A sponge count is performed. Sterile dressings are placed, and an abduction brace or pillow is used during transfer of the patient to the recovery room.

PEARLS AND PITFALLS

- If an ipsilateral rectus abdominus rotational flap is used, be quite sure the inferior epigastric blood supply to the muscle is intact.
- Key to the successful long-term outcome is achieving an adequate surgical margin, which may require resection of all or part of nearby visceral structures. With a saddle prosthesis, imaging artifact will make it more difficult to detect early local recurrence within the pelvis.
- A high speed burr or Kerrison rongeur can be used to create a small groove along the medial ilium or lateral sacrum in order to keep the Gigli saw from sliding off the bone when starting the transection of the ilium.
- If the tumor resection is extensive and requires many hours, consideration should be given to stage the resection and reconstruction on different days to minimize the risk of infection.
- Add heavy suture or tapes around the saddle component and through drill holes in the adjacent ilium to provide resistance to early dislocation.

POSTOPERATIVE MANAGEMENT

If the case is prolonged or there is extensive blood loss, the patient may initially be in the intensive care unit. Appropriate intravenous antibiotics and venous thromboembolism prophylaxis are given. Blood transfusions and replacement electrolytes are given as needed. A careful postoperative neurologic check is performed to assess the status of the femoral and sciatic nerves. The author recommends using a hip abduction brace with hip flexion from 0 to 70 degrees and fixed abduction of approximately 30 degrees (see Fig. 5.2). Unless there is a nerve palsy, free knee and ankle motion is allowed, and the brace includes a footplate to maintain the leg in neutral alignment. The patient works with physical therapy to ambulate with assistive devices on postoperative day No. 2 if medically stable. Depending on how the abductors were reconstructed, the patient either bears weight as tolerated or protects his or her weight bearing for 6 weeks in the brace. Daily attention to the brace is required to prevent pressure sores, which can lead to skin breakdown. The author prefers that wound drains be discontinued before the patient leaves the hospital. After 6 weeks, the brace is removed and the patient works with physical therapy to progress to bearing weight as tolerated. At this time, strengthening of the hip flexors, extensors, and abductors is initiated. Several weeks after surgery, a fibrous pseudocapsule forms around the saddle component of the prosthesis, and this often gradually ossifies, decreasing the likelihood of dislocation.

COMPLICATIONS

The benefits of limb stability, equal leg lengths, and ease of reconstruction compared to other options must be balanced against the 33% to 65% chance of major complications when using the saddle prosthesis in patients with massive bone loss or tumors in the periacetabular region. However, modifications of the Link saddle prosthesis have improved the early design problems to minimize mechanical failures, and other manufacturers have developed new models of pelvic endoprostheses. Given the rarity of this underlying problem and type of reconstruction, the available literature on results and complications is limited.

Infection

Infection is the most common complication after saddle prosthesis reconstruction and occurs 18% to 33% of the time (2–8). Causes include the large dead space after resection of a periacetabular tumor, which the prosthesis cannot fill, in addition to the prolonged surgical time and need for multiple blood transfusions. Average surgical times range from 361 to 600 minutes (2,3,5). The first report of a large series of saddle prostheses described its use after failed total hip replacement and reported 15/72 cases of infection, which led to poor results (7). Local rearrangement of soft tissues or rotational rectus abduminus flaps are used to minimize the dead space to decrease the risk of infection (3).

Prosthesis Dislocation/Dissociation/Migration

Dislocation of the saddle component from the ilium groove occurs in 2% to 22% of patients and the risk is highest in the immediate postoperative period (2–5,7). Prevention of this complication requires optimal soft tissue tension balanced against excessive stretch on the neurovascular structures. Once a pseudocapsule forms and begins to ossify around the saddle component, the risk is minimized unless a traumatic event occurs that puts undue force on this junction. However, if a dislocation occurs, it requires an open reduction due to twisting of the saddle component (Figs. 5.3 and 5.4). Interestingly, the early series of Nieder et al. (7) only had a 2% dislocation rate in 72 cases. A separate complication involves dissociation of the actual prosthetic components, which occurs in 0% to 12% of cases (2,3,5). This can occur when the middle body segment detaches from the hip prosthesis or between the body segment and the saddle component. Progressive proximal migration of the saddle into the ilium occurs in 0% to 25% of cases and has been associated with infection and prior radiation (3–5). This leads to progressive leg shortening, which usually stabilizes by 12 months (3).

Ilium Fracture

The pyramidally thickened bone superior to the acetabulum and along the medial ilium must be maintained to support the saddle prosthesis. Laterally, the bone becomes progressively thinner, and placement of the saddle in this area can lead to a postoperative ilium fracture when the patient starts to bear full weight on the reconstruction (Fig. 5.3). Patients with severe osteoporosis are contraindicated for this reconstruction due to their increased risk of fracture. It is reported in 0% to 20% of series and primarily occurs in the ilium (3,8).

Heterotopic Ossification

Within a few weeks after surgery, the junction of the saddle component with the ilium is surrounded by a fibrous capsule that gradually consolidates into thicker scar tissue or bone, which helps protect against dislocation. Extensive bone formation or heterotopic ossification around the prosthesis is reported in up to 35% of cases (3,8) (Fig. 5.5).

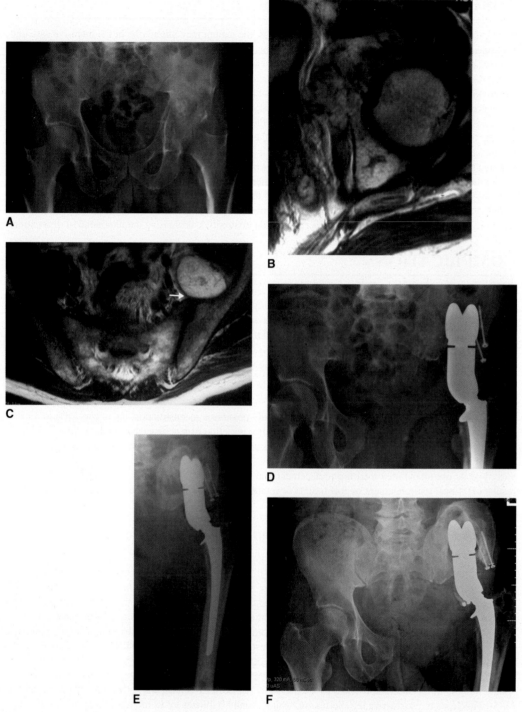

FIGURE 5.3

A: A pelvic radiograph showing a left acetabular grade 2 chondrosarcoma in a 66-year-old man. Note the mixed osteolytic and osteosclerotic appearance. **B:** Axial MRI reveals involvement of the anteromedial acetabulum with soft tissue extension. **C:** Axial MRI through the lower sacroiliac joint showing the proximal extent of the soft tissue mass (*arrow*). This requires the osteotomy to be through the thinner proximal iliac bone. **D:** Postoperative pelvic radiograph with the Link saddle prosthesis in place. A prominent portion of the anterior ilium (ASIS) was removed and used to buttress the prosthesis laterally with two screws. **E:** The patient developed a postoperative ilium fracture, which was managed nonoperatively with protected weight bearing and eventually healed as shown on this left hip radiograph taken 3.5 years postoperatively. **F:** Nine years after surgery, the saddle prosthesis failed between the saddle and body components and required an open revision. The position of the saddle component was maintained. This radiograph is taken 10 years after surgery with a stable prosthesis.

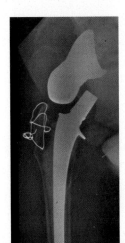

FIGURE 5.4

Example of a Link saddle prosthesis that dislocated between the body component and the stem. This required an open reduction.

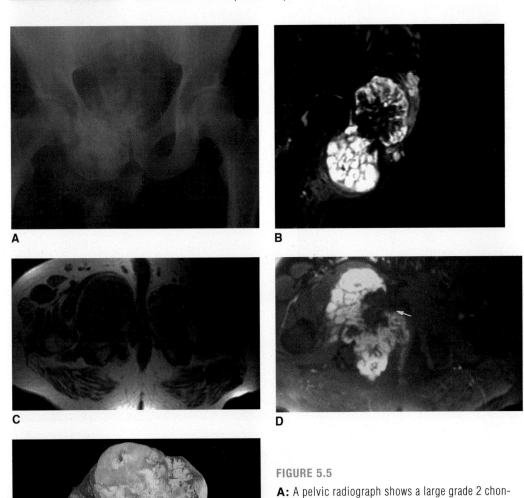

FIGURE 5.5

A: A pelvic radiograph shows a large grade 2 chondrosarcoma in the right periacetabular region in a 55-year-old man. The mass is heavily mineralized. **B:** Coronal T2-weighted, fat saturated MRI reveals the extent of soft tissue extension within the pelvis and distally into the thigh. **C:** Axial T1-weighted MRI reveals the proximity of the mass to the right side of the penis and urethra. **D:** Axial T2-weighted MRI shows the tumor overlapping the symphysis pubis, necessitating osteotomies through the contralateral superior and inferior pubic rami (*arrow*). **E:** The gross specimen with the femoral head remaining in the acetabulum as the tumor extends close to the hip joint.

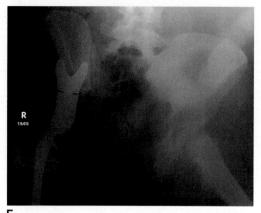

F

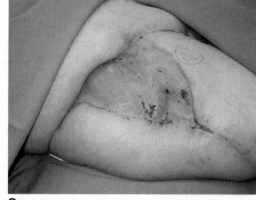

G

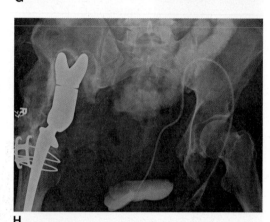

H

FIGURE 5.5 (*Continued*)

F: Postoperative pelvic radiograph after reconstruction with a Link saddle prosthesis. Note the trochanteric osteotomy reattached with a trochanteric claw and cables. **G:** The patient developed postoperative wound drainage due to a deep infection requiring several operative débridements with local soft tissue rearrangement and an eventual skin graft over the anterolateral thigh. The components remained in place and the patient was maintained on suppressive oral antibiotics. **H:** Four years after surgery, a pelvic radiograph shows extensive heterotopic ossification around the saddle component. The patient did not have recurrence of the infection. Note the suprapubic catheter due to a urethral injury at the time of resection.

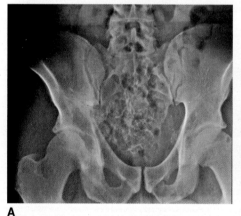

A

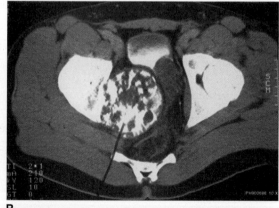

B

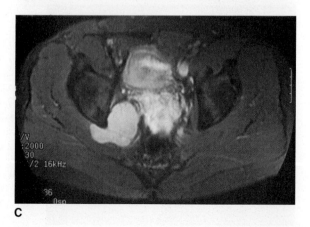

C

FIGURE 5.6

A: A pelvic radiograph in a 44-year-old man with a grade 1 chondrosarcoma along the right medial acetabulum. **B:** CT scan reveals the heavily mineralized medial soft tissue mass extending into the pelvis. The patient refused the appropriate Type 2 pelvic resection and had the chondrosarcoma "shaved" off of the medial wall instead. **C:** Axial MRI 3 years later with a local recurrence of the chondrosarcoma in the posterior pelvic soft tissues.

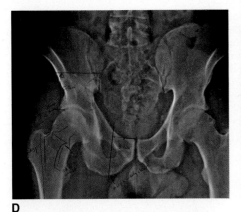

D

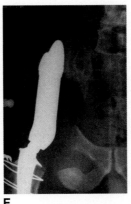

E

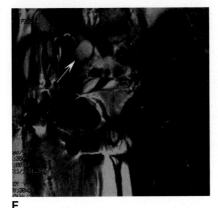

F

FIGURE 5.6 (*Continued*)

D: A pelvic radiograph used to template the appropriate pelvic cuts and saddle prosthesis. **E:** During the second surgery, the recurrent tumor was peeled from the lumbosacral plexus and final pathology revealed that it was now a grade 2 chondrosarcoma. A Link saddle prosthesis was placed after a trochanteric osteotomy. **F:** Eight months later, the patient developed a second local recurrence near the sacroiliac joint (*arrow*), necessitating a hindquarter amputation. He died of metastatic disease 30 months later.

Neurovascular

Neurovascular damage to the sciatic, femoral, or peroneal nerves can occur with transient or permanent palsies in 12% to 20% of patients (2,3,5,8). These complications can occur during the tumor resection or the saddle reconstruction.

RESULTS

Most of the recent series on saddle prosthesis reconstruction involve treatment of patients with primary or metastatic periacetabular tumors. Resection of primary pelvic bone tumors leads to a local recurrence rate of over 19% due to the complex anatomy and proximity of visceral structures (3,9) (Fig. 5.6). The largest series of saddle prostheses for pelvic sarcoma is from Aljassir et al. with 27 cases and a mean follow-up of 45 months. Seven patients had a Type 2 resection while 20 patients had a Type 2/3 resection. The overall survival was 60% at the time of reporting with 22% local recurrence and 22% metastasis. The average MSTS 93 score in their 17 living patients was 50.8% ± 21.7%. This is similar to functional results in other series (2,4,9). The periacetabular region is particularly challenging to reconstruct, given its crucial effect on limb function. Cottias et al. (10) reported fair function in 17 patients after saddle prosthetic reconstruction and surmised that this was due to decreased saddle range of motion and weak abductor strength.

REFERENCES

1. Hugate R Jr, Sim FH. Pelvic reconstruction techniques. *Orthop Clin North Am.* 2006;37:85–97.
2. Aboulafia AJ, Buch R, Mathews J, et al. Reconstruction using the saddle prosthesis following excision of primary and metastatic periacetabular tumors. *Clin Orthop Relat Res.* 1995;314:203–213.
3. Aljassir F, Beadel GP, Turcotte RE, et al. Outcome after pelvic sarcoma resection reconstructed with saddle prosthesis. *Clin Orthop Relat Res.* 2005;438:36–41.
4. Guo W, Li D, Tang X, et al. Surgical treatment of pelvic chondrosarcoma involving periacetabulum. *J Surg Oncol.* 2010;101:160–165.
5. Kitagawa Y, Ek ET, Choong PFM. Pelvic reconstruction using saddle prosthesis following limb salvage operation for periacetabular tumour. *J Orthop Surg.* 2006;14:155–162.
6. Natarajan MV, Bose JC, Mazhavan V, et al. The saddle prosthesis in periacetabular tumours. *Inter Orthop.* 2001;25:107–109.

7. Nieder E, Friesecke C: Mid-term results of 73 saddle prostheses, endomodular, at total hip revision arthroplasty. Seventh International Symposium on Limb Salvage. Singapore, August 23–27, 1993.

8. Renard AJS, Beth RPH, Schreuder HWB, et al. The saddle prosthesis in pelvic primary and secondary musculoskeletal tumors: functional results at several postoperative intervals. *Arch Orthop Trauma Surg.* 2000;120:188–194.

9. Pring ME, Weber KL, Unni KK, et al. Chondrosarcoma of the pelvis. A review of sixty-four cases. *J Bone Joint Surg.* 2001;83:1630–1642.

10. Cottias P, Jeanort C, Vinh TS, et al. Complications and functional evaluation of 17 saddle prostheses for resection of periacetabular tumors. *J Surg Oncol.* 2001;78:90–100.

6 Periacetabular Metastases

Peter F. M. Choong

Metastatic carcinoma is the commonest malignancy of bone and characterizes the behavior of 50% of carcinomas. Carcinomas of the prostate, breast, and lung account for over 80% of lesions with renal and thyroid metastases being less frequent. The most destructive lesions are lytic with carcinoma cells permeating the bone and activating lytic proteases and instigating osteoclastic bone resorption. Lung and renal carcinomas typically invoke osteolysis and a permeative behavior. Sclerotic lesions, in contrast, are dominated by regions of bone formation rather than resorption. The stereotypic carcinoma that incites sclerosis with its metastases is prostate carcinoma. Breast carcinoma is characterized by a mixed sclerotic-lytic picture. Regardless of whether the picture is one of lysis or sclerosis, the quality of bone is poor with disorganized formation interspersed between sheets of neoplastic cells. Pain, pathologic fracture, marrow disturbance, and hypercalcemia are the commonest consequences of metastatic bone disease.

The pelvis is a common site of metastatic disease and frequently the entire area can be involved. Destruction of the periacetabulum has far-reaching implications because of its central role in connecting limb mobility and weight bearing. The periacetabular bone transmits the weight of the torso to the legs and the legs in turn transmit the power of mobility to the body through the hip joint. As such, there is a concentration of forces at the hip joint, which makes it vulnerable to failure in the presence of tumor-induced weakening of bone. Failure of function manifests as a loss of weight-bearing capacity, pain, or both.

In the majority of cases, metastatic pelvic disease is treated with a combination of chemotherapy, radiotherapy, hormonal therapy, bisphosphonate therapy, and regimes of analgesia. These combinations of treatment are effective in reducing pain, preventing fracture, preserving function, and improving the quality of life of most patients with pelvic disease. Until recently, the progressive nature of metastatic disease and the lack of surgical experience with periacetabular reconstruction have deterred many from exploiting operative approaches to managing aggressive periacetabular disease that have had a profoundly detrimental effect on patient mobility and independence. Consequently, many patients with potentially surgically treatable disease have had to endure a painful and infirm end to their lives.

GOALS OF SURGERY

The goals of surgical management of periacetabular metastases are to achieve pain control, maintain hip function and mobility, and permit weight-bearing ability. Achieving these goals will have an enormous impact on the patients' quality of life. To this end, surgery will be directed toward the safe removal of tumor, filling and structurally bypassing the defect, and creating a durable and dependable joint reconstruction. The decision to operate is predicated on the knowledge of the local and systemic extent of the disease, the patient's health status and longevity, and the probability of the reconstruction improving the patients' pain, function, and mobility.

INDICATIONS

Periacetabular reconstruction for metastatic disease is indicated in the following situations.

- When patients have failed conservative nonsurgical treatment including a non–weight-bearing period, radiotherapy, chemotherapy, and potent pain control programs.
- Reconstruction is also indicated when periacetabular destruction presents at an advanced stage when it is clear that nonsurgical treatment is unlikely to improve pain and function.

- Periacetabular surgery is also indicated when other surgery for femoral disease, such as impending or completed fracture, is indicated in the presence of periacetabular disease.
- Patients who are expected to survive with disease for longer than 3 months should be considered for periacetabular reconstruction.

CONTRAINDICATIONS

- The pain and recovery from periacetabular reconstruction and the potential risks of the procedure need to be carefully considered in patients with <2 months survival chance. The justification for surgery in this group may be questionable.
- This procedure may also be contraindicated in patients who have significant visceral disease and who may not tolerate the stress of prolonged surgery or blood loss. In this regard, patients with significant pulmonary disease may be particularly vulnerable to a condition known as pulmonary embolic phenomenon which manifests itself as acute cardiovascular and pulmonary collapse at the time of femoral preparation, cementation, or prosthesis insertion.
- Surgery is also contraindicated when metastatic disease is so extensive as to provide no bony foundation for the attachment of the reconstruction.

PREOPERATIVE PREPARATION

Preoperative preparation is critical for the safe and successful management of patients with metastatic disease. This includes imaging to assess the local and systemic extent of disease, biopsy to confirm the nature of the bone lesion if this is not known, blood tests to assess the general health status of the patient, and other special tests as required. It is recommended that patients are also reviewed by the anesthetic and internal medicine teams to reverse, stabilize, or optimize any comorbidity that may have a negative impact on the patient's intra- and postoperative course.

Plain Radiographs

Plain radiographs of the whole pelvis should be obtained (Fig. 6.1). This would allow an assessment of not only the extent of periacetabular disease from which surgical planning may be undertaken but also involvement of any other part of the pelvis, which may be relevant. There are a number of classifications of acetabular disease based on plain radiographs. More complex reconstructions are required with increasing degrees of destruction. Plain radiographs should also be taken of the full length of the femur to identify the location of any femoral lesions. This is important to avoid the mistake of implanting a femoral prosthesis above the level of the femoral metastasis, which would create an increase in stress that may lead to periprosthetic fracture.

Computed Tomography

Computed tomography (CT) is an excellent modality for assessing cortical and trabecular destruction. This imaging technique is useful for more accurate delineation of periacetabular disease (Fig. 6.2A,B) than plain radiographs. Later-generation software are able to produce excellent three-dimensional reconstructions which can be rotated and manipulated, providing surgeons with different perspectives of the pelvis, which may help to guide their choice of reconstruction (Fig. 6.2C).

CT of the chest, abdomen, and pelvis is a fast and reliable means of determining the extent of visceral spread. This is particularly important for alerting treating teams of the potential for intraoperative pulmonary complications.

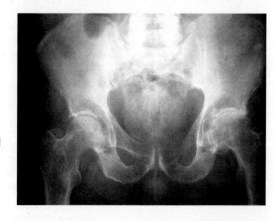

FIGURE 6.1

Anteroposterior radiograph of pelvis from 58-year-old male with metastatic renal carcinoma. Note metastasis in the right femoral neck, right medial wall of acetabulum, left superior pubic ramus, and left iliac crest.

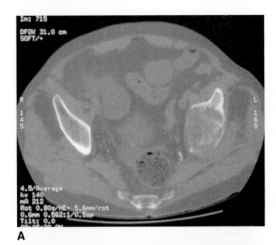

A

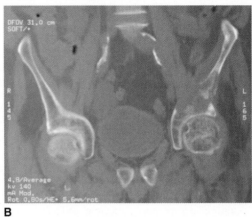

B

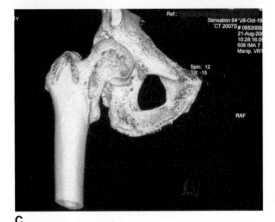

C

FIGURE 6.2

A,B: Axial computed tomographic scan and coronal reconstruction highlighting the mixed lytic sclerotic nature of a periacetabular breast carcinoma metastasis. **C:** Three-dimensional reconstruction of computed tomographic scan of right hip joint demonstrating femoral neck and calcar renal metastasis. Software that permits three-dimensional reconstructions and manipulation of the angle of view facilitates a better spatial understanding of the pathology and the subsequent reconstruction that may be required.

Magnetic Resonance Imaging

Magnetic resonance imaging (MRI) provides unsurpassed soft tissue contrast for clearly delineating any soft tissue extension of the periacetabular tumor (Fig. 6.3A). Further, the marrow extent of disease (Fig. 6.3B) is very clearly seen on magnetic resonance scans and this is important when planning which parts of the pelvis

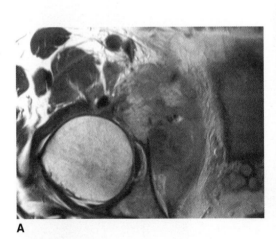

A

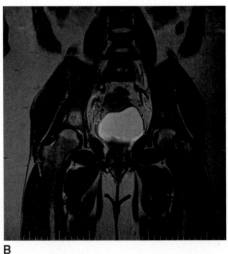

B

FIGURE 6.3

A: T2-weighted axial magnetic resonance image of right acetabulum demonstrating periacetabular metastasis with prominent soft tissue component. Anatomy is clearly defined and assists in the planning of surgical margins. **B:** T1-weighted coronal magnetic resonance image of solitary metastasis from malignant melanoma in the right periacetabulum above the hip joint. Note the dark marrow signal in the vertebrae representing red marrow stimulation.

may be relied upon as stable foundations for transfixing Steinmann pins that are inserted for supporting the acetabular component.

Bone Scans

All patients with metastases should undergo technetium nuclear bone scanning (Fig. 6.4) for the existence of other lesions in the same or other bones because lesions in the other long bones may be exposed to increased stress from having to bear greater amounts of weight in the early postoperative convalescence. Identifying other lesions at risk of fracture may lead to earlier intervention to avoid the pain of fracture and the need for emergent surgery.

Blood Tests

Marrow suppression is common with metastatic disease. Anemia, thrombocytopenia, and neutropenia should be corrected or managed appropriately in order to minimize the potential for complications such as sustained postoperative hemorrhage, infection, and anemia. Post-chemotherapy nadir of blood elements is common and may occur up to 2 weeks after the last dose of chemotherapy. Certain cytotoxic agents are more frequently associated with anemia, thrombocytopenia, and neutropenia. Surgery should be considered after discussions

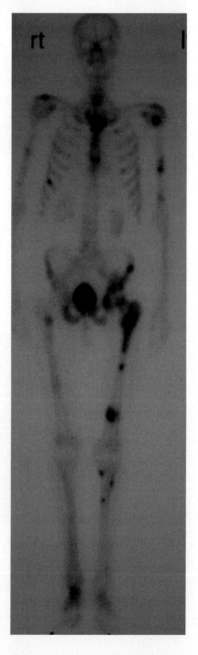

FIGURE 6.4

Technitium nuclear bone scan demonstrating widespread skeletal metastases in a 66-year-old man with metastatic pulmonary carcinoma.

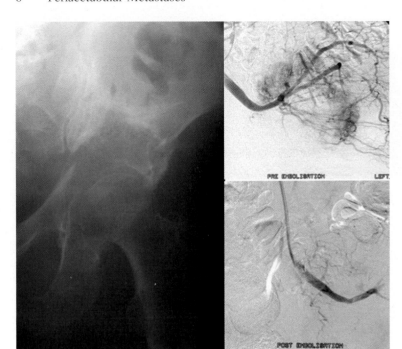

FIGURE 6.5

Large destructive left periacetabular Harrington type III metastatic renal carcinoma. Note very prominent blush of tumor neoangiogenesis which is obliterated following elective embolization of feeding vessel.

with the oncology team regarding the timing of normalization of blood counts. Renal function tests should be performed to exclude incipient renal failure and to correct any pre-renal cause of dysfunction such as dehydration. Liver function tests give an indication of the patient's nutritional state which will have an impact on post-operative healing. Further, liver dysfunction may be associated with coagulopathy that may have a detrimental impact on surgery.

Pulmonary Function Tests

Pulmonary function tests should be performed on all patients with significant pulmonary metastases to determine if there is sufficient pulmonary reserve to undergo surgery and to withstand the effects of pulmonary embolic phenomenon.

Angiography and Embolization

Certain tumors such as renal and thyroid carcinoma can give rise to hypervascular metastases (Fig. 6.5). All tumors, however, are capable of torrential bleeding. As pelvic tumors can be very large, and with feeding vessels arising directly from the iliac system, preoperative angiography is recommended to identify tumors, which have a high risk of bleeding. These can then be embolized between 24 and 36 hours prior to surgery (Fig. 6.5). Delays >72 between embolization and surgery may allow recanalization of embolized vasculature, thus negating the benefit of preoperative embolization.

MULTIDISCIPLINARY TEAM CONSULTATION

The safe management of an oncology patient who is to undergo periacetabular reconstruction requires active input from a variety of teams. These include the internal medicine team who should stabilize and optimize the patients' reversible comorbidities. The oncology team should provide guidance on the timing of surgery and the postoperative chemotherapy. The anesthetic team needs to familiarize themselves with the patient's cardio-pulmonary, hematological, and electrolyte status as well as any factor in the patient's history that will have an impact on the anesthetic technique to be employed.

CLASSIFICATION OF ACETABULAR DEFECTS

Classification systems provide a means of standardizing communications between different practitioners (1,2). This is important because of the complexities of such cases, which may benefit from referral or consultation between practitioners. A good classification system accurately describes the pathology, which in the case of periacetabular metastases is the position and extent of acetabular destruction, provides a gradation of severity,

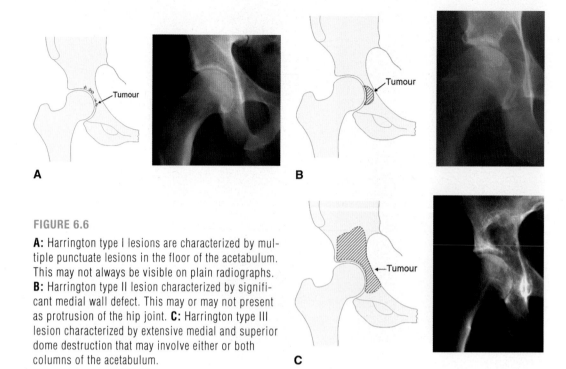

FIGURE 6.6

A: Harrington type I lesions are characterized by multiple punctuate lesions in the floor of the acetabulum. This may not always be visible on plain radiographs. **B:** Harrington type II lesion characterized by significant medial wall defect. This may or may not present as protrusion of the hip joint. **C:** Harrington type III lesion characterized by extensive medial and superior dome destruction that may involve either or both columns of the acetabulum.

and guides the use of specific techniques depending on the grade of disease. The Harrington classification system is a four-grade system which has enjoyed much popularity (1).

- Type I defects are characterized by an acetabulum with intact anterior and posterior columns, superior dome of the acetabulum, and medial wall with only punctuate disease of the floor of the acetabulum (Fig. 6.6A).
- Type II defects are characterized by loss of the medial wall with potential or true migration of the acetabulum medially into the pelvic cavity (Fig. 6.6B).
- Type III defects are the most challenging because of destruction that involves the medial wall, lateral margin, and superior dome of the acetabulum (Fig. 6.6C). One or both columns are often involved too.
- Type IV defects are rare, and were originally classified as solitary lesions that were amenable to en-bloc resection with a curative intention.

TECHNIQUE

Intraoperative Monitoring

Appropriate intraoperative monitoring is required to determine the stability of the patient under anesthesia as well as to rapidly identify changes in the patients that may signal deterioration in their well-being. Invasive monitoring with central venous catheterization allows measurement of right heart performance, while an arterial line permits accurate blood pressure recording. Expiratory carbon dioxide monitoring in conjunction with endotracheal anesthesia will permit an assessment of right to left shunting in the event of cardiopulmonary. Temperature monitoring is important to minimize body cooling that may impact myocardial function. A urinary catheter with a burette should be employed to provide accurate fluid output measurements.

Anesthetic

Postoperative pain management may begin prior to surgery with the insertion of an epidural catheter to allow intraoperative and postoperative instillation of anesthetic. Combining regional anesthesia with a general anesthesia may also allow a lighter general anesthetic to be used. Regional anesthesia alone may be considered safer in patients with pulmonary dysfunction. However, if cardiopulmonary collapse is anticipated, it may be argued that it would be safer to have in position secure endotracheal access from the beginning of the case rather than to attempt an urgent intubation in the middle of surgery with the patient in the lateral position.

Blood Loss

Large-bore intravenous access should be obtained prior to the commencement of surgery. Central venous catheterization is ideal for venous access and intraoperative monitoring. The purpose of such venous access is

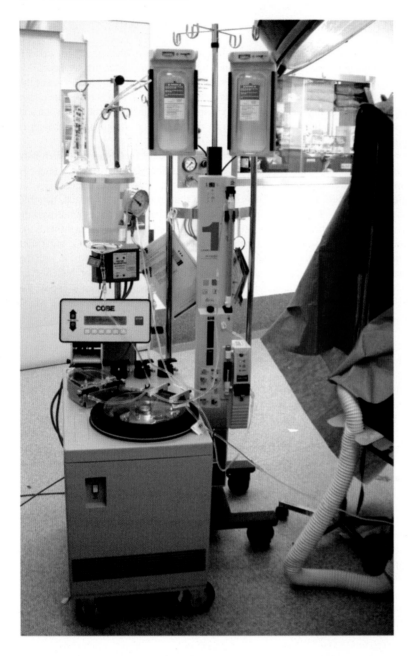

FIGURE 6.7
Rapid fluid transfusion machine (**left**) and rapid heat exchange fluid warmer (**right**).

to be able to provide rapid and high volumes of fluid and blood products should the need arise. Heat exchange systems must be available to allow rapid warming of blood should urgent transfusion be required. Warming prevents the transfusion of high volumes of chilled blood products which may result in a coagulopathy. Customized systems are available to rapidly transfuse fluids of up to 1,500 mL/min (Fig. 6.7). Although unusual, high-volume fluid resuscitation may be required if excessive bleeding from a hypervascular lesion is encountered.

Position and Draping

The patient should be positioned in the lateral position with the pelvis held securely between pelvic rests. All prominences on the downside of the patient should be appropriately padded to avoid pressure necrosis. An axillary support should be in place to elevate the chest wall from the underlying arm to prevent compression of the axillary neurovascular bundle between the chest wall and the upper arm. The downside leg should be positioned in slight flexion to provide stability to the body but it should not be so flexed as to impede venous return in the limb. The use of intraoperative antithrombotic stockings together with sequential calf or foot compression devices on the downside leg may be helpful for minimizing the risk of developing deep vein thrombosis during surgery. The ipsilateral leg should be draped free with the entire iliac crest exposed for the entry of Steinmann pins if required.

Incision and Approach

A slightly curved skin incision is marked out from a point 10 cm below the greater trochanter passing upward through the tip of the greater trochanter to a point 10 cm above and slightly posterior to the greater trochanter (Fig. 6.8). The incision is extended down to the deep fascia which is incised beginning at the lower end of the wound. A finger is passed upward underneath the fascia lata as it is incised and the division between the tensor fascia lata and anterior border of the gluteus maximus is identified from the undersurface of the fascia lata and split. A Charnley initial incision retractor is then deployed to retract the wound and the greater trochanter is seen in the center of the wound.

A transtrochanteric approach may be chosen if the hip has not been subjected to radiotherapy which may impair healing of the trochanteric osteotomy. This approach is also contraindicated if the proximal femur is affected by metastatic disease because a trochanteric osteotomy may not heal, or may be the stress riser for a fracture through pathologic bone. If there is no contraindication to a transtrochanteric approach, then the osteotomy is chosen from a point close to Smith-Peterson point on the lateral surface of the femur passing upward to where the piriform fossa meets the base of the femoral neck. The trochanteric fragment with the attached gluteus medius is then reflected superiorly toward the iliac crest to expose the acetabulum and a considerable amount of the pelvic side wall above the acetabulum. Reflecting the gluteus medius muscle with the trochanteric fragment exposes the underlying hip capsule which is then incised along the neck of the femur up to the acetabular margin and also along the intertrochanteric line. The capsule can then be excised to expose the hip joint proper. This exposure has the benefit of preserving the integrity of the superior gluteal nerve which innervates the gluteus medius muscle and minimizes the risk of a Trendelenberg gait.

An anterolateral Hardinge-type approach aims to split the gluteus medius muscle to gain access to the lateral side wall of the pelvis and acetabulum. With the hip held in slight internal rotation, the gluteus medius muscle buckles upward at its attachment to the greater trochanter. A line approximately 0.75 cm lateral to the musculotendinous junction of gluteus medius is marked out and a subperiosteal dissection of the gluteus medius muscle is made with a coagulating diathermy. As the dissection passes upward along the greater trochanter, a line of dissection is chosen that splits the gluteus medius into anterior one third and posterior two thirds in the line of its fibers. A finger is passed between the fibers at this point and brought down to the edge of the greater trochanter and the subperiosteal dissection is carried up to this point. Then with careful separation of the gluteus medius split, the diathermy is used to continue the dissection down onto the capsule to expose the top of the femoral neck. The capsule is split along the line of the femoral neck all the way to the acetabular margin. The subperiosteal dissection of the gluteus medius muscle off the intertrochanteric line is continued inferiorly until the inferior border of gluteus medius is encountered. The dissection is then carried anteriorly over the front of the femur to complete the gluteus medius release. To help, the muscle is placed on slight tension by adduction and external rotation of the hip. The gluteus minimus muscle and the hip joint capsule may be maintained with the gluteus medius muscle to add substance to the muscle for its later repair.

A standard femoral neck osteotomy is performed after controlled dislocation of the femoral neck and the neck is then retracted out of the way of the acetabulum with a self-retaining retractor (Norfolk-Norwich). Release of the capsule and the psoas tendon at the inferior part of the neck may allow further retraction of the femoral neck and better exposure of the acetabulum. If despite this, the femoral neck still obstructs the inferior part of the acetabulum it is likely that insufficient femoral neck has been excised and this will need to

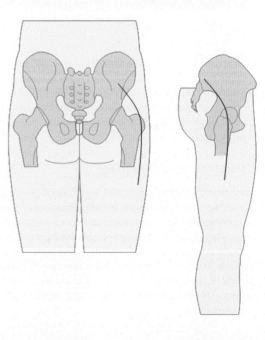

FIGURE 6.8

Incision required to expose the periacetabulum.

be refashioned. Exposure of the acetabulum is critical for adequate excisional curettage of the metastatic lesion and subsequent reconstruction.

Type I Lesions

Type I lesions are those that pepper the floor of the acetabulum with only minimal effect on the walls of the acetabulum. These lesions uncommonly present for surgical intervention. At most, small deposits need specific curettage, but none compromise the integrity of the medial or other walls. Standard acetabular reaming is all that is required, and rarely is medial wall mesh used before cementing of an all-polyethylene acetabular component. Many of these lesions have or will receive palliative radiotherapy, thus precluding the use of cementless devices. Cement provides immediate fixation of the acetabulum and also serves to strengthen the underlying bone by interdigitating between the bony interstices (Fig. 6.9A,B). There is a theoretical advantage of cement which is its thermonecrotic effect on tumor tissue.

Type II Lesions

Type II lesions are characterized by medial wall destruction with the potential for femoral head protrusion. The principle of surgery after removal of the metastatic deposit is to fortify the medial wall, prevent protrusion, and return the hip center to its normal position if required. Once the metastatic deposit has undergone excisional curettage, acetabular reamers are passed to remove the articular cartilage from the remaining acetabular surface. Reamers should be gently and gradually applied to preserve as much bone as possible with the aim of removing only the subchondral bone. The medial wall defect is then reinforced by a layer of medial wall mesh which is fashioned to cover the defect and to extend on to normal acetabular bone (Fig. 6.9C,D).

If the medial wall destruction is severe enough to cause protrusion, a reinforcement cage/ring can be utilized to prevent medial migration of the acetabular component and to transfer the forces from the medial wall to the dome and anterior and posterior columns. In this case, the notch is cleared of the transverse acetabular ligament and the nubbin of residual ligamentum teres to allow seating of the notch hook that is found on a variety of reinforcement cages/rings. Some reinforcement rings have an ischial flange that is designed to be buried into the ischium. These devices need adequate surgical exposure of the posterior column and inferior acetabulum, at times necessitating an additional posterior approach. The obturator externus needs to be cleared from the ischium to allow the ischial flange to be seated in the bone. An appropriately sized reinforcement cage/ring is chosen that matches the diameter of the acetabulum. It does not matter if there is a space between the mesh which lies on the deepest surface of the acetabulum and the reinforcement device as all this will be filled with cement. The reinforcement device is held in place by screws passed from the lateral margin of the acetabulum and directed upward at angle of 35 to 45 degrees and backward 10 to 15 degrees. The line of the pelvis which has to be followed can be appreciated by passing a finger from the superior aspect of the acetabulum along the external surface of the pelvis. Depending on the size of the pelvis, several 4.5-mm cortical screws up to 90 mm in length may be required to hold the reinforcement ring in place.

Type III Lesions

Type III lesions are the most challenging because of the considerable destruction to the medial wall, superior dome, and one or either of the pelvic columns. Curettage of the metastatic lesion is likely to leave a defect that can be alarmingly deep with very little natural bone left to support an acetabular component. Simply filling the defect with cement will fail because there is no structure to transfer the stresses from the acetabulum to the stronger bone of the iliac crest and the thick bone above the sciatic notch. Reconstructions should aim to contain the defect, prevent medial migration, and to enhance the transfer of force across the defect from acetabulum to strong proximal bone. After ensuring as thorough an excision as possible, medial wall mesh is once again used to line the floor of the acetabulum and the cavity of defect which may be deep and extensive (Fig. 6.9E). The defect is then reinforced with Steinmann pins to allow the transfer of force between acetabulum and strong bone of the pelvis, namely the iliac crest that acts like an I-beam, and the bone above the sciatic notch, which leads to the sacroiliac joint. In general, two groups of Steinmann pins are used. One group of pins is drilled from the iliac crest down toward the defect such that the points of the Steinmann pins pass into the defect, then are grasped with forceps and guided to the inferior parts of the defect. It is possible to direct the pins into the ischium for further fixation or forward to the root of the superior pubic ramus. A second group is directed from the lateral margin of the acetabulum and anterior inferior iliac spine through the superior cavity toward the sacroiliac joint. A lattice work of Steinmann pins is thus created deep to and above the level of the true acetabulum to provide support for the reinforcement cage/ring and acetabulum (Fig. 6.9E–G). Once the pins are in place, a reinforcement ring is applied and held with a number of supra-acetabular screws. The cavity with the lattice of Steinmann pins is filled with antibiotic cement under compression before the cup is implanted over the reinforcement cage.

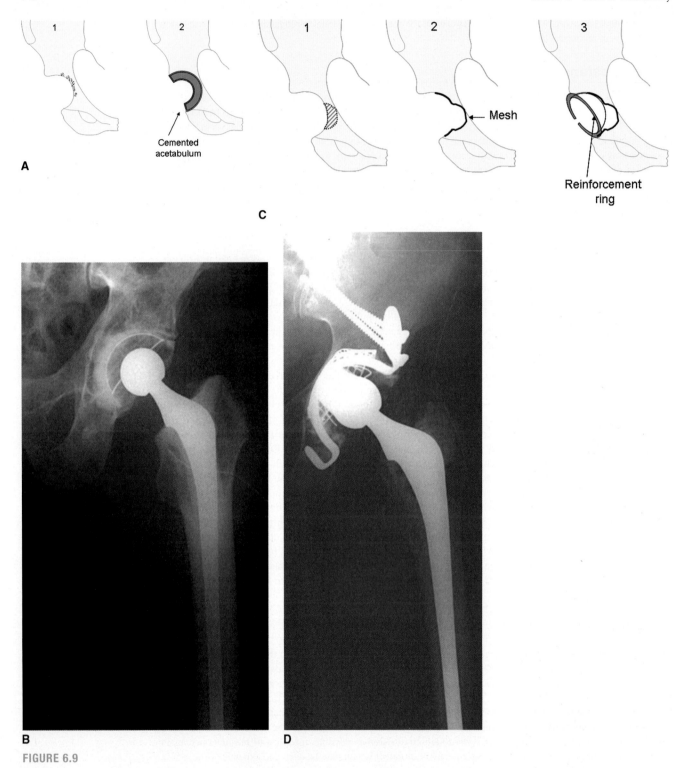

FIGURE 6.9

A: Harrington type I lesions (*1*) may be treated by curettage and cementation (*2*) as part of the implantation of a cemented acetabular component. **B:** Cemented total hip replacement for treatment of Harrington type I lesion. **C:** Harrington type II lesion (*1*) treated by curettage and reinforcement of the medial wall with shaped metal mesh (*2*), then further fortified with a reinforcement ring and a cemented acetabular component (*3*). **D:** Cemented total hip replacement with medial wall fortified by metal mesh and construct reinforced with a reinforcement acetabular ring.

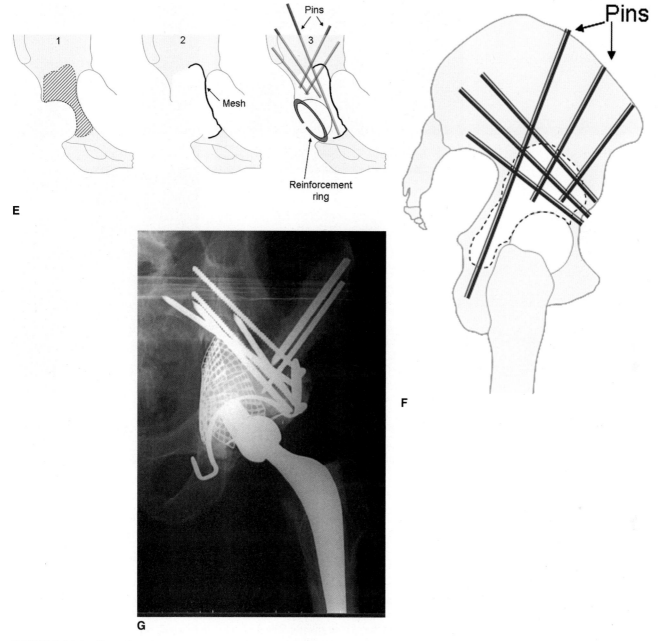

FIGURE 6.9 (*Continued*)

E: Harrington type III lesion with extensive medial wall and superior dome involvement (*1*) may be treated with extensive curettage, reinforcement of medial wall with metal mesh (*2*), then reinforcement of the superior dome with stout pins passing from the iliac crest into the defect and through into supportive bone in the ischium, pubic bone, or sacroiliac joint. A reinforcement ring is then applied and a cemented acetabular component used (*3*). **F:** Cemented total hip replacement with reconstruction of the medial wall and superior dome defect with a combination of metal mesh, bridging Steinmann pins, a reinforcement ring, and a cemented acetabular component.

Pelvic Discontinuity and Total Acetabular Destruction

Occasionally, the acetabulum is completely destroyed or a pathologic fracture has resulted in a grossly unstable pelvic discontinuity that is unlikely to heal or be amenable to rigid fixation. In this situation, reconstruction is best undertaken with a saddle prosthesis. This is discussed elsewhere in this book.

FEMORAL RECONSTRUCTION

The principle of management is that the entire femur should be protected because metastasis is a progressive condition and may arise anywhere along the femur after reconstruction. It would be problematic if a metastasis arose below the tip of a standard prosthesis (Fig. 6.10A). Therefore, no matter what reconstruction is used on

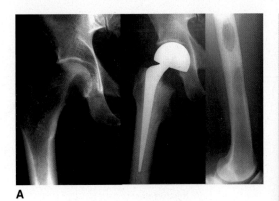

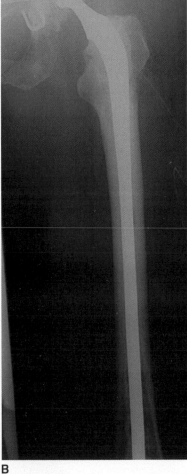

FIGURE 6.10

A: A renal metastasis of the femoral head and neck has been treated with a standard bipolar hip replacement. Shortly afterwards a further metastasis develops at the tip of the standard length prosthesis. **B:** Long-stemmed cemented femoral prostheses should be used where ever possible when managing a metastasis that requires hip arthroplasty. Metastasis is a progressive disease and prophylactic use of a long-stemmed prosthesis affords protection to the length of the femoral shaft should further metastases develop.

the acetabular side, a long-stemmed cemented femoral prosthesis should be employed to provide protection against pathologic fracture (Fig. 6.10B).

RADIOFREQUENCY ABLATION

Radiofrequency ablation is a well-established method for treating a variety of solid tumors. It may have particular value in patients with periacetabular tumors who are deemed to be inoperable because of poor health status or the advanced state of their disease. The goals of radiofrequency ablation are to destroy tumor and to bring about pain relief without open operation. Under intraoperative fluoroscopy or computed tomographic guidance, radiofrequency probes are inserted into the center of metastases and the tumor subjected to thermocoagulation.

PERCUTANEOUS OSTEOPLASTY

Percutaneous osteoplasty is a method whereby osseous lesions are accessed via minimally invasive image guidance and after attempts to evacuate a lytic lesions are made, the lytic cavity is filled with a synthetic material (Fig. 6.11A–E). Historically, this has been polymethylmethacrylate acetate (PMMA), which can be injected under pressure into cavities and after it sets it can sustain high compressive forces, thereby adding strength to weakened bone. Preventing impending fractures, permitting immediate weight bearing, and reducing pain are some of the advantages of using PMMA. An added advantage is the thermonecrotic effect of PMMA on residual tumor tissue as it undergoes an exothermic reaction as it polymerizes where it is capable of raising the local temperature to 90°C. A variety of injectable substances are now available which are able to fill defects and provide immediate strength.

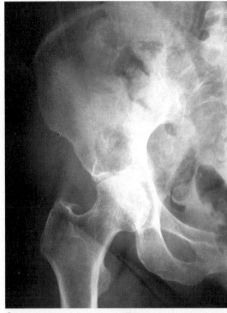

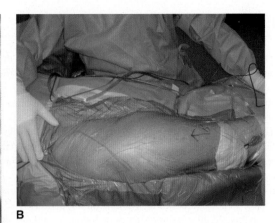

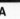

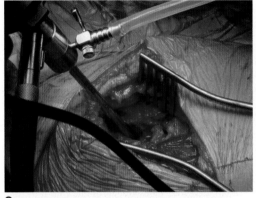

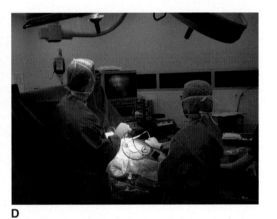

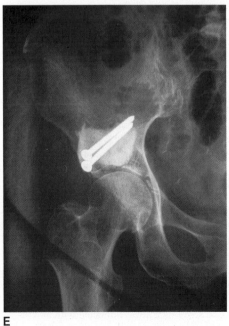

FIGURE 6.11

A: An isolated superior acetabular dome lesion that is amenable to minimally invasive osteoplasty. **B:** Patient is prepared in the supine position with the hip draped free as far as the iliac crest. The operative incision is along a line drawn between the anterior superior iliac spine and the greater trochanter. **C:** The space between the sartorius muscle and the tensor fascia lata is sought and divided and the origin of the straight and reflected heads of rectus femoris are elevated from the bone. A window is created into the bone and the lytic lesion cleared of tumor tissue. **D:** In this case, the cavity is evacuated under endoscopic guidance and tissue cleared using an arthroscopic shaver. **E:** Cavity is then filled with polymethylmethacrylate and two screws passed into the pelvic bone to reinforce the bone cement.

PEARLS AND PITFALLS

- The position of the lateral margin is a valuable guide to the orientation and position of the cup. This is frequently preserved despite significant tumor destruction of the remaining acetabulum. In very late disease, the lateral part of the acetabulum is so involved as to require excision. It is advisable to preserve this anatomic structure as long as possible prior to cementation in order to assist in the final orientation of the acetabular component.
- There are a number of reinforcement rings/cages available in the market. I prefer the cruciform variety with plenty of space between the arms to allow good visualization into the cavity behind the cage. This aids in directing the placement of Steinmann pins after the reinforcement ring has been seated as well as permitting a good flow of cement between the tumor cavity and the acetabulum. The latter ensures that the reinforcement device is truly embedded in the cement. In contrast, some other devices, which are nearly fully formed cups with perforations in their floors, do not permit a free flow of cement between the acetabulum and the cavity behind the reinforcement device, thus potentially allowing unsupported and sizeable voids to remain in the tumor cavity.
- The majority of long-stemmed femoral prostheses are designed for revision hip surgery with a range of bodies that begin at a larger size than their primary counterparts and increase further with increasing stem length. This may hamper treatment in small women with metastatic femoral disease. Unless the correct prosthesis is selected, there is the potential for intraoperative fracture in the preparation of the femur. A number of prostheses are now available on the market with small bodies and a range of stem lengths which covers most individuals. Some also come with the possibility of calcar buildups should there be involvement of the calcar femorale by tumor.

POSTOPERATIVE MANAGEMENT

The management of the patient in the postoperative setting is similar to that following revision hip surgery. Standard precautions are used when mobilizing the patient and an abduction pillow is left in situ in the early days after surgery. Antithrombosis protocols should be maintained until the patient becomes independently mobile. Blood loss is likely to continue after surgery with up to 30% of the intraoperative blood loss volume to be lost again in the first 24 hours after surgery. Regular hemoglobin and other blood examinations should be made and coagulation screens should be performed until this has normalized.

The patient should be mobilized out of bed as soon as possible to avoid the complications of prolonged recumbency. By day 2 the discomfort is usually well enough controlled to allow the patient to stand or sit out of bed. Weight bearing may commence with the use of walking aids such as a frame or crutches and weight bearing through the limb may be increased as tolerated by the patient. Drainage tubes are left in place until the rate of flow is <10 mL/h for 3 consecutive hours when the drainage tubes may be removed. Staples are left in situ for 3 weeks if radiotherapy has been previously used in the operative field. If no radiotherapy has been used, then removal at 2 weeks is permissible. Check radiographs are performed according to surgeon preference.

COMPLICATIONS

- Intraoperative hemorrhage is the main complication to be anticipated. Bleeding from the diseased bone and tumor surface during curettage is common and usually continues until all tumor has been removed. This is usually controllable by tamponade with packs if bleeding becomes heavy. The amount of blood loss may be deceptive because the flow is constant throughout the operation. It is important that the anesthetic team performs regular intraoperative assessments of hemoglobin. Surgery on renal, thyroid, or myeloma deposits are prone to heavy blood loss and preoperative embolism is strongly recommended. Notwithstanding this, any tumor may lead to significant bleeding; therefore, any large tumor should be screened with angiography before surgery for hypervascularity.
- Nerve injury is unusual but may occur in three situations. First, the dissection of the gluteus medius to expose the acetabulum and clearing the pelvis immediately above the acetabulum may traumatize the nerve to gluteus medius, which runs about two finger breadths above the acetabular margin. Second, Steinmann pins or transfixing screws which are directed upward toward the sacroiliac joint from the acetabular margin may emerge anteriorly to the sacroiliac joint and injure the lumbosacral plexus. This is uncommon and can be avoided if the entry points for Steinmann pins or screws are sited anteriorly or laterally on the margin and are directed upward and posteriorly. Third, screws to hold the reinforcement ring/cage may accidentally be directed into the sciatic notch. Ensuring that the drill bit and screws are always directed with an upward inclination rather than straight backward should avoid sciatic notch complications.
- Infection is a major risk following prolonged and complex surgery in an immunocompromised patient whose operative site has undergone irradiation. Frequent lavage is recommended to ensure that any bacterial

contamination is diluted and at the end of the procedure, prolonged pulsatile lavage with several liters of isotonic fluid is recommended. Addition of antiseptic fluids such as Betadine and chlorhexidine to the intra-operative wash may help to minimize bacterial colonization. Antibiotic cement should be used. Our practice is to prescribe intravenous vancomycin and a third-generation cephalosporin for the first 48 hours following surgery. Continuation of antibiotics is then guided by surgeon preference.

• Dislocation is an uncommon complication of periacetabular reconstruction for metastatic disease. This can be minimized by ensuring the appropriate placement and orientation of the acetabular component. This may be difficult if there has been a considerable amount of bone destruction with the loss of the usual anatomic landmarks. This is why preservation of the lateral margin of the acetabulum is critical to defining the correct position of the acetabulum. Another important landmark is the acetabular notch which needs to be cleared and its location identified as this will also help with the seating and orientation of the acetabular component.

• Pulmonary embolic phenomenon can occur during any stage of femoral manipulation from creating a pilot hole, to passing the initial fluted reamer, to reaming and broaching, trialling, and finally cementing the prosthesis. The surgeon should always warn the anesthetist prior to commencing any of these steps. Should this phenomenon occur, it usually does so within 30 seconds of the particular step. In the awake patient with regional anesthesia, pulmonary embolic phenomenon is heralded by a bout of coughing or spluttering as the lung becomes irritated by marrow products. The anesthetist who is ready would have ensured that the patient is well hydrated and oxygenated during the case, and is ready to deliver a further volume load. Intravenous vasopressors are kept at the ready and should be injected at the first signs of this condition because hypotension is a common occurrence. The surgeon can help to minimize this by careful preparation of the femur including trying to avoid fast plunging strokes when using an intramedullary instrument.

RESULTS

Improvement of Symptoms

Reconstructive surgery for metastatic disease of the periacetabulum is a complex procedure. Removal of tumor and fortification of periacetabular bone with Steinmann pins before hip arthroplasty consistently produces good symptomatic relief and improvement in hip function and weight-bearing status (3–7). In the majority of cases, these reports confirm the longevity of patients (mean >18 months), which justifies the application of this complex procedure. However, the longevity of patients also underscores the importance of a durable reconstruction.

Complications

The incidence of complications is high in the majority of reports (up to 30%) (4,5,7–10). The more common complications include infection and dislocation. The former is most likely due to the prolonged operative time and the need for wide dissections, which may also be compounded by the use of chemotherapy and radiotherapy. Dislocation is noticeably high and may be due to the orientation of the acetabular component. With the destruction of the periacetabular bone, it is vital that key landmarks are preserved to allow appropriate referencing and orientation of the acetabular component (3).

Osteoplasty

Some periacetabular metastases in the pubic rami or superior dome lesions do not involve the acetabulum although their proximity to the hip joint may cause symptoms. These may be candidates for minimally invasive osteoplasty (11–18) or radiofrequency ablation (15,19–23). Greater sophistication of imaging modalities, advances in the development of radiofrequency probes and the percutaneous or minimally invasive approaches that are possible should permit more frequent and repeated use of this technique in patients who are not candidates for complex resections, who are unsuitable for anesthesia, or whose main problem is the palliative control of pain.

REFERENCES

1. Harrington KD. The management of acetabular insufficiency secondary to metastatic malignant disease. *J Bone Joint Surg Am.* 1981;63:653–664.
2. Levy R, Sherry H, Siffert R. Surgical management of metastatic disease of bone at the hip. *Clin Orthop.* 1982;169:62–69.
3. Kunisada T, Choong PF. Major reconstruction for periacetabular metastasis: early complications and outcome following surgical treatment in 40 hips. *Acta Orthop Scand.* 2000;71:585–590.
4. Marco RAW, Sheth DS, Boland PJ, et al. Functional and oncological outcome of acetabular reconstruction for the treatment of metastatic disease. *J Bone Joint Surg Am.* 2000;82A:642–651.

5. Nilsson J, Gustafson P, Fornander P, et al. The Harrington reconstruction for advanced periacetabular metastatic destruction—good outcome in 32 patients *Acta Orthop Scand*. 2000;71:591–596.

6. Tillman RM, Myers GJC, Abudu AT, et al. The three-pin modified 'Harrington' procedure for advanced metastatic destruction of the acetabulum. *J Bone Joint Surg Br*. 2008;90B:84–87.

7. Wangsaturaka P, Asavamongkolkul A, Waikakul S, et al. The results of surgical management of bone metastasis involving the periacetabular area: Siriraj experience. *J Med Assoc Thai*. 2007;90:1006–1013.

8. Abudu A, Grimer RJ, Cannon SR, et al. Reconstruction of the hemipelvis after the excision of malignant tumours—complications and functional outcome of prostheses. *J Bone Joint Surg Br*. 1997;79B:773–779.

9. Papagelopoulos PJ, Galanis EC, Greipp PR, et al. Prosthetic hip replacement for pathologic or impending pathologic fractures in myeloma. *Clin Orthop Relat Res*. 1997;341:192–205.

10. Stark A, Bauer HCF. Reconstruction in metastatic destruction of the acetabulum—Support rings and arthroplasty in 12 patients. *Acta Orthop Scand*. 1996;67:435–438.

11. Cotten A, Deprez X, Migaud H, et al. Malignant acetabular osteolyses—percutaneous injection of acrylic bone-cement. *Radiology*. 1995;197:307–310.

12. Hierholzer J, Anselmetti G, Fuchs H, et al. Percutaneous osteoplasty as a treatment for painful malignant bone lesions of the pelvis and femur. *J Vasc Interv Radiol*. 2003;14:773–777.

13. Hoffmann RT, Jakobs TF, Trumm C, et al. Radiofrequency ablation in combination with osteoplasty in the treatment of painful metastatic bone disease. *J Vasc Interv Radiol*. 2008;19:419–425.

14. Kamysz J, Rechitsky M. Pubic bone cement osteoplasty for pubic insufficiency fractures. *J Vasc Interv Radiol*. 2008;19:1386–1389.

15. Kelekis A, Lovblad KO, Mehdizade A, et al. Pelvic osteoplasty in osteolytic metastases: technical approach under fluoroscopic guidance and early clinical results. *J Vasc Interv Radiol*. 2005;16:81–8.

16. Langlais F, Lambotte JC, Lannou R, et al. Hip pain from impingement and dysplasia in patients aged 20–50 years. Workup and role for reconstruction. *Joint Bone Spine*. 2006;73:614–623.

17. Masala S, Konda D, Massari F, et al. Sacroplasty and iliac osteoplasty under combined CT and fluoroscopic guidance. *Spine*. 2006;31:E667–E669.

18. Yamada K, Matsumoto Y, Kita M, et al. Clinical outcome of percutaneous osteoplasty for pain caused by metastatic bone tumors in the pelvis and femur. *J Anesth*. 2007;21:277–281.

19. Callstrom MR, Charboneau JW, Goetz MP, et al. Image-guided ablation of painful metastatic bone tumors: a new and effective approach to a difficult problem. *Skeletal Radiol*. 2006;35:1–15.

20. Maruyama M, Asano T, Kenmochi T, et al. Radiofrequency ablation therapy for bone metastasis from hepatocellular carcinoma: case report. *Anticancer Res*. 2003;23:2987–2989.

21. Papagelopoulos PJ, Mavrogenis AF, Soucacos PN. Evaluation and treatment of pelvic metastases. *Inj Int J Care Injured*. 2007;38:509–520.

22. Pawlik TM, Vauthey JN, Abdalla EK, et al. Results of a single-center experience with resection and ablation for sarcoma metastatic to the liver. *Arch Surg*. 2006;141:537–543; discussion 543–544, 2006.

23. Schaefer MP, Smith J. The diagnostic and therapeutic challenge of femoral head osteoid osteoma presenting as thigh pain: a case report. *Arch Phys Med Rehabil*. 2003;84:904–905.

7 Sacrectomy

Peter S. Rose, Franklin H. Sim, and Michael Yaszemski

Curative treatment of most primary sacral malignancies requires en bloc sacrectomy. Surgery in this area is challenging due to the complexity of the pelvic anatomy, adjacent visceral and vascular structures, and frequent compromise of spinopelvic continuity.

INDICATIONS

- The most common indication for sacrectomy is primary sacral malignancy requiring resection for cure.
- More rarely, sacrectomy is indicated for patients with primary or recurrent pelvic visceral tumors (most commonly colorectal carcinoma with sacral involvement by direct extension) and no evidence of metastatic or nodal disease.
- The techniques described may be adapted to intralesional treatment of benign tumors (e.g., osteoblastoma, aneurysmal bone cyst) in a less aggressive fashion.
- Select benign aggressive sacral tumors may be considered for en bloc resection, particularly if small or recurrent.

CONTRAINDICATIONS

- The presence of disseminated malignancy is a strong relative contraindication for sacrectomy. The procedure is of such magnitude and generally entails deliberate neurologic defects with frequent loss of bowel, bladder, sexual, and potentially lower extremity function that it is usually inappropriate to pursue without curative intent.
- We have noted that patients with tumor thrombus in the iliac veins or vena cava by sarcoma predictably have a rapid development of metastatic disease and demise. The suggestion of this on preoperative imaging prompts catheter-directed biopsy at our institution, and its finding at time of surgery prompts abortion of resection (Fig. 7.1).

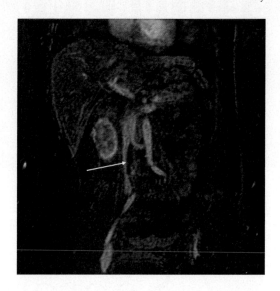

FIGURE 7.1

Malignant clot demonstrated in the vena cava (*arrow*) of an 18-year-old patient with sacropelvic osteosarcoma.

- The inability to obtain a tumor-free margin of resection is similarly a relative contraindication. However, we are aggressive in pursuing this with frequent en bloc resections encompassing the pelvis, lumbar spine, rectum, urogenital, and vascular structures to obtain en bloc tumor resection.
- The medical fitness of the patient for surgery also frequently enters into the calculation of surgery. Patients receiving chemotherapy frequently require alterations in their chemotherapy schedules to allow for surgery of this magnitude. All patients are subject to an intense preoperative medical evaluation including a dobutamine stress echocardiogram for (a) anyone with known cardiovascular disease; (b) men over age 40; or (c) women over age 50.

PREOPERATIVE PLANNING/GENERAL CONSIDERATIONS

Staging and accurate diagnosis are key in the evaluation of patients with sacral malignancy. Systemic staging includes CT of the chest, abdomen, and pelvis and bone scan for all patients; the role of PET-CT in staging is currently evolving. Local tumor imaging is best provided by MR scan. All tumors are biopsied prior to surgery by CT-guided needle biopsy in or near the midline to facilitate biopsy tract removal.

Tumor imaging is accomplished using contrast-enhanced MR. Sagittal images and coronal oblique images (coronal images in the plane of the sacrum) are key to localizing tumor extent and adjacent structure involvement. Selected patients benefit from CT angiography to evaluate the pelvic vasculature (Fig. 7.2).

Resections at or below the level of the S2 neuroforamen are generally resected through a posterior approach unless there is involvement of pelvic visceral or vascular structures. Given the need to obtain an oncologic margin, this generally implies lesions at or below the S2/3 vestigial disc.

Lesions cephalad to this or involving pelvic structures are treated first with anterior mobilization of pelvic structures, vessel ligation, and unicortical anterior sacral osteotomy. It is our practice to harvest a pedicled myocutaneous rectus abdominus flap and tuck it into the abdomen with the anterior procedure. Tumor resection

FIGURE 7.2

Specific imaging techniques. **A:** T1-weighted coronal oblique images demonstrate tumor invasion (*black arrow*) of the left S3 foramen by sacral chordoma. **B:** CT angiography demonstrates near encasement of the external iliac artery (*white arrow*) by sacral chondrosarcoma.

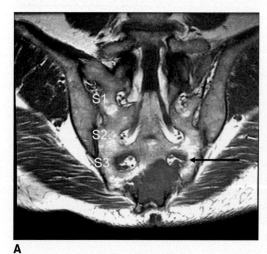

A   B

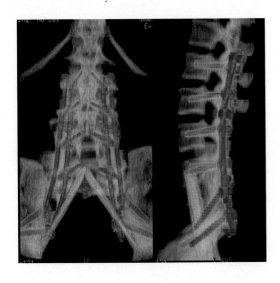

FIGURE 7.3

"Cathedral" technique of spinopelvic reconstruction. Fibula strut grafts are used to recreate the anterior column function of the sacrum while pedicle screw instrumentation provides fixation across the junction.

is then completed through a posterior approach, and the rectus flap is pulled through the abdomen and rotated to assist in wound closure and reconstruction of the posterior abdominal wall. Unless the rectum is devascularized and requires resection with the tumor specimen, we separate the anterior and posterior stages by 48 hours.

Resections cephalad to the S1 neuroforamen require spinopelvic reconstruction. Our preferred method involves a "cathedral" technique using fibula autografts or allografts and posterior spinal instrumentation to be described below (Fig. 7.3). Allograft fibulae are used unless the patient has had prior radiotherapy, in which case consideration is given to vascularized fibula transfer.

Biopsy tracts are excised in continuity with the surgical specimen. In the case of posterior-only resections, gluteal V-Y advancement flaps are commonly used to facilitate wound closure. Ureteral stents are placed preoperatively in all patients undergoing anterior procedures. Patients are at risk of venous thromboembolic disease but also at risk of significant perioperative bleeding. In patients undergoing dorsal-only resections, we place a removable Inferior Vena Cava filter preoperatively. If anterior and posterior procedures are needed, the IVC filter is placed between the anterior and posterior stages so as not to interfere with vena cava mobilization.

All patients complete a bowel preparation preoperatively. If resection will predictably erase meaningful hope of bowel continence, we strongly advise patients to undergo colostomy as part of their anterior procedure (1,2,3).

ANTERIOR TECHNIQUE—RESECTIONS ABOVE S2 OR INVOLVING PELVIC VISCERA

Positioning and Landmarks

The patient is positioned supine on a regular operating table. Critical landmarks for anterior exposure are the sacral promontory, the anterior sacral foramina, the sacroiliac joints, and the sciatic notches. Resections requiring anterior exposure are usually performed through the S1 segment or higher, so the sacral promontory provides adequate localization. Large tumors frequently require inclusion of the medial iliac bones with the specimens to predictably remove the sacroiliac joints without violation. These joints can be palpated and osteotomies begun at the sciatic notches and brought cephalad.

Surgical Technique

Bilateral ureteral stents are placed to facilitate ureteral identification. A midline laparotomy incision is made with planned harvest of a vertical rectus abdominus myocutaneous flap. The timing of flap harvest is at the discretion of the plastic surgeon. It is most efficiently harvested at the conclusion of the anterior procedure to minimize risk of pedicle avulsion during the case. In rare cases, a transverse rectus abdominus flap is raised when a very large posterior soft tissue defect is expected (the TRAM flap has greater bulk).

The abdomen is approached by transperitoneal approach in most cases (in cases of hemisacrectomy, a retroperitoneal approach may be used). The rectum is mobilized or transected as indicated by tumor extent. The pelvic vasculature is identified. If thrombus is palpated, venotomy is made and the specimen analyzed. If tumor is found, the procedure is aborted; if bland, thrombectomy is performed and the procedure continues. The middle sacral vein and the internal iliac artery and vein (and all accessible branches) are ligated. If necessary, a plane between the tumor and the pelvic sidewall is developed. The location of sacral and/or pelvic osteotomies is localized using anatomic landmarks and lateral radiography as necessary. The L5/S1 disk is a reliable landmark, and sacral neuroforamina can be counted down from this.

We prefer a 5- or 6-mm round diamond burr to perform osteotomies. This instrument has a low likelihood of wrapping up soft tissue and cauterizes the bony surface as it cuts to minimize bleeding. The 5- or 6-mm diameter bit allows use of a 3-mm Kerrison rongeur in its kerf for delicate extension of the osteotomy. Iliac osteotomies are generally made completely or nearly so on the anterior approach as no dangerous structures are posterior to them; sacral osteotomies are unicortical to prevent inadvertent tear of the dura from the anterior approach. Section of the psoas may be necessary to access the ilium for osteotomy, but the femoral nerve is carefully protected along its length. We have found it useful to implant a small fragment screw in the bone just cephalad to the osteotomy so it can be located with fluoroscopy during the posterior procedure to verify level of resection. This is usually a 12-mm screw placed unicortically (Fig. 7.4).

Once all visceral and vascular mobilization is complete and the anterior osteotomies performed, a sterile silastic sheet is placed between the tumor mass and the mobilized structures to protect them during the posterior approach. The pedicled rectus abdominus flap is harvested and tucked into the wound just superficial to the silastic sheet, and the laparotomy is closed (Fig. 7.5). If indicated, a colostomy is developed.

POSTERIOR TECHNIQUE

Positioning

Prone positioning is via a radiolucent Jackson spine frame with a Wilson attachment to provide for appropriate sacral exposure and hip flexion. The head is placed in Gardner-Wells tongs and suspended using 15 lb of traction. Surgical prep is wide to allow for gluteal flap mobilization and harvest of sural nerves as needed for cauda equine reconstruction. The anus is sewn shut to minimize the risk of fecal contamination. The patient is maintained in maximum reverse Trendelenberg during the case to minimize intraocular pressure (Fig. 7.6).

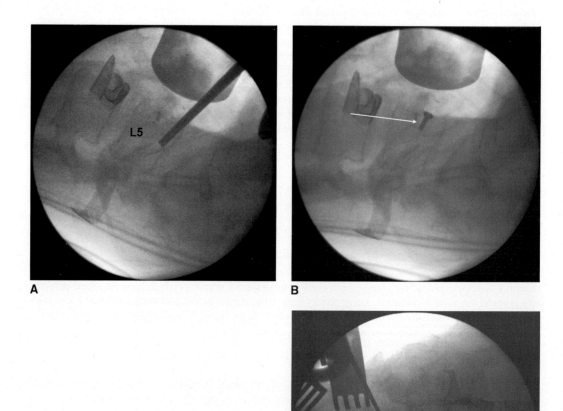

FIGURE 7.4

Localization techniques. **A:** Anterior unicortical osteotomy is made through L5 for total sacrectomy. **B:** Small fragment screw marks the site of osteotomy (*arrow*). **C:** During posterior approach, marker screw is readily visualized on fluoroscopy (*arrow*) to guide the trajectory of the posterior osteotomy to meet the anterior one.

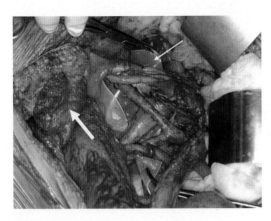

FIGURE 7.5

Silastic sheet (*small arrow*) is placed between the tumor mass and the vascular structures. Pedicled VRAM flap (*large arrow*) is tucked into the wound before closure of the laparotomy.

Landmarks

Key posterior resection landmarks include the L5 spinous process, dorsal sacral foramina, inferior sacroiliac joints, and sacrospinous and sacrotuberous ligaments. It is our practice to expose the sacrum from the L5 spinous process to the coccyx and demarcate the dorsal sacral foramina of all levels not involved by tumor. The caudal aspect of the sacroiliac joint almost always falls between the S2 and S3 levels (this is verified on preoperative imaging studies). The sacrospinous and sacrotuberous ligaments are critical landmarks in identifying the pudendal and sciatic nerves. Lateral fluoroscopy is used to verify posterior landmarks and localization if necessary. If an anterior procedure has been done with a marker screw left at the level of the osteotomy, lateral fluoroscopy can visualize this.

Surgical Technique

A midline incision is made from the L5 spinous process down to the coccygeal region, ellipsing out the biopsy tract. Dissection comes down to the fascia. Depending upon the extent of the tumor, it may or may not be possible to come through the fascia to expose the posterior sacrum. We have found that a Charnley retractor adapted from hip procedures works quite well to help with exposure.

Localization begins cephalad to minimize any risk of going too far down into tumor mass. We identify the dorsal neural foramina. On lateral fluoroscopy, the lumbosacral junction can also be visualized. In cases of anterior approach, the screw that is placed near the anterior osteotomy is well visualized to guide resection. A dorsal sacral laminectomy is performed to expose the most cephalad nerve roots, which will be preserved. Preoperative imaging studies will indicate the level at which the thecal sac ends, but it is usually at the S2 segment. If the thecal sac requires transection, it is doubly ligated with 0 silk suture. Exposure then comes out laterally beyond the edge of the sacrum and any associated soft tissue masses.

Once full exposure is obtained, osteotomy is performed at the appropriate level. Again we utilize a diamond burr with a 5- or 6-mm round bit to perform the initial osteotomy cuts as it has a nice effect cauterizing the bony edges to minimize bony bleeding and will allow the use of a 3-mm Kerrison rongeur for more delicate extension. Care is taken to preserve the gluteal vessels as they exit the sciatic notch if at all possible as they are the dominant supply to the gluteal muscles, which form a portion of the flap closure.

As the osteotomy is completed, the specimen is carefully delivered from proximal to distal; this allows protection of the lowest nerve roots, which are being saved. Other nerve roots that go through the tumor mass are sectioned to prevent them from being pulled out and potentially spreading tumor cells in this area. If at all possible, the pudendal nerves are preserved as a part of the resection. These are found accompanying the sacrospinous and sacrotuberous ligaments. These ligaments are strong structures, which require sectioning as the specimen is delivered dorsally and removed. Finally, transection is made through the anococcygeal ligaments

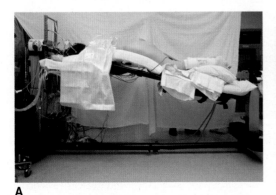

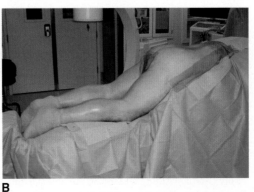

A   **B**

FIGURE 7.6

Prone positioning. **A:** Patient is placed on a Wilson frame on the Jackson table in maximum reverse Trendelenberg position; the head is suspended by 15 lb of skull traction. **B:** Final prepping allows wide access for resection, reconstruction, and harvest of nerve and fibula grafts.

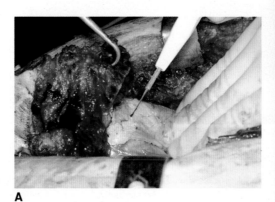

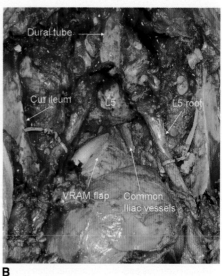

FIGURE 7.7

Tumor delivery. **A:** Tumor is delivered proximal to distal to allow preservation of the most caudal free nerve roots. **B:** View of the operative field immediately after posterior resection of the sacrum.

A   **B**

to free the specimen out. If the rectum is excised en bloc with the tumor, dissection proceeds in a different plane ventral to the rectum and the anus and anal sphincter are excised with the tumor (Fig. 7.7).

Once the tumor is delivered, it is subject to radiography and pathologic analysis to verify that appropriate margins have been obtained. Hemostasis is obtained during this time frame. After this, the decision is made as to whether the patient requires an instrumented spinopelvic reconstruction. Our practice is to pursue this in resections that are proximal to the S1 neural foramina based upon anatomic and biomechanical experiments by Dr. Gunterberg as well as Dr. Hugate (4 and 5).

Spinopelvic Reconstruction Technique

If instrumented reconstruction is needed, pedicle screw instrumentation is performed in usually the remaining three to four vertebral body sites. The Wilson frame is flattened out to restore lumbar lordosis prior to instrumentation. Pedicle screws are placed aggressively to extend to the anterior cortex or even bicortically with appropriate caution in this setting. Usually after the sacrum is removed, a hand can be placed ventral to the spine to feel the pedicle screws as they come through to allow for safe bicortical placement. Screws are placed in the remaining ilium, ideally two long screws upon each side. "Docking sites" are placed for fibula strut grafts in the supraacetabular region. A burr is used to place these from behind. If the level of iliac resection prohibits this, the ischium is usually an appropriate site for docking stations as well. Once this is done, fibula strut grafts are placed as described by Dickey et al. in a "cathedral fashion," struts are placed in the supraacetabular region and then end in the last remaining vertebral segment here (6). Appropriate rods are placed after the strut grafts are positioned, and compression is achieved across these to lock the fibula grafts in. If the patient has undergone prior pelvic radiation, consideration is given to using vascularized fibular grafts. This significantly extends the operative time and may require staging to a further day (Fig. 7.8).

Soft Tissue Closure

Once the tumor is removed and any necessary reconstructions have formed, the final soft tissue reconstruction is performed. It has been our practice to use an Alloderm membrane to reconstruct the posterior abdominal wall to prevent posterior visceral hernia (Fig. 7.9). The pedicled vertical rectus abdominous flap (if harvested at an anterior procedure) is brought through and inserted into the tumor defect to close the wound. If the procedure is done through a posterior only resection, bilateral gluteal advancement flaps are used to help mobilize and close the soft tissue defect over drains. If instrumentation is placed, we remove drains usually by 72 to 96 hours postoperatively, which are near the instrumentation. If no instrumentation is placed, drains are usually left in a more liberal fashion until output trends are below 30 mL per shift.

POSTOPERATIVE MANAGEMENT

Postoperatively patients go on a pressure-relieving specialty air mattress for a period of 5 to 10 days. After that they are mobilized as tolerated. Usually, this encompasses slide board transfers to a medichair as well as the use of a tilt table for patients who retain lower extremity function for ambulation. Generally, their sitting protocol involves initially sitting for only 30 minutes at a time four times a day and advancing to more extensive periods. Once patients can be out of bed for up to 3 hours a day, they are transferred to the inpatient rehabilitation service

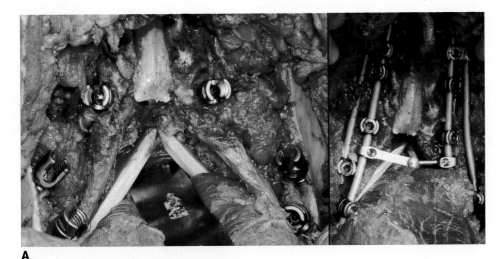

A

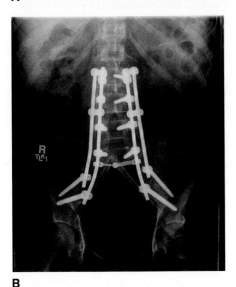

B

FIGURE 7.8

Instrumented spinopelvic reconstruction **A:** Once fibulas are placed into the lowest remaining vertebral body, the spine is compressed across the rods onto the pelvis to lock these in place. Dual rods decrease the risk of catastrophic instrumentation failure. **B:** Radiograph of reconstruction.

for further aggressive rehabilitation. In patients undergoing a unilateral reconstruction, we limit weight bearing on the affected side until evidence of bony healing is seen on radiographs (usually 6 to 8 weeks for patients not on chemotherapy and 12 weeks for patient on chemotherapy or requiring radiotherapy to the area).

Pharmacologic DVT prophylaxis is instituted as soon as felt medically prudent. Until that time frame, the patient's IVC filter minimizes the risk of symptomatic thromboembolic disease to the lungs. Antibiotics are maintained for 24 hours perioperatively only. Ureteral stents (in patients undergoing anterior procedures) are removed approximately 1 week postoperatively when it is clear that the patient has not suffered any complications from the anterior exposure.

One thing we have noted in patients who have undergone high resections into the lumbar spine (at the level of L3 or higher) is a risk of lymphatic leak postoperatively. In these patients, we institute TPN (total parenteral nutrition) postoperatively. Once the diet is advanced, we are careful to use a low fat diet for the first 2 weeks

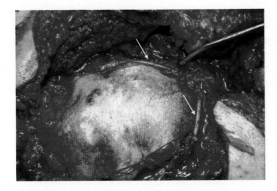

FIGURE 7.9

Alloderm mesh reconstruction of the posterior abdominal wall. Note preserved nerve roots (*arrows*).

postoperatively to minimize the risk of symptomatic lymphatic leak. Lymphatic leak has not shown itself to be a clinical problem in patients who undergo resections at lower levels.

Oncologic surveillance for local or distant recurrence begins at 4 months with axial imaging studies of the chest and operative site.

POSTOPERATIVE COMPLICATIONS

- Sacral surgeries are accompanied by significant perioperative complications. In patients undergoing dorsal sacrectomy only, complications are modest and usually restricted to difficulties with wound healing and superficial infection owing to the proximity of the anus and fecal contamination of the wound. We have often used a wound Vacuum assisted closure to seal off the wound for a period of 1 week postoperatively to minimize the risk of fecal contamination until initial epithelialization is in place. When wound healing difficulty occurs, it is usually able to be treated by local measures only.
- High sacrectomies, which do not require spinopelvic reconstruction, have an increased set of complications due to the increased magnitude of the procedure. Wound healing complications are more frequent but are usually managed with the vertical rectus abdominous flap with local care only. Because of a high risk of thromboembolic disease in these patients, we have placed an IVC filter prophylactically in all patients. The greatest complications are seen in those patients who undergo a resection requiring reconstruction of spinopelvic continuity. In our experience, this surgery is of quite significant magnitude (7). In 44 consecutive patients, 20 required reoperation for wound healing difficulties. Five patients (11%) died in the perioperative period. The most common cause of perioperative mortality was myocardial infarction due to previously silent coronary artery disease. For this reason, we now employ dobutamine stress echocardiography in the preoperative evaluation of almost all of these patients. Deep infection is seen in approximately 40% of patients undergoing instrumented spinopelvic reconstruction owing to the high rate of wound healing difficulty. At mean 3-year follow-up, late instrumentation failure has been seen in approximately 10% of patients.
- Patients with high-grade sarcomas will require resumption of chemotherapy postoperatively. Ideally, this is accomplished by postoperative day 21 in patients undergoing more traditional resections. It has been our experience that it is rarely possible to resume perioperative chemotherapy this rapidly in patients undergoing such aggressive resections. Our goal is to resume chemotherapy approximately 1 month postoperatively. A careful discussion is made with the appropriate medical or pediatric oncologist preoperatively regarding the timing of surgery and the resumption of chemotherapy postoperatively.

RESULTS

Oncologic results are most favorable when complete en bloc excision of the tumor is obtained. It is best illustrated by the data of Fuchs et al. reporting the operative management of sacral chordoma (8). In a series of 52 patients undergoing surgery, complete survival was seen in all patients in whom a wide margin was achieved at the time of surgery. In contrast, the majority of patients with less than a wide resection succumb to disease. Results of more aggressive tumors depended heavily upon the response to chemotherapy.

Neurologic function after major sacrectomy has been examined by Gunterberg as well as Todd. Preservation of bilateral S2 nerve roots and a unilateral S3 nerve root or unilateral S2/3 and 4 nerve roots is required for predictable maintenance of bowel and bladder function.

In those patients undergoing major spinopelvic reconstruction, our experience in a cohort of 44 patients at mean 34-month follow-up has been as follows (7):

- 20 of 44 no evidence of disease
- 6 of 44 alive with disease
- 5 of 44 with perioperative demise
- 11 of 44 dead of disease
- 2 of 44 dead of other causes

Of the 26 surviving patients, 19 were independent in their activities of daily living. About 20 of 44 patients required early operation for wound healing, and 16 of these 20 patients had a deep infection. In the patients requiring reoperation, a mean of three reoperations were necessary. Four patients in this cohort have been revised for instrumentation failure.

These results pertain to very large resections, which disrupt spinopelvic continuity; much fewer complications and more favorable results are seen with lesser sacral resections provided appropriate margins are obtained (9).

CONCLUSIONS

Sacrectomy is a large procedure performed for the treatment of malignancies for which few if any other curative treatment options exist. Posterior-only resections can be performed for tumor up to the S2/3 vestigial disk level. Higher resections require a combined anterior and posterior approach. It has been our practice to stage these resections. An instrumented spinopelvic reconstruction can be performed in high surgeries, which disrupt spinopelvic continuity. Complications are frequent and vary with the extent of resection. However, these surgeries offer a chance of survival for patients who would otherwise have a very dismal prognosis.

REFERENCES

1. Gunterberg B, Kewenter J, Petersen I, et al. Anorectal function after major resections of the sacrum with bilateral or unilateral sacrifice of sacral nerves. *Br J Surg.* 1976;63:546–554.
2. Gunterberg B, Norlen L, Stener B, et al. Neurologic evaluation after resection of the sacrum. *Invest Urol.* 1975;13:183–188.
3. Todd L, Yaszemski M, Currier B, et al. Bowel and bladder function after major sacral resection. *Clin Orthop Rel Res.* 2002;397:36–39.
4. Gunterberg B. Effects of major resection of the sacrum: clinical studies on urogenital and anorectal function and a biomechanical study on pelvic strength. *Acta Orthop Scand.* 1976;162:1–38.
5. Hugate R, Dickey I, Phimolsarnti R, et al. Mechanical effects of partial sacrectomy: when is reconstruction necessary. *Clin Orthop Rel Res.* 2006;450:82–89.
6. Dickey I, Hugate R, Fuchs B, et al. Reconstruction after total sacrectomy: early experience with a new surgical technique. *Clin Orthop Rel Res.* 2005;439:42–50.
7. Rose P, Yaszemski M, Dekutoski M, et al. Classification of spinopelvic resections: oncologic and reconstruction implications. *International Society of Limb Salvage Meeting.* Boston, MA, 2009.
8. Fuchs B, Dickey I, Yaszemski M, et al. Operative management of sacral chordoma. *J Bone Joint Surg Am.* 2005;87:2211–2216.
9. Zileli M, Hoscuskun C, Brastianos P, et al. Surgical treatment of primary sacral tumors: complications associated with sacrectomy. *Neurosurg Focus.* 2003;15:1–8.

8 Amputative Sacral Resections

Panayiotis J. Papagelopoulos, Andreas F. Mavrogenis, Peter S. Rose, and Michael J. Yaszemski

 mputative sacral resections are an extension of the sacrectomy techniques described in Chapter 7. These are complex oncologic procedures performed for curative resection of sacral malignancies, which extend into the pelvis.

INDICATIONS

- To determine the need for external hemipelvectomy coupled with sacral resection, one carefully defines the extent of the tumor. Tumors may require such a resection if their epicenter is within the ilium but disease extends across the sacroiliac joint, or if their epicenter is in the sacrum but removal requires resection of the femoral nerve as well as the lumbosacral trunk or the lumbosacral trunk as well as the hip joint articulation.
- In general, when patients require resection, which disrupts spinopelvic continuity and either resects both the lumbosacral trunk and femoral nerve or the lumbosacral trunk and hip joint, the ultimate function of the limb is so poor that external hemipelvectomy is often indicated in conjunction with the sacral resection. This technique also allows the maximal oncologic margin to be obtained and provides for healthy and robust flap coverage from the limb.

CONTRAINDICATIONS

- Contraindications are as outlined in the chapter on sacrectomy. These center on carefully assessing patients for any evidence of metastasis, as procedures of this magnitude are generally considered too great to be considered for noncurative intent. Similarly, surgeons should have a strong plan in place to obtain a tumor-free margin of resection. This frequently requires resection of adjacent visceral organs.
- The medical fitness of the patient for a surgery of this magnitude should be carefully considered before proceeding with these resections.

PREOPERATIVE PLANNING/GENERAL CONSIDERATIONS

Tumor staging, diagnosis, and imaging are as outlined in the Chapter 7 on sacrectomy. We have classified major spinopelvic resections in four types (Fig. 8.1). Type 1 and 2 resections (total sacrectomy, hemisacrectomy) may proceed as outlined in Chapter 7 (Sacrectomy). Type 3 and 4 resections (partial and total sacretomies in conjunction with external hemipelvectomy) are the subject of this chapter.

The amputative part of the procedure is performed in a single setting. Patients undergoing type 3 resections are considered for an instrumented spinopelvic arthrodesis to the remaining limb if >50% of the lumbosacral articulation is resected. It is our preference to perform this fusion procedure in a second operation staged approximately 48 hours after the amputation to allow time for final margins to be ascertained and to minimize the physiologic impact on the patient. In type 4 resections, the amputative resection is carried out in a single stage and the tumor-free portion of the amputated femur is stored sterilely in a liquid nitrogen freezer until a second stage of the surgery at which time an instrumented fusion between the remaining lumbar spine and remaining limb is performed.

Careful consideration is given preoperatively to the flap, which will allow closure after the amputation. In the majority of cases, the buttock flap is contaminated by the presence of tumor extending in and around the sciatic notch and the gluteal vessels. However, in most cases, the external iliac vessels are free of tumor allowing a flap based upon the quadriceps of the amputated femur pedicled off the external iliac/femoral artery system to provide for robust closure. In rare cases, tumor extent is such that either free flap coverage or vascular bypass techniques are necessary because of compromised soft tissue in the flap or tumor encasement of both the internal and external iliac vessels.

Similar to patients who are undergoing conventional sacral resections, patients undergoing amputative sacral resections are at high risk for thromboembolic complications. We prefer to place a removable inferior vena cava (IVC) filter after the index surgery. This is deliberately not placed prior to the index surgery to allow maximum mobilization of the vena cava without risk of luminal injury.

TECHNIQUE

Positioning

Ureteral stents are placed preoperatively, and patients complete a bowel preparation. The anus is sewn shut and prepped into the field only if it is to be excised as part of the tumor resection. After robust vascular access is obtained, patients are positioned in a very sloppy lateral position on the operating table. We have found that rather than using a conventional beanbag positioner, it is more successful to place a large sandbag both in front of and behind the patient's chest to allow them to be rolled to a near supine and a near prone position during the procedure.

SURGICAL TECHNIQUE

The surgical incision goes midline over the sacrum and then courses up and around the posterior iliac crest to come over the lateral aspect of the pelvis to the anterior superior iliac spine (Fig. 8.2). The incision curves down distally over the greater trochanter down to the lateral epicondyle of the knee. The line of dissection then crosses the front of the distal femur just proximal to the patella, over to the intermuscular septum, and courses up the medial aspect of the thigh to the harvest of the entire quadriceps group as an anterior flap. We initially

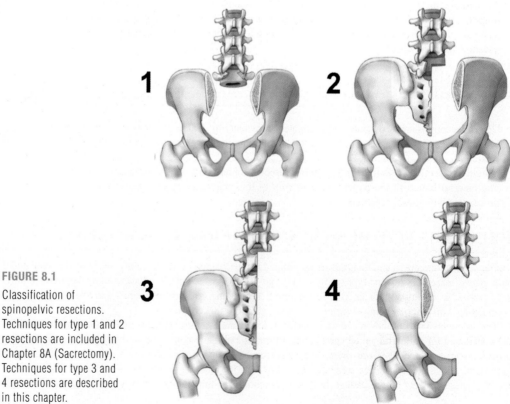

FIGURE 8.1

Classification of spinopelvic resections. Techniques for type 1 and 2 resections are included in Chapter 8A (Sacrectomy). Techniques for type 3 and 4 resections are described in this chapter.

begin by mobilizing the anterior thigh flap as it provides robust access to the pelvis once this is lifted up in conjunction with the pelvic/iliac incision (Fig. 8.3). The dissection is taken sharply down through tumor-free areas to isolate the quadriceps mechanism and ligate the femoral vessels as they come through Hunter's canal. This large muscle mass is then lifted proximally to the level of the inguinal ligament. As dissection proceeds around the iliac wing, the abdominal wall muscles are sharply transected and tagged to assist the ultimate closure. The incision extends around to the posterior-superior iliac spine allowing maximal access to the pelvis and tracing of the vascular system. The ureter is protected by the stent, which has been placed preoperatively. The external iliac vessels and femoral nerve are located and traced proximally into the pelvis. We try hard to preserve the inferior epigastric artery to maintain perfusion to the rectus abdominous muscle as this can be used as a rescue flap if any area of the wound becomes a matter of concern postoperatively.

In cases of hemisacrectomy (type 3 resections), the dissection can generally be performed entirely in a retroperitoneal fashion. Vascular mobilization proceeds up to the level of the common iliac vessels with ligation of the internal system and mobilization of the distal aspect of the aorta and vena cava overlying the lower lumbar spine as necessary for tumor dissection and osteotomies in this region. For the majority of type 3 resections, a purely retroperitoneal approach can be used provided the sacral osteotomy can be performed at the midline. However, in cases requiring either total sacrectomy (type 4 resections) or in which there is a very large pelvic mass preventing safe access, the medial aspect of the incision used to harvest the anterior flap can be extended up the midline of the abdomen to allow reflection of the entire abdominal wall proximally and a transperitoneal approach can be used to provide full access to the pelvis for resections, which cannot be reached through the retroperitoneal approach alone. Strong efforts are made to preserve the femoral nerve throughout the course of dissection such that the flap will be sensate for the patient.

Once the flap has been developed and the vascular dissection is complete, the pubic symphysis is transected with either an osteotome or a Gigli saw. The incision is then extended down over the midline of the sacrum and traced posteriorly around the ischium and through the perineum to meet the anterior incision to provide for the amputative nature of the resection.

The sacral resection is approached as outlined in Chapter 7 (Sacrectomy). We deliberately leave the sacral dissection until the lateral half of the procedure as there is often vigorous bleeding from the epidural veins, which would otherwise ooze continuously throughout the procedure. Once the sacral osteotomy is performed, further dissection is made around the perineum and through the ischiorectal fossa to complete the amputation and deliver the specimen. It is important to preserve the integrity of the rectum throughout this procedure. In addition, care is taken to maintain the flap moist and not on tension.

Soft tissue closure then proceeds at the conclusion of specimen delivery. In the case of a type 3 resection, dissection is usually entirely retroperitoneal. The anterior thigh flap provides for good muscle coverage and often excess skin. When necessary, surplus skin can be trimmed and the distal quadriceps muscle flap tucked

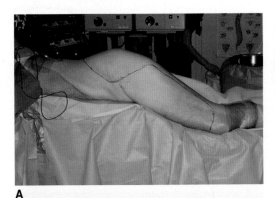

A

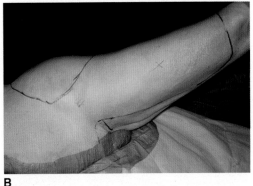

B

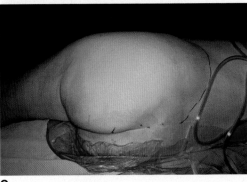

C

FIGURE 8.2

A–C: Surgical incision allows access to the sacrum, pelvis, and harvest of the anterior thigh flap. The medial incision in panel **(B)** can be extended proximally if a transperitoneal exposure is needed.

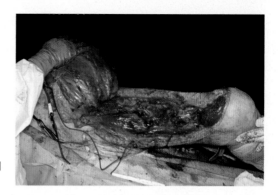

FIGURE 8.3

Raising of the anterior thigh flap pedicled on the femoral vessels.

in to help fill the dead space of the wound (Fig. 8.4). In the case when a transperitoneal approach becomes necessary, an Alloderm mesh or similar tissue is often used to confine the abdominal contents (Fig. 8.5). As reoperation is often necessary as a planned part of staged reconstructive procedures or for unplanned treatment of infection, we mark the area on the flap where the femoral vessels lie close to the incision with either a tattoo of methylene blue or a stitch in the skin. This decreases the risk that during reopening of the wound the femoral vessels feeding the flap will be injured.

Assuming a type 3 resection, colostomy is usually not a part of the procedure as the patients are expected to have a high likelihood of maintaining continence. In type 4 resections, a colostomy and resection of the anus and rectum are generally considered part of the procedure.

Spinopelvic Reconstruction Technique: Type 3 Resection

The need for an instrumented spinopelvic reconstruction after a type 3 resection (external hemipelvectomy coupled with hemisacrectomy) is controversial. In our experience, if the majority of the lumbosacral articulation is resected, patients likely benefit from instrumented fusion across the spinopelvic junction. This is generally performed in a second stage approximately 48 hours after the index surgical procedure. It is usually simple to reopen the wound (and probably advantageous to wash out the inevitable degree of hematoma which develops). Reconstruction is performed using spinopelvic instrumentation from L4 through the ilium on the retained side. There is usually excellent exposure to perform a diskectomy of the remaining disk at the L5-S1 segment and provide an anterior interbody graft at this junction. Depending on the vascular mobilization achieved in

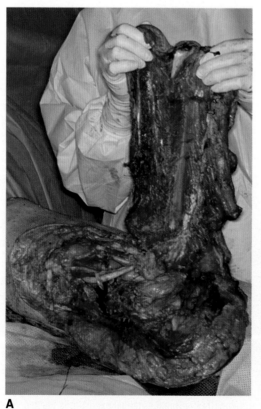

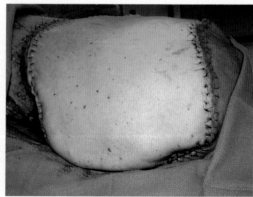

FIGURE 8.4

A,B: Insetting of anterior thigh flap in a type 3 resection.

A   B

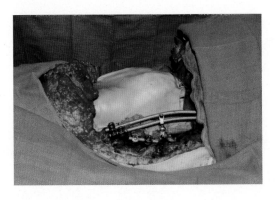

FIGURE 8.5

Use of Alloderm mesh to sequester abdominal contents in a type 4 resection closure.

the index procedure or desired in the secondary procedure, similar anterior lumbar interbody fusion can be performed at the L4-5 level as well (Fig. 8.6).

Spinopelvic Reconstruction Technique: Type 4 Procedure

In the case of a type 4 resection (total sacrectomy external hemipelvectomy) it is necessary to provide reconstruction between the remaining lumbar spine and remaining hemipelvis and limb. Because of the very large magnitude of the oncologic resection, these procedures are staged at least 48 hours and oftentimes longer after the index surgical procedure once the patient is physiologically recovered appropriately.

Key aspects of the reconstruction of a type 4 procedure include centralizing the remaining hemipelvis and limb under the lumbar spine as well as providing a robust autograft strut between the lowest remaining vertebral body and the hemipelvis. At the time of the index resection for patients with type 4 procedures, a portion of the femur of the amputated limb, which is largely free of tumor, is saved sterilely in a liquid nitrogen freezer. This provides a strut graft to bridge the gap between the remaining lumbar spine and pelvis on the retained side.

Pedicle screw instrumentation is performed into at least the lowest three segments of the lumbar spine on the remaining side. Screw fixation is obtained in the bone stock of the remaining ilium avoiding the hip joint (Fig. 8.7). In performing the type 4 reconstruction, two key factors are involved. The first is externally rotating the pelvis and similarly "centralizing" the remaining lumbar spine over the remaining pelvis such that the patient's center of gravity is relatively uniform. Second, it is often necessary to perform a foraminotomy of the lowest one or two lumbar segments remaining to avoid too much traction on the lumbar nerve roots to the remaining leg from this maneuver.

Once the instrumentation is in place, the femoral autograft from the resected limb is used as a strut graft between the supraacetabular pelvis and the remaining lumbar spine. Rods and screws allow for fixation and compression across this graft. An Alloderm or similar membrane is used to sequester the abdominal contents away from the instrumentation (Fig. 8.5). Similar to the type 3 resection, the anterior thigh flap is inserted to close the soft tissue defect. As type 4 resections commonly involve resection of the anus and genital structures, the amount of skin defect may require the full aspect of skin from the quadriceps flap.

POSTOPERATIVE MANAGEMENT

Postoperative management is similar to that described for patients with sacrectomies; however, because of the amputative nature of the procedure, the rehabilitation requirements for these patients are more challenging.

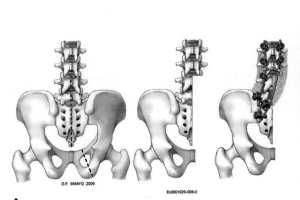

A

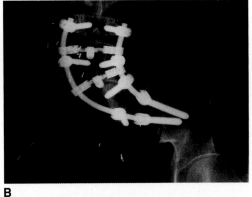

B

FIGURE 8.6

Type 3 reconstruction. **A:** Schematic. **B:** Radiograph.

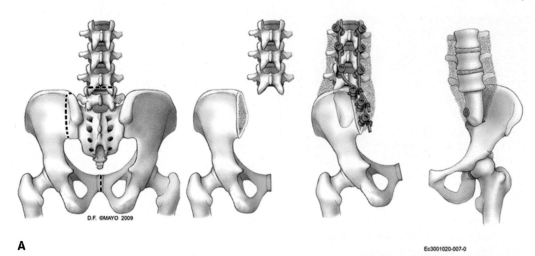

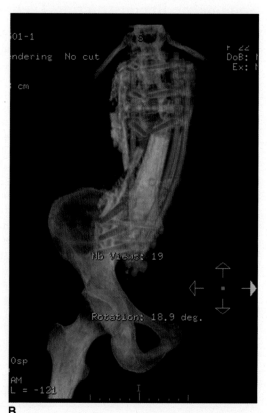

FIGURE 8.7

Type 4 reconstruction. **A:** Schematic. **B:** CT scan. **B**

Just as with standard large sacrectomy procedures, patients are maintained on a suspension air mattress for approximately 5 to 10 days. Mobilization then proceeds with the use of a tilt table and progresses to standing. In patients undergoing type 4 resections, the magnitude of the surgical insult usually prohibits aggressive postoperative mobilization for approximately 2 weeks after the reconstructive procedure.

Drains remain in place until output trends are below 30 mL per shift. An effort is made not to have the drains directly adjacent to instrumentation. If drains are necessary directly adjacent to implants, a strong attempt is made to remove them by 72 to 96 hours. We generally use an incisional wound vacuum device set on the lowest setting to keep the wound sterilely sealed and distribute any tensile forces across it. This is changed approximately every 4 days.

The remainder of the postoperative management is similar for patients undergoing large more conventional spinopelvic resections.

COMPLICATIONS

- The most common complications following amputative sacral resections are infection and wound healing difficulties. Given the large magnitude of the resection, infection/wound breakdown rates of approximately

50% are observed. These are generally well managed with early reoperation for irrigation and debridement of any nonviable or questionable areas.

RESULTS

Results parallel those outlined in the chapter on sacrectomies for large spinopelvic resections. The 16 patients in our surgical experience undergoing amputative sacrectomies are included in the summary of results presented there.

CONCLUSIONS

Amputative sacral resections are rare procedures performed for locally advanced malignancies without evidence of disseminated disease. Innovative techniques allow successful tumor resection of these challenging patients, with a chance for survival in patients who otherwise have little prospect for cure.

REFERENCES

1. Dickey I, Hugate R, Fuchs B, et al. Reconstruction after total sacrectomy: early experience with a new surgical technique. *Clin Orthop Rel Res*. 2005;439:42–50.
2. Fuchs B, Dickey I, Yaszemski M, et al. Operative management of sacral chordoma. *J Bone Joint Surg Am*. 2005;87: 2211–2216.
3. Gunterberg B, Kewenter J, Petersen I, et al. Anorectal function after major resections of the sacrum with bilateral or unilateral sacrifice of sacral nerves. *Br J Surg* 1976;63:546–554.
4. Gunterberg B, Norlen L, Stener B, et al. Neurologic evaluation after resection of the sacrum. *Invest Urol*. 1975;13: 183–188.
5. Gunterberg B. Effects of major resection of the sacrum: clinical studies on urogenital and anorectal function and a biomechanical study on pelvic strength. *Acta Orthop Scand*. 1976;162:1–38.
6. Hugate R, Dickey I, Phimolsarnti R, et al. Mechanical effects of partial sacrectomy: when is reconstruction necessary. *Clin Orthop Rel Res*. 2006;450:82–89.
7. Marvogenis AF, Patapis P, Kostopanagiotou G, et al., Tumors of the sacrum. Orthopedics, 2009; 32(5):342.
8. Rose P, Yaszemski M, Dekutoski M, et al. Classification of spinopelvic resections: oncologic and reconstruction implications. *International Society of Limb Salvage Meeting*. Boston, MA, 2009.
9. Todd L, Yaszemski M, Currier B, et al. Bowel and bladder function after major sacral resection. *Clin Orthop Rel Res*. 2002;397:36–39.
10. Zileli M, Hoscuskun C, Brastianos P, et al. Surgical treatment of primary sacral tumors: complications associated with sacrectomy. *Neurosurg Focus*. 2003;15:1–8.

9 General Considerations

Peter F. M. Choong

Resections and reconstructions of the proximal femur are usually performed for malignant disease (1–7). Non-neoplastic conditions may also require similar resections and reconstructions (8–10) and these include complications of total hip arthroplasty including gross loosening with bone loss, periprosthetic fracture, and failed conventional treatment of proximal femoral fractures. The nature of the resection and hence the reconstruction will depend on the etiology of the condition. Regardless of the indication, the challenges that unite the treatment of these conditions are the potential for resection of considerable lengths of bone, loss of important soft tissue attachments, instability of the joint, and alteration in the normal function of the hip.

INDICATIONS

Primary Malignancies of Bone

The proximal femur and the femoral diaphysis are common locations for a number of primary bone malignancies. These include chondrosarcoma, Ewing sarcoma, and osteosarcoma. The surgical management of primary tumors mandate adherence to certain principles of oncologic surgery that aim to maximize the local control of disease. The most important aspect of tumor resection is to ensure oncologically sound margins (11–15). Intralesional margins that breach the tumor capsule should be avoided at all costs. Marginal excisions that pass through the edematous zone of areolar tissue immediately adjacent to the tumor capsule should only be employed if a vital neurovascular structure is at risk of injury, and under this circumstance marginal margins should only be utilized in the setting of adjuvant chemotherapy or radiotherapy. Wide margins are preferred and constitute at least 2 cm of tumor-free bone either side of the tumor in the longitudinal direction and at least one named soft tissue layer in the radial direction from the tumor-bearing bone. Radical margins that are seldom used necessitate resection of the entire tumor-bearing compartment, which in the case of the femur is the entire bone. The quality of the surgical margin is judged by the least adequate margin achieved. For example, a tumor resected with wide margins except for one location where the tumor was breached is regarded

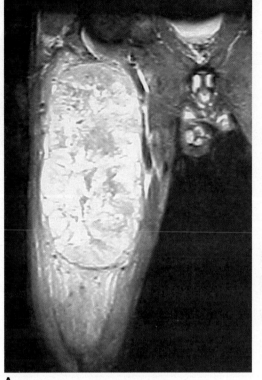
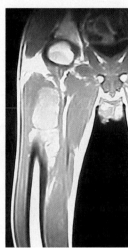

FIGURE 9.1

A: 21-year-old man with an extensive extraosseous soft tissue component from an Ewing sarcoma of his proximal femur. **B:** Marked reduction in the size of the soft tissue component after neoadjuvant chemotherapy.

as a contaminated wide margin which has the same effect as an intralesional or marginal margin only unless immediate remediation is undertaken with wide re-excision and copious intraoperative lavage (11,14).

Resections of such large lengths of bone will inevitably impact on the surrounding soft tissue. Specifically, the abductor and extensor attachments are vulnerable to excision, which has obvious implications for joint function and stability. The tumor may alter following neoadjuvant therapy and the nature of this change has to be considered carefully prior to planning resection margins (16). For example, Ewing sarcoma is often characterized by a large soft tissue component with associated edema (Fig. 9.1A). Following neoadjuvant chemotherapy, there can be substantial reduction in the extent of the soft tissue component (Fig. 9.1B) such that the post-chemotherapy margins may not resemble the margins originally anticipated at the time of diagnosis. Further, the intraosseous extent of the tumor may also reduce quite markedly with chemotherapy, requiring less bone resection. In principle, an excellent response to chemotherapy as judged by complete reduction in tracer avidity on functional nuclear scans like positron emission tomography, or near-complete reduction in the size of the soft tissue component should allow a determination of the required wide surgical margin based on the post-chemotherapy imaging of the tumor. In contrast, a Ewing tumor with a poor response to neoadjuvant chemotherapy should always have its surgical margins determined on the pre-treatment imaging. As the periphery of an Ewing tumor is typically the site of the most viable cells, wide margins are mandatory. A similar approach can be employed for osteosarcoma. Chondrosarcoma, however, is not conventionally treated with chemotherapy or radiotherapy (Fig. 9.2A–D). Under this circumstance, wide margins should be planned from the outset based on the initial staging studies (Fig. 9.2E).

Secondary Malignancies of Bone

The commonest malignant tumor of bone is a metastasis from carcinoma. The likely primary carcinomas that metastasize to bone include the midline paired organs such as breast, lung, thyroid, kidney, and prostate. The femur is a common location for metastasis and surgeons are frequently called upon to consider the surgical management of an impending or completed fracture. Pain is a major feature of metastatic bone disease and surgery is an important option for management. Femoral resection is often only considered when the extent of tumor involvement or its likelihood to progress in a single site is so great as to make intramedullary rod fixation or internal plate and screw fixation impractical or perilous (Fig. 9.3A–E).

Isolated lesions are uncommon but may occur in relation to thyroid and renal metastases. Occasionally, late presentation of breast carcinoma metastases many years after the treatment of the primary may present as a solitary lesion. In all these cases, en-bloc resection may be attempted with locally curative intent. More often, however, disease arises in multiple sites within a single bone and any solution should seek to protect the entire bone. While the systemic treatment of bone metastasis has improved, its success is generally regarded as temporary

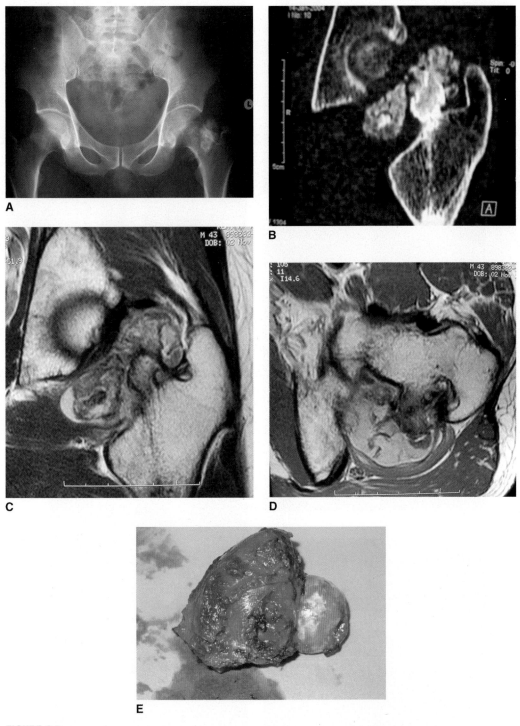

FIGURE 9.2

A: 36-year-old man with reduced flexion and rotation of his left hip and increasing groin and knee pain. Plain anteroposterior radiograph demonstrating a flocculent, calcific lesion in the periarticular area of the left hip. **B:** Computed tomographic scan of the lesion in **(A).** Demonstrating a pedunculated lesion arising from the posterior aspect of the femoral neck. This mass is characterized by a lobulated appearance with the cortex of its stalk being continuous with that of the posterior aspect of the femoral neck and the trabeculae of the stalk crossing into that of the femur. **C:** Proton density weighted coronal magnetic resonance image demonstrating cartilaginous nature of femoral neck mass. **D:** Proton density weighted axial magnetic resonance image demonstrating very thick cartilage cap on pedunculated mass on posterior aspect of left femoral neck. **E:** En-bloc resection of proximal femoral mass with sacrifice of the proximal femur. Subsequent histologic examination confirmed a conventional chondrosarcoma.

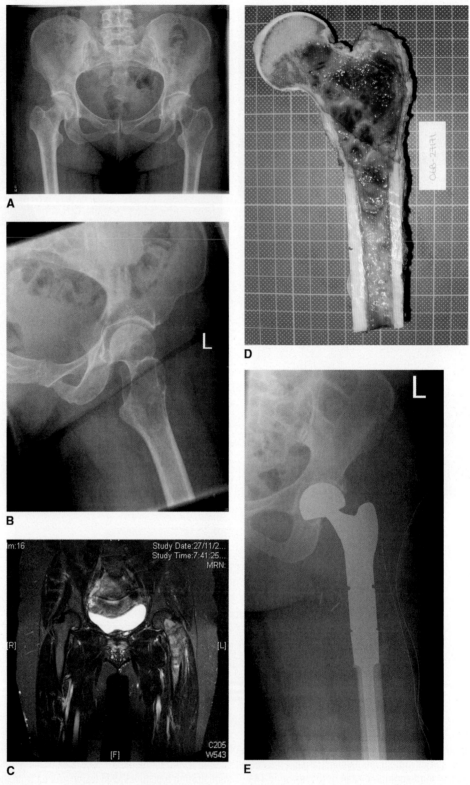

FIGURE 9.3

A: Anteroposterior radiograph of the pelvis of a 46-year-old woman demonstrating an extensive area of lysis in the intertrochanteric region of the left proximal femur. Subsequent needle biopsy confirmed the presence of a metastatic breast carcinoma. The markedly lytic nature of the lesion and the extent of its location threatens impending fracture of the left femur and contraindicates simple plate or rod fixation. **B:** Lateral radiograph of the left hip demonstrating the extent of lysis in the proximal femur. **C:** Fat-suppressed contrast-enhanced T2-weighted coronal magnetic resonance image demonstrating a moderately enhancing lesion in the proximal left femur with extraosseous extension of the tumor. **D:** Operative specimen confirming the extensive destruction of proximal femoral bone. **E:** Reconstruction of the left proximal femur with a modular tumor endoprosthesis and a bipolar femoral head component. Note the prominent shoulder on the prosthesis which is designed to allow easier attachment of the abductors.

rather than curative. Therefore, in providing a surgical solution to metastatic bone disease, the expectation should be one of disease progression that compels a need for a durable reconstruction. Further, the longevity and status of the patient at the time of the surgery needs to be considered when planning an appropriate response to disease.

Complications of Hip Prostheses

Total hip arthroplasty has been one of the most successful procedures in orthopedics. Advances in prosthetic design and materials manufacture and a better understanding of tribology has permitted greater patient activity and improved prosthetic longevity. One of the key advances in arthroplasty has been the recognition of the need for improved revision techniques to address prosthetic complications such as loosening, periprosthetic fracture, dislocation, and infection.

Like the management of bone tumors, the complexity of proximal femoral reconstruction when revising failed hip joint arthroplasty arises when there has been absolute loss of significant amounts of femoral cortical bone or the quality of bone stock is too poor to accept a standard prosthetic replacement (8–10). This can be seen in gross loosening of a cemented prosthesis where motion of the prosthesis has caused expansile remodeling of the proximal femur, or migration of the prosthesis into a varus position with or without breach of the lateral cortex by the tip of the prosthesis, or markedly comminuted periprosthetic fractures. In all cases, conversion to a specialized megaprosthesis, enhancement of the native femur by allograft, or a combination of an allograft prosthetic composite (17–20) will require careful consideration of the appropriate surgical approach and technique. Using the same prostheses or techniques as employed in tumor surgery will also require surgeons to address the need for safe exposure, good soft tissue attachment, joint stability, and creation of a durable construct.

Complications of Proximal Femoral Fracture

Highly comminuted fractures or nonunion of comminuted proximal femoral fractures may be treated with megaprosthetic reconstructions. This device provides immediate stability and permits early weight bearing in the setting of someone who may otherwise require prolonged protected weight bearing to allow bone union (Fig. 9.4A–E).

INVESTIGATIONS

Plain Radiographs

Biplane radiography is important in all orthopedic procedures. Specifically, radiography provides information required for templating the acetabulum and femoral canal when selecting the appropriate prosthesis. Hard-copy radiographs of the whole femur should be acquired if possible. While digital imaging has many advantages, the lack of digital templating and the difficulty in producing 1:1 magnification of images hampers preoperative planning of prosthetic requirements. This may be particularly important in situations where abnormally large or small sizes of implants are required as these may not be present on the standard inventory of equipment and prostheses and may have to be especially requested. Radiographs are also important for assessing the symmetry of the pelvis and hips, and the status of the lumbar spine prior to revision joint arthroplasty. Recognizing the extent of femoral and acetabular bone loss and implant migration is critical for preoperative planning of reconstruction in revision joint arthroplasty.

Radiographs are important for initial screening of malignant tumors. In this regard, whole bone radiographs are required to ensure that disease at the limits of the radiograph is not missed. The nature of the primary or secondary bone tumor will determine the appropriate surgical approach and reconstruction. The relative existence of lytic and sclerotic lesions in metastatic disease will also be a factor in determining the appropriate management of metastatic disease of the femur. It should be noted that radiographs on their own may not be sufficient to account for all malignant disease in a bone because the loss of 30% or more of bone is required before a lytic lesion becomes obvious on plain radiographs.

Nuclear Scintigraphy

Nuclear scintigraphy with bone-targeting tracers is an excellent modality for identifying areas of increased bone turnover that may represent malignancy, prosthetic loosening, or periprosthetic fracture. Unlike plain radiography which requires at least 30% of bone loss to clearly identify a bone abnormality, scintigraphy may detect subtle increases in bone activity. More recently, co-registration of nuclear scans with multislice computed tomography (CT) has facilitated greater specificity and accuracy in the interpretation of results. Nuclear tracers such as thallium and glucose-6-phosphate that can detect metabolic activity may also be useful for identifying areas of increased metabolic activity (21). This is pertinent when assessing the nature of a malignancy because areas of increased metabolic activity may be targeted for biopsy, or the changes in tracer avidity between prechemotherapy/radiotherapy and postchemotherapy/radiotherapy may be important for determining response to treatment. Response to treatment can have significant bearing on the choice of surgical margin when planning resection of a malignant tumor.

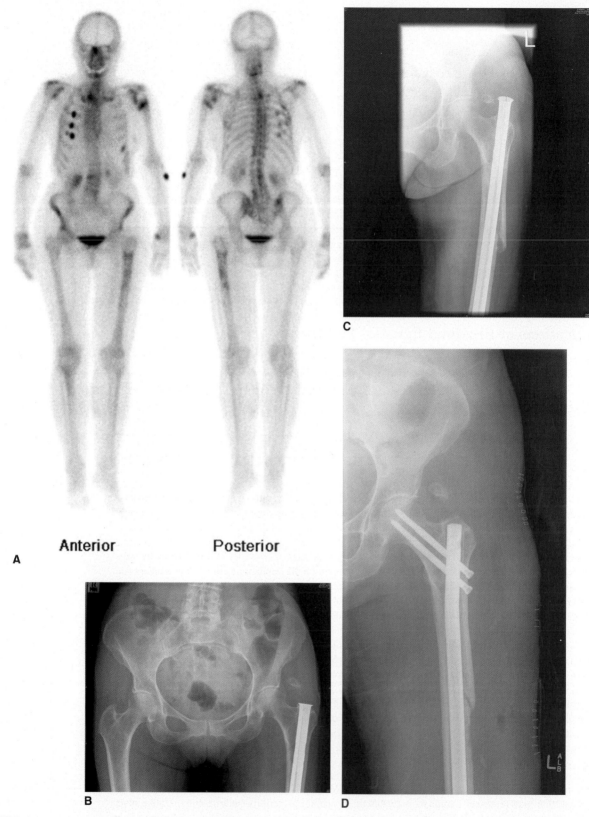

FIGURE 9.4

A: Technetium bone scan demonstrating an area of heterogeneous nuclear uptake in the left proximal femur of a 68-year-old lady with metastatic breast carcinoma. **B:** Prophylactic non–cross-bolted intramedullary rod fixation of the left femur and postoperative radiotherapy. **C:** Six months after radiotherapy the patient experiences increasing left hip pain, loss of weight-bearing capacity through the left hip and a significant limp. Plain radiograph of the hip demonstrates a fracture of the proximal femur with proximal migration of the intramedullary rod as the proximal fragment deviates into varus. **D:** Exchange procedure to replace the previous intramedullary rod with another intramedullary device that permits proximal and distal cross bolts to control the fracture.

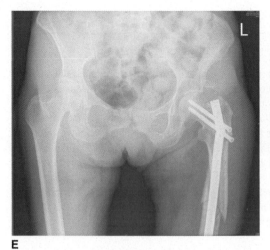
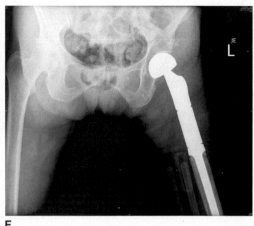

E   F

FIGURE 9.4 (*Continued*)

E: Nonunion and fragmentation of the proximal femoral fracture fragment results in catastrophic failure of the intramedullary rod with fracture of the device and displacement of the fracture. **F:** Radionecrotic fracture fragments excised after removal of intramedullary rod and reconstruction with a modular proximal femoral tumor endoprosthesis and a bipolar femoral head.

Computed Tomography

CT is an excellent modality for delineating cortical and trabecular bone. Thus, CT has an important role in identifying bone loss of any cause including fracture, tumor, or periprosthetic lysis. Multiplanar and three-dimensional reconstructions may be invaluable for providing spatial information when planning reconstruction. Loss of extensive areas of cortical bone may require selection of bulk allografts or alternately segmental mega-prostheses for reconstruction. Similarly, defects of the acetabulum may also require allograft or prosthetic supplementation prior to acetabular component implantation. Image degradation is encountered when CT scans are performed through metallic devices. The ability of sophisticated CT software to subtract the prosthetic image or suppress the metal artifact of an existing prosthesis allows better delineation of periprosthetic lysis.

Magnetic Resonance Imaging

Magnetic resonance imaging (MRI) provides unsurpassed soft tissue contrast allowing excellent delineation between tissues of differing hydration. This modality may also provide greater information with the addition of contrast enhancement. The specific value of MRI scans is in staging tumors where the extra- and intraosseous extent of tumor is required for planning operative margins. The artifact from ferrous materials is significant and degradation of image quality by large prostheses makes the use of this modality less valuable in revision surgery. Titanium implants, however, cast a smaller image artifact and MRI may still be useful for identifying soft tissue abnormalities in the setting of an existing prosthesis. This may be relevant when trying to determine the presence of a local recurrence of tumor.

Angiography

Angiography may be indicated when involvement of the superficial femoral artery and its profunda branch is suspected. This is relevant when dealing with proximal femoral tumors that have a large soft tissue component that is medially directed. Under such a circumstance, ligation and division of the profunda femoris vessels is usually required. Displacement of the vascular tree by a medially directed soft tissue component may distort the anatomy making it more difficult to secure the profunda femoris artery as it leaves the main artery in a posteromedial direction. Therefore, preoperative delineation of the arterial tree is indicated. CT angiography or MR angiography has now revolutionized the visualization of the vascular tree and in most circumstances has supplanted standard angiography for this purpose.

Angiography is imperative when dealing with large metastatic bone lesions. Metastases such as renal and thyroid metastases and myeloma which are characterized by hypervascularity may require preoperative embolization to minimize potentially life-threatening intraoperative hemorrhage. Conventional angiography by percutaneous puncture and catheterization of the vascular tree is the preferred route when embolization is being considered. It is also important to conduct surgery within 36 hours of embolization as there is a high risk of revascularization of the tumor after this time. The size, number, and extent of the vascular lesions within a bone may be important when deciding on whether resectional surgery or excisional curettage will be employed and also the type of implant to be used in any reconstruction.

ANATOMIC CONSIDERATIONS

Hip Capsule

The anatomy of the hip capsule becomes important when planning an extra-articular resection of the hip joint. This may be indicated when primary tumors of the femur or acetabulum involve the joint. This may occur following intracapsular femoral neck fractures (Fig. 9.5A and B), invasion into the joint via the ligamentum teres, or extension of tumor through the roof and medial wall of the acetabulum. The medial wall of the acetabulum is not a thick structure and early joint involvement, is a feature of sarcomas within this region. Involvement of the joint should be suspected if there is a joint effusion, alteration in the normal signal intensity of the ligamentum teres, or alteration in the normal fat signal of the fat pad at the floor of the acetabulum. An extra-articular resection requires that the joint capsule is not breached during the resection. On the acetabular side osteotomies through the pubic rami and another beginning at the sciatic notch and extending to the anterior inferior iliac spine will preserve the margin of the acetabular capsular attachment. On the femoral side an osteotomy below the lesser trochanter will avoid breaching the joint capsule which extends to the level of the lesser trochanter anteriorly. The psoas bursa may also communicate with the joint capsule anteriorly. MRI scans should be closely scrutinized to confirm the integrity of the joint when there is a risk that the bursa may be involved.

Parafemoral Musculature

The anterior compartment musculature is closely applied to the proximal femur. Specifically, the vastus medialis, lateralis, and intermedius arise from the anterior two thirds of the surface of the proximal femur. Their position provides an excellent barrier to expanding tumors of the proximal femur. Sacrifice of these muscles will result in weakness of knee extension. The rectus femoris muscle, however, arises from the pelvis and lies as the most superficial of the four quadraceps muscles. As such, the rectus femoris is rarely involved with primary tumors of the femur and surgical plans may include an attempt at preserving this muscle for knee extension. If it is required, transfer of either the medial or lateral hamstring into the quadriceps tendon may improve the power of knee extension. Lateral hamstring transfers may be associated with a greater tendency for lateral patellar subluxation. The hamstring muscles can usually be preserved in resections of the proximal femur. The adductor brevis muscle and at times the upper portion of the adductor magnus muscle will require division from the proximal femur. Division of these muscles is often performed once the osteotomy of the femur is completed because osteotomy allows retraction of the proximal femur out of the wound and rotation from side to side, which provides a much better view of the two adductor muscles that are thus placed on tension. Division of the psoas tendon is required to finally release the proximal femur and is best done when all other attachments have been divided. The posteromedial position of the psoas tendon may make division of this structure difficult unless all other stuctures have been divided.

The gluteus maximus muscle is the most superficial of the gluteal muscles and attaches to the iliotibial tract (Fig. 9.6A–F). The deeper portion of the muscle also attaches to the gluteal tuberosity on the posterior aspect of

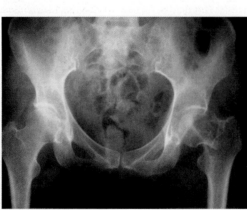
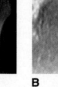

A   **B**

FIGURE 9.5

A: Anteroposterior radiograph of the left hip demonstrating an intracapsular pathologic fracture through a malignant fibrohistiocytoma of bone with contamination of the hip joint. **B:** Contrast-enhanced fat-suppressed T1-weighted axial magnetic resonance image demonstrating intra-articular extension of tumor. Note effusion which should raise suspicions of intra-articular involvement with tumor.

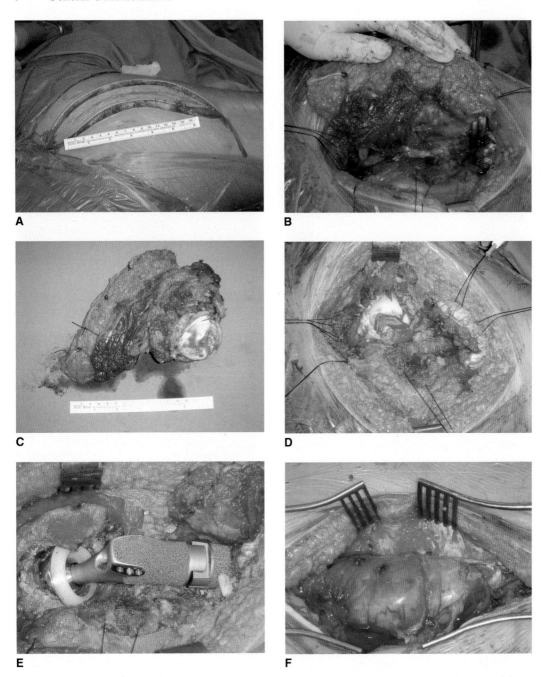

FIGURE 9.6

A: Excision of biopsy tract used for diagnosis of proximal femoral chondrosarcoma. **B:** En-bloc resection of proximal femur with previous operative scar, gluteal attachments, and proximal parts of femoral musculature. **C:** Surgical specimen. **D:** Following removal of the proximal femur, tags are applied to the gluteus medius muscle belly (**far left**), gluteus maximus tendon and muscle (**bottom sutures**), psoas tendon (**top right**), and adductor brevis (**far right**). **E:** Proximal femoral prosthesis with bipolar head reduced into position. Capsule reconstructed around bipolar head. **F:** Tagged muscles and tendons are sequentially sutured to and around the prosthesis.

the proximal femur. Preservation or ensuring reattachment of this part of the gluteal insertion will aid in maintaining the strength of hip extension. This is particularly relevant when proximal femoral resection is usually associated with loss of other bulk movers.

Competence of the gluteus medius is important for stability of the hip joint and normalization of the gait pattern. Loss of gluteus medius function by soft tissue resection, loss of its femoral attachment into the greater trochanter, or superior gluteal nerve injury will lead to a Trendelenberg gait and may require supplementary techniques to increase the stability of the hip joint itself. Preservation of the hip abductor mechanism is preferred unless this would compromise the safe achievement of oncologic margins. In the setting of proximal femoral resection, abductor preservation can be difficult. Techniques such as trochanteric osteotomy with reattachment

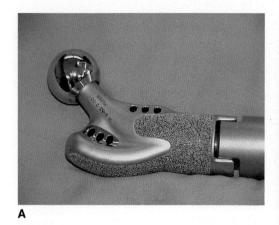

A

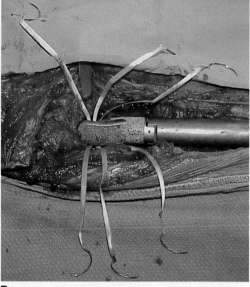

B

FIGURE 9.7

A: Typical proximal femoral modular prosthesis with holes for attachment of abductor and medial femoral musculature. **B:** Large double-ended needles on Dacron tape that are threaded through the attachment holes on the trochanteric shoulder of the prosthesis for attachment of the abductor musculature. **C:** Abductors sequentially sutured to proximal femoral component using Dacron tape. Remaining femoral musculature can be sutured to the abductor reconstruction.

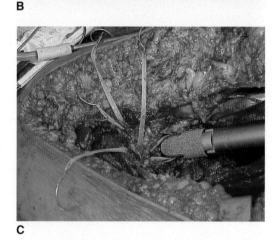

C

of the trochanteric fragment to the megaprosthesis or femoral allograft, and soft tissue transfer (Fig. 9.7A–C) or mesh supplementation may assist in situations where the alternative is complete abductor loss.

Neurovascular Structures

The superficial femoral artery passes quite medially to the femur as it bisects the femoral triangle to enter Hunter's canal. The main trunk of the artery is usually not encountered in resections of the proximal femur unless there is a very large medial soft tissue component. If so, this may tent the vascular tree and care has to be taken to ensure that this is not injured during the dissection. Preoperative angiography should be performed if there is a suggestion that the normal anatomy may be perturbed by extension of the tumor medially. The largest branch of the superficial femoral artery is the profunda femoris artery which is the main arterial supply to the thigh. It leaves the superficial femoral artery on its posterior or lateral surface within the femoral triangle before diving deeply into the thigh, being separated from the main trunk by the adductor longus muscle. Because its course brings it towards the femur, it may be complicated by the extraosseous extension of tumor. The profunda femoris artery passes next to the femur, giving off perforating arteries that wrap themselves around the posterior aspect of the femur. Proximal femoral resections that extend beyond the lesser trochanter may involve any number of branches of the profunda femoris and plans should therefore include the possibility of ligating and dividing the profunda femoris at its takeoff on the superficial femoral artery to avoid troublesome hemorrhage during the dissection. The obturator artery that emerges from the obturator foramen is usually not a problem unless the dissection extends towards the pelvis. If so, it is important to look for this vessel and to ligate it under direct vision as retraction of the vessel behind the obturator muscle or back into the pelvis may be problematic. The lateral and medial circumflex arteries are branches of the profunda femoris and pass into the upper parts of the vastus lateralis and medialis muscles and the quadratus femoris from their medial borders. Ligation of these vessels is not difficult and can be done under direct vision once the femoral osteotomy is completed, which allows manipulation of the proximal femur into more favorable positions for dissection. The femoral vein lies medial to the artery and its position is confirmed once its partner artery has been identified.

The femoral nerve is the largest branch of the lumbar plexus. It enters the femoral triangle lateral to the femoral artery by passing under the inguinal ligament. The majority of its branches are given off within the femoral triangle. Two branches, the nerve to vastus medialis (motor) and the saphenous nerve (sensory) travel with the femoral artery and vein as they traverse the adductor canal in the middle section of the thigh. Dissections that approach the femur from its lateral aspect with preservation of the vastus musculature usually allow preservation of femoral nerve and its branches. Dissections that enter the adductor canal should be performed carefully to preserve the motor branch of vastus medialis.

Anesthetic Considerations

Tumor resections and revision arthroplasty can cause significant physiologic stress on patients. Although expeditious treatment of malignancy is important, and early surgery for prosthetic complications is preferred, these should not occur at the expense of good preoperative preparation. It is imperative that all patient comorbidities are stabilized and optimized prior to surgery. Good communication should be encouraged between the surgical, anesthetic, internal medicine, and nursing teams.

- Appropriate and adequate intraoperative monitoring is mandatory because of the prolonged nature of surgery in patients who are compromised through either chemotherapy or age. This should include invasive intra-arterial blood pressure, central venous pressure, blood oxygen saturation, and exhalation carbon dioxide monitoring. A urinary catheter and core temperature probe should also be in place. Intraoperative cooling should be avoided with the use of body warming devices. Transfusion of warmed blood is also preferred to minimize the development of a coagulopathy.
- Management of blood loss and pain are the major intra- and postoperative anesthetic challenges. Intravenous access via wide bore cannulization into the internal jugular or subclavian veins allows rapid transfusion of blood products, colloid, and crystalloid fluids. Significant hemorrhage may be deceptive if it occurs as a slow ooze over a sustained intraoperative or postoperative period, which is usually the case with complicated revision arthroplasty. Hemorrhage is usually brisk if it occurs during tumor resections and may be torrential if major branches of the iliac veins or the profunda femoris vessels are avulsed. Up to one third of the volume of intraoperative blood loss may be anticipated to occur in the first 24 hours after tumor resection. Appropriately placed drainage tubes will assist in estimating the amount of postoperative blood loss. These should be of wider bore than usual to ensure that they are not occluded by blood clot from heavy bleeding.
- Deep vein thromboprophylaxis is recommended and should include a combination of physical and chemotherapeutic modalities. Intraoperative application of static and sequential calf compression devices may be useful in this regard. Postoperatively, low molecular weight heparin is recommended although the specific type, dose, and frequency are institution specific. In general, chemical thromboprophylaxis is usually withheld for 12 hours after surgery to ensure that any heavy intraoperative blood loss or coagulopathy is not exacerbated by the effects of thromboprophylaxis. Epidural catheters and large drains should be removed 12 hours after the last dose of chemothromboprophylaxis to avoid the complication of hemorrhage.
- Adequate and appropriate pain relief is important to encourage early patient mobilization and ease of care. Regional anesthesia such as by epidural anesthesia or femoral nerve catheterization is an excellent modality for controlling postoperative pain. Femoral nerve and epidural catheters may be left safely in situ for up to 5 days. Careful monitoring, however, is required to maximize analgesia while minimizing motor block. Patient-controlled analgesia (PCA) is an effective means of pain control but an important disadvantage is the reduction in its efficacy when used in patients who are obtunded or who have a poor understanding of the use of this modality. After 3 to 4 days, most patients are able to receive adequate analgesia via oral or intramuscular method routes.

Patient Positioning

Patients are usually fixed with rests in the lateral position. This position may be held over a prolonged period. Therefore, it is imperative that pressure care is provided during surgery. Specifically, this includes the shoulder, the greater trochanter, the lateral knee and ankle of the downside limbs. An axillary roll is important to ensure that the weight of the body is supported at the level of the upper chest wall to minimize compression of the axillary neurovascular structures as they pass between the chest wall and the upper arm at the level of the axilla. The head needs to be carefully positioned to avoid too much lateral flexion that may result in a traction plexopathy of the brachial plexus.

The pelvic supports should be secure and the draping should be wide enough to permit an extensile approach to the hip joint if required. The operated limb should be draped free to allow ease of intraoperative positioning. A sandbag fixed to the operating table in front of the flexed downside leg should prevent intraoperative movement of the downside limb, which will improve stability of the body and also provide the surgeon with a fixed reference from which to estimate leg length discrepancies. Placement of a second back rest at the level of the scapula may assist in keeping the upper body steady and preventing intraoperative rolling of the torso that may confound attempts at accurately positioning the acetabular component.

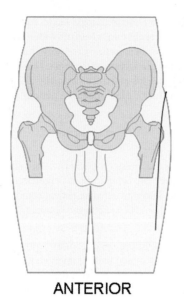 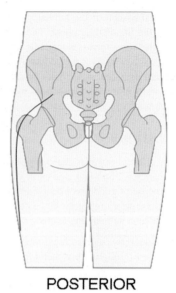 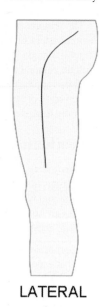

ANTERIOR   POSTERIOR   LATERAL

FIGURE 9.8

Extended universal incision for the exposure of the proximal femur. Incision may be extended proximally in a straight line or curved gently backward.

Incisions

The universal incision that allows exposure to the upper femur for tumor resection and revision arthroplasty (Fig. 9.8) passes upward along the midlateral aspect of the thigh to the greater trochanter, then extends proximally while curving backwards slightly. Any biopsy should be performed in the line of this incision, thus allowing excision of the biopsy tract when formally creating the operative incision. A more posterior approach may be selected for revision arthroplasty. The universal approach permits clear exposure of the greater trochanter and the insertion of the gluteus medius muscle. A trochanteric osteotomy may be performed if required. This incision also permits rotation of the limb internally and externally to view the postero- or anteromedial aspects of the femur where access to the femoral vasculature may be required. If an extra-articular resection of the hip joint is required, the interspace between gluteus maximus and tensor fascia lata is found and the incision may be extended to the iliac crest between these two muscles and then posteriorly along the iliac crest to create a posteriorly based buttock flap. Such an extensile exposure permits access to the sciatic notch and also the supra-acetabular region. Detaching the hamstrings from the ischium exposes the site of an ischial osteotomy and dissection along the superior ramus will expose the site of its osteotomy which is necessary to complete an extra-articular resection.

COMPLICATIONS

- Dislocation is the most common complication following proximal femoral resection (Fig. 9.9). The longer the resection length, the greater the risk because the more extensive the detachment of soft tissue restraints. This risk may be lower in nonmalignant cases where the resection of soft tissue is much less with a greater potential for repair of tendonous and muscular attachments. The most important restraint to dislocation,

FIGURE 9.9

Dislocated proximal femoral tumor endoprosthesis. Deficient abductors and poorly reconstructed capsule may contribute to joint instability. It is common to lengthen the limb to increase the tension in the soft tissue envelope that helps to keep the joint enlocated.

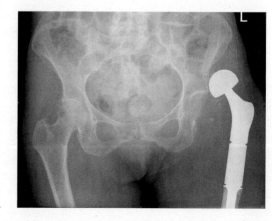

however, is the preservation or reconstruction of the hip capsule. Supplementing this by suturing the remnant of psoas or pectineus to the anterior capsule may also facilitate the development of a stronger restraining force. The use of a bipolar head will also facilitate stability as will preservation of the abductor mechanism. If the abductor mechanism cannot be reconstructed, then lengthening of the femoral component may be required to increase soft tissue tension to hold the joint enlocated. Patients must be forewarned of this complication and the various steps that may be required to achieve stability.

● Infection is a real risk with operations that are prolonged, where soft tissue trauma is extensive and where large prostheses or allografts are employed. Prophylaxis includes preoperative broad spectrum antibiotics such as cephalosporins. In immunocompromised patients a combination of cephalosporin and an antimicrobial that targets staphylococcal species may be used. For example, vancomycin 1 g intravenously every 12 hours and cefotaxime 1 g every 12 hours may be prescribed. The duration of antibiotic therapy is frequently empirical and institution specific. We prefer to maintain intravenous antibiotics until the removal of all wound suction catheters. We then continue oral antibiotics until the removal of skin staples or sutures. Antibiotics against Gram-negative organisms are given at the time of insertion and removal of urinary catheters. Antibiotic-loaded cement should be considered when cemented fixation is chosen. Frequent irrigation with copious amounts of pulsatile saline lavage may also help to dilute the development of bacterial contamination. Minimizing wound hematomas by the judicious use of drainage catheters, careful obliteration and closure of soft tissue dead spaces, and careful application of compressive bandaging may also add to the prevention of infection.

● Patients who are undergoing femoral resection for metastatic disease are vulnerable to the condition of cardiopulmonary collapse that follows a pulmonary embolic phenomenon (22,23). These patients are observed to experience sudden hypotension and oxygen desaturation with intramedullary reaming, cementation, or insertion of a femoral component. If this cardiopulmonary upset is not quickly reversed, the patient may progress to cardiac arrest. The cause of this is thought to be a combination of embolism of marrow components or tumor cells into the pulmonary circulation which causes an activation of the complement system rather than a pure structural blockade of the pulmonary system by a massive embolus. In support of this, reversal of the hypotension and oxygen desaturation by the injection of adrenaline or vasopressor and the delivery of high-flow oxygen are not followed by persistently raised right heart pressures. This complication should be preempted by the anesthetic team who should be made familiar with this complication prior to the commencement of surgery. During surgery, good communication between the anesthetic and surgical team should exist where any manipulation of the intramedullary space should be brought to the attention of the anesthetist prior to commencement of the procedure. The anesthetic team should ensure that the patient is well hydrated intraoperatively with intravenous inotropes or vasopressors ready for deployment. Early detection of hypotension is fundamental to successful management of the case, therefore intra-arterial monitoring of blood pressure is highly recommended.

REFERENCES

1. Ahlmann ER, Menendez LR, Kermani C, et al. Survivorship and clinical outcome of modular endoprosthetic reconstruction for neoplastic disease of the lower limb. *J Bone Joint Surg Br.* 2006;88B:790–795.
2. Choong PF, Sim FH. Limb-sparing surgery for bone tumors: New developments. *Semin Surg Oncol.* 1997;13:64–69.
3. Damron TA. Endoprosthetic replacement following limb-sparing resection for bone sarcoma. *Semin Surg Oncol.* 1997;13:3–10.
4. Donati D, Zavatta M, Gozzi E, et al. Modular prosthetic replacement of the proximal femur after resection of a bone tumour—A long-term follow-up. *J Bone Joint Surg Br.* 2001;83B:1156–1160.
5. Gosheger G, Gebert C, Ahrens H, et al. Endoprosthetic reconstruction in 250 patients with sarcoma. *Clin Orthop Relat Res.* 2006;450:164–171.
6. Sanjay BK, Moreau PG. Limb salvage surgery in bone tumour with modular endoprosthesis. *Int Orthop.* 1999;23:41–46.
7. Shin DS, Choong PF, Chao EY, et al. Large tumor endoprostheses and extracortical bone-bridging: 28 patients followed 10–20 years. *Acta Orthop Scand.* 2000;71:305–311.
8. Clarke HD, Berry D, Sim FH. Salvage of failed femoral megaprostheses with allograft prosthesis composites. *Clin Orthop Relat Res.* 1998;356:222–229.
9. Parvizi J, Sim FH. Proximal femoral replacements with megaprostheses. *Clin Orthop Relat Res.* 2004;420:169–175.
10. Parvizi J, Tarity TD, Slenker N, et al. Proximal femoral replacement in patients with non-neoplastic conditions. *J Bone Joint Surg Am.* 2007;89:1036–1043.
11. Enneking W, Maale GE. The effect of inadvertent tumor contamination of wounds during the surgical resection of musculoskeletal neoplasms. *Cancer.* 1988;62:1251–1256.
12. Enneking WF, Spanier S, Goodman MA. A system for the surgical staging of musculoskeletal sarcoma. *Clin Orthop Relat Res.* 1980;153:106–120.
13. Enneking WF, Spanier S, Malawer MM. The effect of the Anatomic setting on the results of surgical procedures for soft parts sarcoma of the thigh. *Cancer.* 1981;47:1005–1022.
14. Virkus WW, Marshall D, Enneking WF, et al. The effect of contaminated surgical margins revisited. *Clin Orthop Relat Res.* 2002;397:89–94.

15. Wolf R, Enneking WF. The staging and surgery of musculoskeletal neoplasms. *Orthop Clin North Am*. 1996;27:473–481.

16. Picci P, Sangiorgi L, Rougraff BT, et al. Relationship of chemotherapy-induced necrosis and surgical margins to local recurrence in osteosarcoma. *J Clin Oncol*. 1994;12:2699–2705.

17. Gitelis S, Heligman D, Quill G, et al. The use of large allografts for tumor reconstruction and salvage of the failed total hip arthroplasty. *Clin Orthop Relat Res*. 1988;231:62–70.

18. Harris AI, Gitelis S, Sheinkop MB, et al. Allograft prosthetic composite reconstruction for limb salvage and severe deficiency of bone at the knee or hip. *Semin Arthrop*. 1994;5:85–94.

19. McGoveran BM, Davis AM, Gross AE, et al. Evaluation of the allograft-prosthesis composite technique for proximal femoral reconstruction after resection of a primary bone tumour. *Can J Surg*. 1999;42:37–45.

20. Springer BD, Berry D, Lewallen DG. Treatment of periprosthetic femoral fractures following total hip arthroplasty with femoral component revision. *J Bone Joint Surg Am*. 2003;85-A:2156–2162.

21. Hicks RJ, Toner G, Choong PF. Clinical applications of molecular imaging in sarcoma evaluation. *Cancer Imaging*. 2005;5:66–72.

22. Barwood SA, Wilson JL, Molnar RR, et al. The incidence of acute cardiorespiratory and vascular dysfunction following intramedullary nail fixation of femoral metastasis. *Acta Orthop Scand*. 2000;71:147–152.

23. Choong PF. Cardiopulmonary complications of intramedullary fixation of long bone metastases. *Clin Orthop Relat Res*. 2003;415:S245–S253.

10 Megaprosthesis for Non-Neoplastic Conditions of the Proximal Femur

Javad Parvizi, S. M. Javad Mortazavi, Tim van de Leur, and Panayiotis J. Papagelopoulos

With the rise in the number, and to some extent the complexity, of revision hip surgery, continuous challenges need to be met. One of these challenges is the reconstruction of femur with extensive bone loss. Although a number of options exist, there are some patients in whom the best option is replacement of the proximal femur with a so-called megaprosthesis. Megaprosthesis has been available in the armamentarium of orthopedic surgeons for a few decades. The problems with the earlier generation of megaprosthesis were twofold. First, these prostheses did not provide flexibility for restoration of limb length and soft tissue tension. The second problem is related to the proximal surface of these prostheses that did not allow reattachment of soft tissues or ongrowth of bone. In recent years, modular megaprostheses (Fig. 10.1A) have been introduced that intended to address the shortcomings of the first-generation megaprosthesis. The modularity has allowed reconstructive surgeons to more accurately restore limb length, soft tissue tension, and subsequently reduce the incidence of instability that was seen with the older megaprostheses. In addition, the introduction of constrained cups (Fig. 10.1B) has been very effective in reducing dislocation following the use of megaprosthesis.

INDICATIONS

Due to concomitant advances in alternative reconstruction methods and increased use of cortical strut grafts to augment host bone, the indications for the use of the megaprosthesis have narrowed. Recent evidence, however, does point to the fact that in select cases with severely compromised bone stock where the use of a conventional prosthesis is precluded, proximal femoral replacement is a viable choice for reconstruction (7).

The indications for megaprosthetic use include older patients with extensive femoral bone loss that may have occurred as a result of

- Infection (Fig. 10.2A)
- Osteolysis (Fig. 10.2B)
- Periprosthetic fracture (Fig. 10.2C)
- Multiple previous surgeries (Fig. 10.2D)
- Nonunion of proximal femur despite multiple attempts for osteosynthesis
- Reconstruction of femur following resection arthroplasty

In younger and more active patients, reconstruction of deficient proximal femur may be attempted by an allograft prosthetic composite (See Chapter 12). An important and critical prerequisite for the use of

FIGURE 10.1

A: Photograph of modular megaprosthesis with different stem, body, and neck length that allow more accurate restoration of offset, limb length, and soft tissue tension that in turn lead to reduced instability. **B:** Constrained liners, being used in conjunction with megaprosthesis on occasions, have also played an extremely important role in prevention of instability following the use of megaprosthesis.

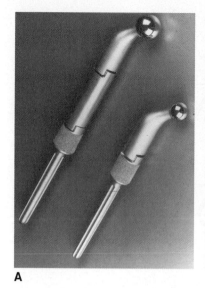

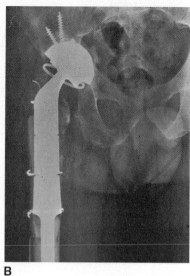

A

B

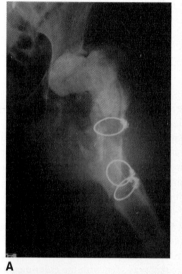

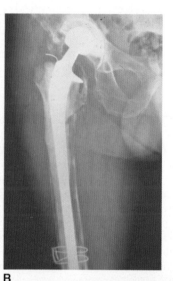

A

B

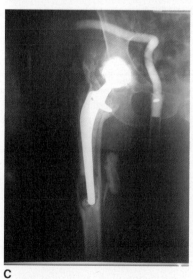

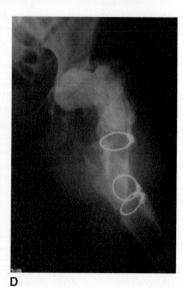

C

D

FIGURE 10.2

Proximal femoral replacement is utilized to reconstruct the proximal femur with extensive bone loss that may have occurred as a result of infection **(A)**, osteolysis **(B)**, periprosthetic fracture **(C)**, or multiple previous surgeries **(D)**.

proximal femoral replacement is that there is sufficient distal femoral length (>10 cm available for secure fixation of the prosthesis). When distal bone is inadequate, consideration for total femoral replacement must be given.

CONTRAINDICATIONS

- The presence of superficial or deep infection around the hip
- Uncooperative patient
- Vascular insufficiency of the limb
- Malnutrition
- Skin disorders with active lesions or ulcers
- Significant medical comorbidities precluding administration of anesthesia

PREOPERATIVE PLANNING

Preoperative planning is an important aspect of hip reconstruction particularly during revision surgery. Patients requiring proximal femoral replacement have often had numerous previous surgeries making preoperative evaluation and templating critical. The purpose of the preoperative templating is mainly to determine (a) if sufficient length of distal femur is available to allow fixation of the proximal femoral replacement and (b) the approximate length of the prosthesis that will be needed. The templating also allows the surgeon to determine the site of transverse osteotomy and the diameter of distal femur. During templating, the quality of the distal bone is also assessed and decision is made regarding the use of cemented versus uncemented prosthesis (Fig. 10.3). For cementless fixation, adequate bone stock must be present to allow either creation of a 4-to 5-cm tube of bone of a specific diameter into which a porous stem may obtain a scratch fit or a tapered geometry into which a tapered, splinted stem may be placed for axial and rotational loading. If the remaining bone stock is deemed inadequate because of osteopenia or extremely patulous and capacious, cemented fixation should be used.

Most patients undergoing megaprosthesis reconstruction have had multiple previous hip procedures. Therefore, it is imperative to examine the incision site carefully for the presence of skin lesions that may predispose or increase the rate of infection and to determine the appropriate previous scar to be utilized. A new incision may occasionally have to be used if the previous scars are inappropriately placed. On occasion, involvement of plastic surgeons may be necessary to evaluate the status of the soft tissues in case local or free flaps may be required for reconstruction.

Thorough examination of the hip with particular attention to the status of the abductors and the limb length should also be carried out preoperatively. Clinical and radiographic (standing films) assessment of the limb length is carried out and recorded. Patients should be counseled about the possibility of limb length discrepancy that may result from surgery. In our opinion, lengthening of the limb up to 4 cm can be carried out safely. Any lengthening beyond this point is likely to place the neurovascular structures at increased risk. Intraoperative monitoring of the sciatic and femoral nerves should be performed in patients in whom extensive (>4 cm) limb lengthening is anticipated.

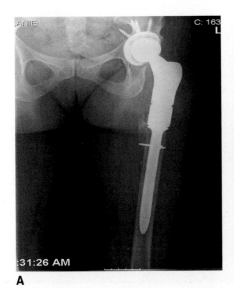
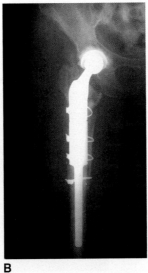

FIGURE 10.3

Good cortical thickness of the distal femur **(A)** allowed the use of an uncemented stem versus cemented stem **(B)** that was used in another patient with poor distal cortical bone undergoing proximal femoral replacement.

It is paramount to rule out infection. We always order a white blood cell count with differential, C-reactive protein, and erythrocyte sedimentation rate for this purpose. Based on clinical and radiographic examinations and the result of serology, hips with a high index of suspicion are also preoperatively aspirated to rule out deep infection. At the time of surgery, multiple (usually odd numbers) tissue samples should be sent for culture.

All patients should receive a thorough medical examination with appropriate laboratory investigations to ensure their fitness for surgery. Revision hip arthroplasty with megaprosthesis involves extensive soft tissue dissection and unusually long operative times; moreover, large volumes of blood loss place immense physiological demand on the patient.

Preoperative templating to select the appropriate stem length and diameter is essential for operative success. Problems with the removal of existing hardware, specific needs for acetabular reconstruction, and the potential need for insertion of constrained liners should be anticipated and addressed appropriately. Despite the most accurate preoperative measurements, a variety of prosthetic sizes should be available in the operating room as intraoperative adjustments often lead to changes in the anticipated size of prosthesis. The megaprosthesis manufacturing company representative should be contacted and be present in the operating room for assistance. Experienced operating room personnel, particularly the scrub person, should be available and assist with this procedure. An experienced anesthesia team should administer anesthesia as invasive monitoring in these, often elderly and frail, patients is warranted.

SURGICAL TECHNIQUE

Anesthesia

Regional anesthesia is preferred in these patients, and intraoperative blood salvage (cell saver) should be used. The anesthesia team should be warned about possible large volume loss and encouraged to monitor this closely. Invasive monitoring with the use of arterial lines or pulmonary catheters may be necessary in the appropriate patients.

Position and Draping

We place the patient in the supine position and use a hip bump to position the patient (Fig. 10.4). Nonpermeable U-drapes are used to isolate the groin. The distal one third of the extremity is also isolated from the field using impermeable drapes. It is very important to preoperatively assess limb length and to have an idea where the patient lay straight on the table in order to accurately assess limb length adjustments. Extension of the incision and arthrotomy of the knee to address intraoperative problems such as fractures extending distally is not uncommon. The skin is scrubbed with betadine solution for at least ten minutes and Duraprep applied prior to application of Ioband to the skin.

Incision and Exposure

We use the direct lateral approach (Hardinge) to gain access to the hip and maintain a low threshold to extend the incision as needed (Fig. 10.5). When extensile exposure of the femur is needed, a vastus slide as described by Head et al. (1) mobilizes the anterior abductors, vastus lateralis, and vastus intermedius muscles anteriorly in unison and exposes the anterior and lateral aspects of the femur (Fig. 10.6). Meticulous soft tissue handling helps the tissues to heal and minimizes postoperative complications. Deep tissue specimens for frozen section and culture are obtained routinely in all cases. Meticulous debridement of the hip is carried out to remove previous metal debris and hardware around the femur.

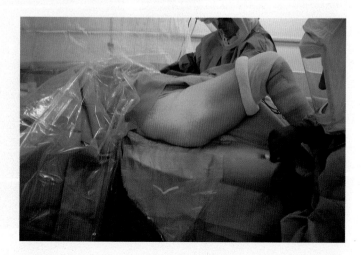

FIGURE 10.4

A patient in supine position.

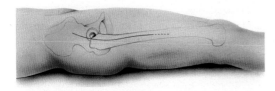

FIGURE 10.5

Diagram showing the placement of incision.

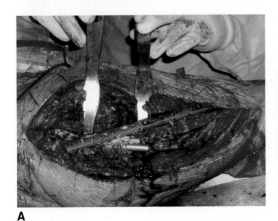

A

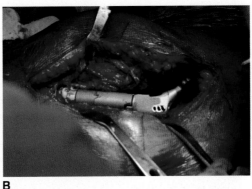

B

FIGURE 10.6

A: Intraoperative picture showing the exposure of femur in a patient who has sustained periprosthetic fracture. **B:** Transverse osteotomy.

Femoral Reconstruction

Proximal Femoral Replacement   An extended osteotomy to split the proximal femur may be required in order to facilitate the removal of the previous prosthesis and hardware. A transverse osteotomy is first made in the host bone at the most proximal area of circumferential adequate quality bone (Fig. 10.6B). Because the outcome of this procedure is influenced directly by the length of the remaining femur, maximum length of the native femur is maintained at all costs (4). We then prefer a longitudinal Wagner type of coronal plane osteotomy to split the proximal femur with poor bone quality. Soft tissue attachments to the proximal femur, particularly the abductor mechanism—if present, should be retained if at all possible. Once the femur is exposed, the distal portion of the canal is prepared by successive reaming/broaching. Preserve the cancellous bone, when present, for better cement interdigitation. After completion of femoral preparation and determination of the size of best-fit, trial components are inserted and the stability of the hip is examined. A distal cement restrictor is used whenever possible. The restrictor is introduced and advanced distally to allow for at least two centimeters of bone cement at the tip of the stem. The cement is pressurized and the final component implanted ensuring that the porous coated portion of the stem is placed directly and firmly against diaphyseal bone with no interposing cement. The prosthesis can be assembled and then cemented into the distal part or the distal segment cemented first and then the body assembled onto it. In any case, extreme care needs to be exercised to prevent rotational malpositioning (Fig. 10.7). To mark the rotation, we use electrocautery once the trial component is appropriately positioned; furthermore, the rotation of the component cannot be changed once the distal stem is cemented in place.

Determination of Limb Length

The length of the femoral component is determined through careful preoperative planning and intraoperative assessment. Two methods may be used for proper leg length determination. The first method is to apply traction to the limb with measurement from the cup to the host bone osteotomy site (for the proximal femoral

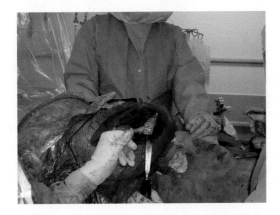

FIGURE 10.7

Intraoperative picture demonstrating how the rotational positioning/version of the femoral component is determined. The version of the femoral stem is judged by appropriate positioning of the knee.

replacement cases). The second and preferred method is to place a Steinmann pin in the iliac crest to measure a fixed point on the femur before dislocation. With the long-stem trial prosthesis in place, proper leg length can be accurately restored. For patients with total femur replacement, radiographs of the opposite and normal femur may be obtained preoperatively and used for accurate templating of length. The length of the prosthesis usually equals the length of the bone being resected, although in many of these patients the integrity of the bone has been breached and the anatomy markedly altered. Ultimately, the femoral prosthesis length depends on the soft tissue tension about the hip. Balancing tension, restoration of the limb length, and avoiding excessive tension on the sciatic nerve are of utmost importance if complications are to be avoided.

Acetabular Reconstruction

The acetabulum is exposed at the beginning of the operation and examined carefully. If a previous acetabular component is in place, the stability and positioning of the component is scrutinized. If the component is appropriately placed and stable, it is left in place and the liner is exchanged. If a previous acetabular component is not in place, a new component is inserted in a press-fit manner with screw augmentation if necessary. More complex acetabular reconstructions such as the use of antiprotrusio cages may occasionally be needed. The type of acetabular liner is determined after completion of the femoral reconstruction, because constrained liners may have to be utilized in patients with poor soft tissue tension and instability. If instability is a concern, a constrained liner is used, and it may be cemented into a well-fixed acetabular shell. In these cases, the inner side of the shell should be scored with a burr. Several longitudinal (grooves are also cut into the back of the liner). The liner is needed to be sufficiently small to allow for 1 to 2 mm of cement mantle. Some commercially available poly is pregrooved, which is cement friendly and no burring is required.

The constrained liners can be either snap-fit or cemented into the shell, depending on the type of the acetabular component implanted. In our experience, constrained liners are required in approximately one half of patients undergoing a megaprosthesis procedure. Our absolute indication for the use of constrained liner is for patients with properly positioned components and equal or near equal leg length who have intraoperative instability secondary to soft tissue deficiency.

Closure

The femur, however poor in quality, is retained and wrapped around the megaprosthesis at the conclusion of implantation. The muscle-tendon attachments are preserved whenever possible. The soft tissues, and in particular the abductors if present, are meticulously secured to the prosthesis (Fig. 10.8). Multiple loops of nonabsorbable sutures are passed around the trochanter remnant and the attached soft tissue. The leg is brought to abduction and the trochanter firmly fixed onto the proximal portion of the prosthesis by passing the sutures through the holes in the prosthesis or around the proximal body and the deep tissues. We occasionally suture the abductors to the vastus lateralis, the tensor fascia latae, or the host greater trochanter, if available (Fig. 10.9). Surgical drains are inserted before closure of the wound in layers using interrupted resorbable sutures. Meticulous skin closure, with excision of hypertrophic prior scar, if necessary, is carried out to minimize postoperative wound drainage.

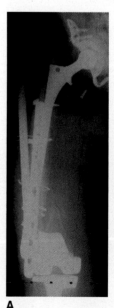
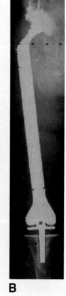

FIGURE 10.8

A: Preoperative radiograph of a 78-year-old patient with failed hip arthroplasty who has a knee arthroplasty in place. The distal femoral bone length and quality was deemed too poor for femoral stem fixation. **B:** Total femoral replacement was performed in this patient.

A   B

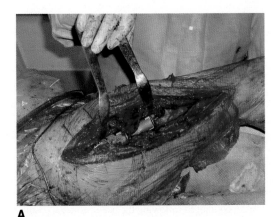

A

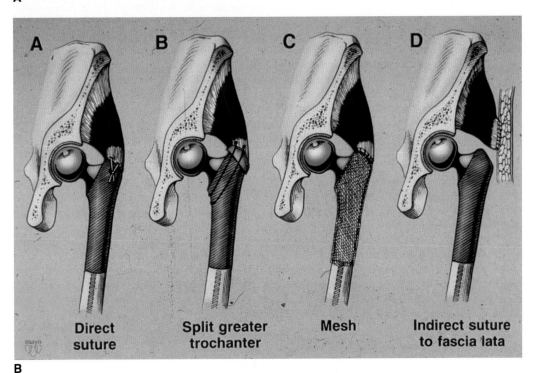

B

FIGURE 10.9

A: Intraoperative picture demonstrating soft tissue closure around the femoral stem. Proximal bone and soft tissue, however poor in quality, needs to be reapproximated to the stem as meticulously as possible. **B:** Various methods of soft tissue reapproximation to the femoral stem.

POSTOPERATIVE MANAGEMENT

Intravenous prophylactic antibiotics are given and maintained until final cultures are obtained (usually 5 days). Thromboembolic prophylaxis for 6 weeks is also administered. Patients are allowed to commence protective weight bearing on postoperative day 1. We recommend the use of abduction orthosis for all patients and protective weight bearing for 12 weeks until adequate soft tissue healing occurs. Patients are usually able to ambulate with the use of walking aids during this time. Daily physical therapy for assistance with ambulation and range of motion exercise for the knee are recommended.

RESULTS

The use of megaprosthesis after tumor resection was encouraging (9), and this led to the expansion of the surgical indications in patients with failed hip prosthesis and severe bone loss for which the only viable option was resection arthroplasty. The initial reviews revealed that the mode of failure of megaprosthesis is similar in patients with or without neoplastic conditions. There was not any significant difference in the outcome of megaprosthesis with respect to failure, incidence of radiographic lucency, limp, pain relief, and the use of walking aids in these two groups.

The initial use of megaprosthesis for reconstruction of proximal femur in nonneoplastic conditions was reported in 1981 (8). Although all 21 patients had significant pain relief, there were two failures. One patient required acetabular component revision, and the second patient needed revision of the femoral component for recurrent instability.

Another retrospective study reported the outcome of 50 revision hip arthroplasties using prosthetic femoral replacement in 49 patients with nonneoplastic condition (4). All patients had massive proximal bone loss, and some patients had multiple failed attempts with other reconstructive procedures. The mean follow-up was 11 years. The mean preoperative Harris hip scores of 43 ± 13 points improved significantly to 80 ± 10 points at 1 year and improved to 76 ± 16 points at the latest follow-up. Before surgery, 86% of the patients had moderate to severe pain. Pain relief was achieved in 88% of patients at 1 year and 73% of the patients at the latest follow-up. There was significant improvement in gait and the ability to ambulate. However, there was some deterioration in all parameters with time.

Detailed radiographic analysis revealed an increase in the incidence of progressive radiolucent lines on the femoral and acetabular sides. Progressive radiolucency was seen around 37% of the acetabular components and 30% of the femoral components. Aseptic loosening constituted the main reason for revision surgery. Using revision as an end point, overall survivorship in the aforementioned series was 64% at 12 years. The most common complication was dislocation, with an overall rate of 22%.

Dislocation and loosening remain the major complications encountered following the use of a megaprosthesis, and the etiology of instability in this group of patients appears to be multifactorial. Again, these patients often have had multiple previous reconstructive procedures that have lead to compromised abductor function; furthermore, the inability to achieve a secure repair of the residual soft tissues to the metal prosthesis predisposes these patients to instability (3). The problem is additionally exacerbated in patients in whom the proper leg length and appropriate soft tissue tension is not attainable.

We have implemented three major changes into our practice to minimize instability. Namely, the use of constrained cups in selective cases, routine fitting and application of a postoperative abduction brace, and, thirdly, augmentation of the proximal bone with the use of strut allograft imparts more rigidity for soft tissue attachment. It is conceivable that the problem of soft tissue to metal attachment may be better addressed in the future with the use of trabecular metals such as tantalum, with its excellent potential for soft tissue on growth; however, at present, this is not a reality.

The relatively high rate of loosening both on the acetabular and femoral side is another common complication of megaprosthesis reconstruction in the majority of reported studies. The reason for this complication lies in the biomechanical aspect of this reconstructive procedure. The diaphyseal cement fixation predisposes the bone-cement-prosthesis to high torsional and compressive stresses leading to early loosening. Cemented long-stem revision implants are known to have limited success and currently are recommended for elderly and sedentary patients (5). As would be expected, the incidence of radiolucency after the use of press-fit or proximally or extensively coated ingrowth stems is, in comparison with megaprosthesis, markedly less (2,6).

The incidence of radiolucency after megaprosthesis reconstruction at our institution has declined somewhat in the latter years, and this is most probably due to third-generation cementing technique. Another and potentially more likely reason for the reduction in the incidence of radiolucency is that we have narrowed the indications for the use of megaprosthesis to elderly and sedentary patients who place lower demands on their prosthesis

PEARLS AND PITFALLS

- Examine patients thoroughly. Note various previous scars, status of abductors, and the limb length.
- Communicate with the patient and help make his or her expectations realistic.
- Perform detailed preoperative templating. Have the company representative available to review your templating and to ensure correct components, and neighboring sizes, are available on the day of surgery.
- Ensure that thorough medical optimization of the patient has been carried out.
- Ask for experienced scrub and anesthetic team.
- Minimize soft tissue dissection off the native bone and retain as much of the host bone as possible.
- Restore appropriate leg length and soft tissue tension.
- Have a low threshold for the use of constrained liners.
- Ensure good hemostasis and perform a meticulous wound closure.

CONCLUSIONS

Despite all of the discussed complications and concerns, the use of a megaprosthesis is a valuable tool for the reconstructive hip surgeon to possess as he is often left to deal with cases of extensive bone loss at the end stage of revision. This prosthesis will have an unacceptably high failure rate if the indications are expanded to include the younger, more active patient. It is in these later cases that other reconstructive options should be exploited.

REFERENCES

1. Berry DL, Chandler HP, Reilly DT. The use of bone allografts in two-stage reconstruction of failed hip replacements due to infection. *J Bone Joint Surg.* 1991;73A:1460–1468.

2. Berry DJ, Harmsen WS, Ilstrup D, et al. Survivorship of uncemented proximally porous-coated femoral components. *Clin Orthop.* 1995;319:168–177.

3. Gottasauner-Wolf F, Egger EL, Schultz FM, et al. Tendons attached to prostheses by tendon-bone block fixation: an experimental study in dogs. *J Orthop Res.* 1994;12: 814–821.

4. Malkani A, Settecerri JJ, Sim FH, et al. Long-term results of proximal femoral replacement for non-neoplastic disorders. *J Bone Joint Surg.* 1995;77B:351–356.

5. Mulroy WF, Harris WH. Revision total hip arthroplasty with the use of so-called second-generation cementing techniques for aseptic loosening of the femoral component: a fifteen-year average follow-up study. *J Bone Joint Surg.* 1996;78A:325–330.

6. Paprosky WG. Distal fixation with fully coated stems in femoral revision: A 16-year follow-up. *Orthopedics.* 1998;21: 993–995.

7. Parvizi J. proximal femoral replacement in patients with non-neoplastic conditions. *J Bone Join Surg Am.* 2007;89: 1036–1043.

8. Sim FH, Chao EYS: Hip salvage by proximal femoral replacement. *J Bone Joint Surg.* 1981;63A:1228–1239.

9. Sim FH, Chao EYS. Segmental prosthetic replacement of the hip and knee. In: Chao EYS, Ivins JC, eds. *Tumor Prostheses for Bone and Joint Reconstruction: The Design and Application.* New York, NY: Thieme-Stratton; 1983:247–266.

11 Megaprosthesis After Tumor Resection

Peter F.M. Choong

The femur is a common site for primary and secondary malignancies of bone. In the majority of cases, proximal and distal tumors can be adequately treated by wide resection and prosthetic reconstruction utilizing proximal or distal femoral prostheses. Extensive tumor involvement, however, can give rise to a challenging surgical situation where wide resection of bone is likely to leave insufficient residual bone for safe and stable fixation of standard proximal or distal femoral prosthetic replacements. The minimum length of proximal or distal femur required for fixation of a tumor endoprosthesis is approximately 130 mm. Therefore, extension of a distally located tumor above the lesser trochanter or a proximally located tumor below the diaphysiometaphyseal junction of the distal femur is unlikely to leave adequate bone stock for stem fixation. Diaphyseal tumors such as Ewing sarcoma can also be so extensive as to involve both proximal and distal parts of the femur requiring total femoral resection for safe removal.

Previously, extensive femoral tumor that would normally require total or near total femoral resection would be treated by hip disarticulation. In comparison to femoral resection and reconstruction, hip disarticulation is simpler and the risk of violating tumor margins is considerably less. To reduce the impact of hip disarticulation, biologic reconstructions have been designed to utilize the bone distal to the knee in a reconstruction that converts a hip disarticulation effectively to a through knee or long above knee amputation (1,2). However, patient expectations have increased in the last 2 decades and the functional deficit and the psychosocial impact of amputation are now far less acceptable, particularly, when an alternative surgical solution includes limb sparing surgery.

Advances in diagnostic imaging have improved dramatically and now facilitate the planning of critical surgical margins that underpin limb sparing surgery. Advances in chemotherapy and radiotherapy have also contributed to the success of limb sparing surgery by increasing survivorship and improving local control of disease. Greater sophistication in prosthetic design that incorporates modularization of component parts permits bespoke assembly of total femoral prostheses to fit almost all adult patients. The alternatives for total femoral prosthetic replacement other than amputation include massive osteoarticular allograft transplantation, allograft prosthetic composites, and custom stem prosthesis. These options are dominated by complications that are associated with biologic reconstructions including fracture, nonunion, infection, prolonged restricted weight bearing, and instability, thus making total femoral prosthetic replacement a very attractive option when considering total femoral resection.

INDICATIONS

- Total femoral replacement is indicated after resections of diaphyseal tumors with long proximal and distal intramedullary extension of disease, after resection of proximal or distal tumor with extension to within 130 mm of the opposite epiphysis, and with extensive bone loss from widespread metastasis in patients with stable disease.
- Total femoral resection and replacement may also be indicated in patients with widespread intramedullary or compartmental contamination of primary tumor. For example, a classic situation is seen with the patient who presents with a presumed solitary metastasis who undergoes prophylactic fixation with an intramedullary rod. The preparation of the femur for rod fixation results in the contamination of the marrow cavity and also the soft tissue around the entry portal for the rod (Fig. 11.1).

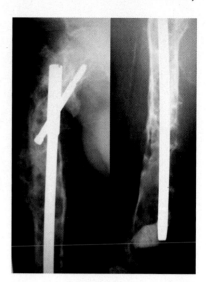

FIGURE 11.1

Intramedullary rod fixation of pathologic fracture through hemangioendothelioma of bone. This was treated with radiotherapy, then total femoral resection with vastus intermedialis, medialis, and part of lateralis. The initial operative wound was also excised en bloc with the tumor.

- Occasionally, this procedure may be further compounded by a pathologic fracture, which results in a contained hematoma that requires wide soft tissue resection as well.
- Some very large soft tissue sarcomas that encircle an extensive length of femur may also be treated by total femoral resection.
- Total femoral resection may also be indicated in patients who have previously been treated with a proximal or distal femoral tumor endoprosthesis who now have the complication of aseptic loosening, periprosthetic fracture, or severe bone lysis.
- Total femoral replacement may be indicated where previous diaphyseal reconstruction has failed (Fig. 11.2A,B).

The versatility of tumor endoprostheses for nononcologic causes is also well known.

- Total femoral replacement may be indicated for patients who have undergone multiple complex revisions and are now left with minimal bone stock in the setting of gross osteolysis, aseptic loosening, or periprosthetic fracture.
- Total femoral replacement may also be indicated in complex comminuted fractures, although this may be more appropriate in the setting of chronic and difficult nonunions of fractures.
- Bone softening diseases such as Paget disease and fibrous dysplasia may result in such deformity and stress fractures that total femoral replacement may be the only option for management.
- Some have suggested that chronic osteomyelitis may be an indication for resection and reconstruction. This should be considered with great caution in light of the very high risk of reinfection that may necessitate subsequent amputation.

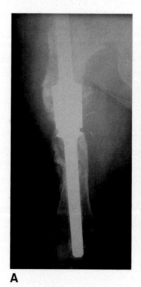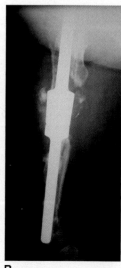

FIGURE 11.2

A,B: Disintegration and lysis of periprosthetic bone around an intercalary prosthesis. Note concertina effect of proximal femur with protrusion of prosthesis stem through greater trochanter. Removal of prosthesis will not leave sufficient bone for stemmed implants.

A   B

CONTRAINDICATIONS

- Total femoral resection is contraindicated for primary malignancies when either contamination or extraosseous tumor growth is so extensive as to make oncologically sound margins difficult to achieve.
- This procedure is also contraindicated in patients who have widespread metastatic disease from sarcoma.
- A total femoral prosthesis relies on stability at the hip and knee joint for proper functioning. The inherent instability of the prosthesis at the knee may be significantly exacerbated by femoral nerve palsy. Therefore, involvement of this nerve may preclude total femoral reconstruction.
- Tumor resection that includes total quadriceps excision causes weakness in extension in much the same way as femoral nerve palsy. Inability to hold the knee in extension can lead to a loss of support in extension and collapse of the affected limb when trying to bear weight. An alternative solution would be the use of custom devices that arthrodesed the knee while permitting hip arthroplasty (3).
- Femoral vessel compromise by tumor is a relative contraindication because these structures may be resected with the tumor and reconstructed by end-end anastamosis or bypass operations. However, major arterial and venous reconstructions are also associated with significant morbidity and limb loss from obstructive complications must be recognized as a potential risk of the operation.
- Prosthetic reconstruction is contraindicated in the setting of systemic or regional sepsis. Delay in surgery is advocated until sepsis is overcome. If persistent limb sepsis prevents safe resection and reconstruction then amputation should be considered to minimize interruptions to systemic chemotherapy.

PREOPERATIVE PREPARATIONS

Total femoral resection is a complex procedure with many associated risks. The purpose of preoperative assessment is to exclude a contraindication to surgery, to define the surgical anatomy, and to plan the surgical margins in oncologic cases. In the setting of previous surgery or radiotherapy, significant fibrosis, thickening, and tethering of neurovascular structures may occur and should be anticipated. Vulnerable areas such as the popliteal fossa and around the femoral neck should be carefully imaged and closely inspected.

Plain Radiographs

Plain radiography is important for preselecting a range of hip and knee sizes for this procedure (Fig. 11.3A). Templating using 1:1 radiographs allows a close estimation as to the appropriate sizes of prosthesis to have

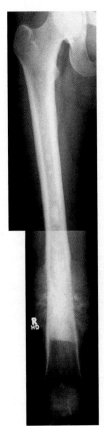
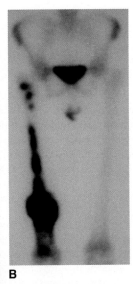
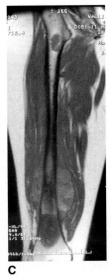

FIGURE 11.3

A: A 16-year-old girl with distal femoral metaphyseal osteosarcoma. Multiple intraosseous metastases extending proximally from distal tumor. **B:** Technitium bone scan confirming extensive femoral diaphyseal involvement of osteosarcoma with intertrochanteric skip lesions. **C:** T1-weighted coronal magnetic resonance image demonstrating involvement of entire diaphysis of femur with osteosarcoma.

available during the procedure. It is important to ascertain if extremes of sizes (very small or very large) are required. With the move toward digital imaging, true size images may be difficult to obtain in certain settings. Plain radiographs may also give an indication of intraosseous spread of tumor (Fig. 11.3B).

Nuclear Medicine Imaging

Technetium methylene diphosphonate is an excellent screening test for identifying skip lesions in adjacent bones such as the pelvis and tibia (Fig. 11.3C). While some skip lesions may be able to be included in the resection, for example, proximal tibial skip lesions, other skip lesions such as in the pelvis may preclude total femoral resection and reconstruction. Newer investigational equipment now combine nuclear with computed tomographic scanning. This permits co-registration of functional and anatomic imaging for greater specificity of diagnosis and more accurate targeting for image guided biopsy. Tests for the presence of acute and chronic infections is critical for avoiding postoperative perioprosthetic infections.

Functional Nuclear Imaging

Thallium and PET scanning are two modalities that assess the metabolic activity of tumor tissue. When obtained at the time of diagnosis, the results form a good baseline measure against which to assess the response to neo-adjuvant therapy. This is important because a poor response to chemotherapy for bone sarcomas requires far wider margins than those with an excellent response.

Computed Tomography

This technique is excellent for assessing the degree of cortical bone loss in metastatic carcinoma. If the extent of destruction is considered to be significant, a decision may be made to undertake total femoral resection and prosthetic reconstruction. Computed tomography is excellent also for assessing trabecular destruction, which can be subtle. Marrow extension or infiltration can be detected by the change in the marrow signal. Fat in the marrow provides an excellent contrast against which to highlight marrow deposits. Pulmonary scans should always be obtained as pulmonary metastases may preclude a major resection and reconstruction procedure.

Magnetic Resonance Imaging

This modality allows unsurpassed soft tissue contrast, which is capable of highlighting the subtle changes that may accompany any extraosseous extension, which is critical for planning surgical margins (Fig. 11.3D). This is also an excellent modality for scrutinizing any potential skip lesions. The excellent contrast between fat and tumor tissue together with contrast enhancement should allow delineation of any suspicious lesions. Careful attention should be paid to the pelvis and periacetabulum.

Angiography

Information on the course of the superficial femoral artery and vein and their significant branches through the thigh is critical when planning a total femoral resection and reconstruction. The vessels pass close to the femur at a number of locations such as the femoral neck, in the adductor canal, and through the hiatus in the distal part of adductor magnus. The profunda femoris vessels also tether the trunk proximally. Expansion of a soft tissue component may cause compression at any of these points leading to vascular obstruction and thrombosis. Advice on the quality of patent vessels should be sought and the potential for bypass surgery identified early.

Bladder Function

In the majority of cases, bladder catheterization is performed to allow urinary measurements and bladder care during and after surgery. Patients who have received thigh radiotherapy, particularly to the adductor compartment or proximal femur, may develop urethral stenosis at the bladder neck. This may result in difficult and traumatic catheterization. In some cases, endoscope-assisted catheterization may be required to safely pass a urinary catheter prior to surgery. Patients who are developing an acute stricture will describe impairment of urinary flow and if suspected, urodynamic studies done prior to surgery are advisable. Resolution of urethral stenosis prior to definitive limb surgery will minimize bacteremia of traumatic catheterization and reduce the risk of hematogenous infection.

PREPARATION

Position and Draping

Access to the hip and the knee is required for total femoral resection (Fig. 11.4). Unlike proximal femoral resection, which can be performed in the lateral position, additional knee resection and reconstruction requires

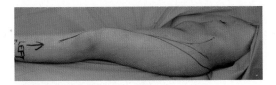

FIGURE 11.4

Preparation of entire limb for surgery with exposure from above iliac crest. Patient is in the supine position with a sandbag underneath the buttock.

the patient in the supine position to allow access to both sides of the knee to achieve adequate dissection of the popliteal neurovascular structures and also to facilitate preparation of the tibia to receive the tibial component.

The patient is prepared in the supine position with no lateral support. A foot rest is used to keep the knee flexed at about 90 degrees and a sandbag is placed under the ipsilateral buttock to lift the buttock and trochanter off the operating table. The patient is draped with the lower limb completely free from the iliac crest down.

Anesthetic Considerations

Total femoral resection and reconstruction is likely to be a long procedure. All precautions are taken to ensure that all pressure points are well padded prior to the commencement of surgery. Sequential calf/foot compression devices should be employed to enhance venous flow in the nonoperated limb. Preoperative antibiotics should be used to minimize the risk of infection. Vancomycin and a third-generation cephalosporin should provide adequate cover against Gram-positive cocci, Gram-negative organisms, and anaerobes.

Venous access should include central lines, and arterial access is very useful to maintain continuous blood pressure monitoring.

Although most centers would induce general anesthesia, some centers may elect to provide regional anesthesia alone or in combination with general anesthesia. The value of including regional anesthesia is the opportunity to continue limb analgesia postoperatively with the use of an epidural catheter. The disadvantage of regional anesthesia is the potential for disguising a nerve plasy or compartment syndrome.

Anatomic Considerations

The hip abductors should be protected where possible. These add to the stability of the hip joint and improve the functionality of the reconstruction. If the greater trochanter is not affected by tumor, then a transtrochanteric approach to the hip should be utilized to enhance the reattachment of the abductors to the prosthesis. Most prostheses have an ingrowth surface on the shoulder of the prosthesis where the greater trochanter may be held using cables and a trochanteric grip. If the tendinous insertion of the abductors is to be elevated off the greater trochanter or divided from the tendon of insertion, these can be reattached using a prosthesis with a high profile trochanter.

Hip Capsule and Psoas Tendon

The hip capsule should be detached from the femur as close to the femoral bone as oncologically possible. This facilitates reconstruction of the capsule after reduction of the hip joint to improve the stability of the joint. The pectineus and psoas tendon may be sutured to the capsule to reinforce the capsular repair. If the psoas tendon is long, this may be attached to the calcar region of the prosthesis via suture holes that are often located at this point. This not only improves stability of the hip joint but may also aid in flexing the hip. However, not reconstructing this should not be regarded as detrimental to the reconstruction.

Quadriceps Muscles

Total femoral resection and prosthetic reconstruction leave the hip and the knee joints unstable. Preserving the power and coordination of muscles that cross these joints improves limb function and gait. Often, the vastus intermedialis is sacrificed with the tumor but in lesions where there is a large soft tissue component, the vastus medialis or lateralis may be included in the resection. Rectus femoris is the most superficial of the quadriceps and is most protected from the underlying tumor. Preservation of this allows weak but useful extension of the knee. Some prostheses are designed with the flexion-extension axis behind the weight-bearing axis of the knee joint. This allows the prosthesis to easily come into extension when weight bearing with a back knee movement in patients who have no quadriceps function.

SURGICAL TECHNIQUE

Incision

The incision passes from the tip of the greater trochanter to the lateral epicondyle of the femur before crossing the proximal tibia below the tibial tuberosity (Fig. 11.5A). A gluteal extension of the incision passes upward

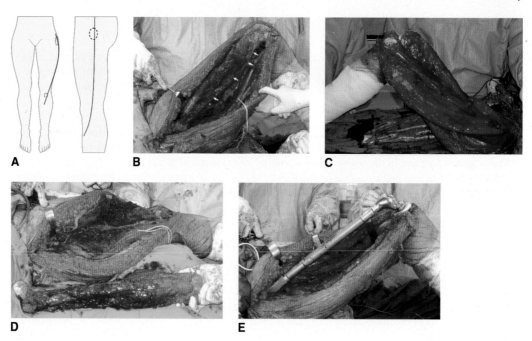

FIGURE 11.5

A: Universal incision passing laterally from above the greater trochanter distally to the lateral epicondyle, then sweeping anteriorly distal to tibial tuberosity. Separate medial incision may be made over the distal femur to allow dissection of large medial soft tissue mass or excision of medial biopsy tract. **B:** Lateral approach allows good exposure of the popliteal fossa after division of the lateral intermuscular septum (*white arrows*). The sciatic nerve and its distal divisions can be easily found (*yellow ligature*) with the popliteal vessels deep to and medial to the sciatic nerve. **C:** A large medial distal femoral soft tissue component may require dissection of a flap that begins on the medial side of the femur with elevation and dislocation of the quadriceps mecha nism to the lateral side of the femur. **D:** With the entire quadriceps mechanism dislocated medially, the femoral vessels can be seen emerging through adductor magnus hiatus from the adductor canal. **E:** Total femoral prosthetic replacement in-situ.

from the tip of the greater trochanter to the interval between the tensor fascia lata and the gluteus maximus muscle. The incision should not curve posteriorly into the buttock as retraction may be made more difficult if the gluteus maximus muscle or the buttock adipose layer is very deep. This incision preserves the blood supply to the anterior quadriceps skin, which arises from the medial side of the thigh. Further, this incision allows excellent exposure to the proximal femur and yet allows a large flap to be created distally, which can be retracted over the distal femur to allow exposure of the medial side of the thigh and femur (Fig. 11.5B). In some cases, a second medial incision is required in the distal part of the thigh to allow dissection of a tumor with a large soft tissue component and also to gain access to the popliteal neurovascular structures. The skin is dissected off the front of the knee to allow visualization of the joint either side of the patella tendon. It is important that the dissection of the skin off the patella should pass through the bursa to preserve the fascia between skin and patella, which minimizes prepatellar skin necrosis.

Isolating and Detaching the Abductors

With the skin incision widely retracted using a Charnley initial incision retractor, the abductor attachment to the greater trochanter should be easily seen. If possible a segment of the greater trochanter is detached with the abductors. First, the anterior border of the gluteus medius is found and lifted with a retractor. The femur is then internally rotated and the posterior extent of the gluteus medius identified and also elevated. The osteotomy of the greater trochanter is then marked out with a coagulating diathermy and with two sharp Hohmann retractors in place anteriorly and posteriorly to the greater trochanter with their points in the pyriform fossa, the greater trochanter is osteotomized a safe distance from the tumor. With a bone hook applied to the cut surface of the osteotomized segment of the greater trochanter, the abductors are reflected superiorly and separated from the gluteus minimus muscle. If the greater trochanter cannot be osteotomized, the abductors are divided with as much of the tendon as possible to retain a resilient part to allow later resuture to the prosthesis.

Elevating the Quadriceps Muscle

The vastus lateralis is swept off the fascia lata with a finger and followed down to its attachment to the lateral intermuscular septum. The vastus lateralis is at its thinnest at its most proximal attachment along the intertrochanteric line. With careful dissection using the coagulating diathermy, the vastus lateralis may be lifted from its proximal attachment and gently detached from the lateral intermuscular septum as the dissection goes inferiorly. Soon, the plane between the vastus intermedialis and the vastus lateralis is found and the lateralis muscle is separated from the intermedialis, which is kept with the femur as a boundary around the tumor. This is followed distally until the conjoint quadriceps tendon is encountered. The intermedialis is detached from this to allow the vastus lateralis and medialis to be lifted away from the femur. Just above the patella, the suprapatellar pouch is encountered and the joint entered if there is no contraindication. The vastus lateralis is lifted off the joint capsule distally as it sweeps to insert into the upper and lateral portion of the patella. Lifting it away from the knee, the arthrotomy at the suprapatellar pouch is then continued laterally along the lateral condyle of the femur down to the patella ligament.

The proximal dissection of the vastus lateralis muscle at its medial extent needs to be performed carefully as the main arterial supply to the muscle crosses the vastus intermedialis at its upper extent. This can be seen, protected, and kept with the vastus lateralis muscle as it is reflected medially.

The vastus intermedialis muscle is continuous medially with the vastus medialis muscle and some part of the bulk of the vastus medialis muscle is usually sacrificed with the femur. Following the upper surface of the vastus intermedialis, the dissection is carried around the medial side of the femur and through the vastus medialis to reach the medial intermuscular septum. Penetrating the vastus medialis distally is safe, but more proximally, care should be taken to avoid injury to the femoral vessels within the adductor canal.

In certain circumstances, the primary incision may need to pass across the front and then the medial part of the thigh. The muscle flap can then be developed from the medial side with elevation of the vastus medialis off the medial intermuscular septum before dislocating the entire quadriceps mechanism laterally off the femur (Fig. 11.5C).

Accessing the Posterior Compartment of the Thigh

A breach in the lateral intermuscular septum is created close to its attachment to the femur distally. Here the muscle bulk is minimal and the septum swings laterally from its more posterior position as it passes from the linea aspera posterior to the supracondylar ridge where it is easily appreciated. Once the septum has been incised a finger is admitted through the slit and the posterior compartment structures lying against the septum can be swept aside. With the finger as a protective barrier, the lateral intermuscular septum is incised proximally with a coagulating diathermy until the femoral attachment of the gluteus maximus tendon is encountered. A branch of one of the proximal perforators is closely related to the gluteus maximus tendon and division of the tendon should be done under direct vision with a coagulating diathermy being ready to clamp the bleeder if encountered.

The posterior compartment of the thigh is now exposed with the long head of biceps most prominent laterally. This is followed down to its tendon, which inserts into the head of the fibula. The gap between the biceps tendon and the iliotibial tract is identified and incised. Just deep to this and behind the lateral femoral condyle is the common peroneal nerve, which can be seen to pass forward deep to the biceps tendon before emerging below its lower border above the lateral head of gastrocnemius, winding its way lateral and then anterior to the neck of the fibula. It is advisable to place a loop around the common peroneal nerve in the popliteal fossa to allow quick identification. The short head of biceps arises from the femur and this should be separated from its origin. The tendon of the lateral head of gastrocnemius is carefully identified, isolated, and then retracted from the posterior condyle with a curved forcep before being divided under direct vision. At this point, the peroneal nerve may be injured if not clearly marked and protected.

Disarticulation of the Hip

The capsule is incised around the neck of the femur passing anteriorly and medially along the intertrochanteric line as far as the lesser trochanter. Externally rotating the hip assists in this part of the dissection. The hip is then internally rotated to place the short external rotators on tension and these are detached from their femoral insertions. The posterior capsule is exposed and divided along its attachment to the posterior femoral neck with a coagulating diathermy. The main arterial supply to the femoral head is through the posterior capsule so active bleeding may be encountered. The capsulotomy is extended medially to the calcar. There is always a medial strip of capsule, which cannot be divided until the hip joint is dislocated and retracted laterally. Sometimes the head is held enlocated tightly by the ligamentum teres, which may need to be divided separately. The artery within the ligamentum teres usually bleeds actively and will require clamping with a long curved artery forcep and cauterized. Once the most medial part of the capsule is identified and put on tension, this can be divided with cautery revealing the underlying psoas tendon as it attaches to the lesser trochanter. The psoas tendon is tagged with some strong sutures and then divided across its tendon. The hip joint should now be dislocated.

Disarticulation of the Knee

The lateral part of the knee is already exposed. After division of the lateral collateral ligament, the capsulotomy is extended posteriorly around the tibial margin. With the lateral head of gastrocnemius and the biceps tendon retracted further posteriorly and distally, the popliteal surface of the capsule can be seen. The cruciate ligaments are then divided from the front allowing separation of the femur and tibia to expose the inner surface of the joint capsule. Once the inner and posterior surfaces of the capsule are identified, this can be divided under direct vision approaching from the lateral side. With the patella dislocated laterally, the medial capsule is divided from its tibial attachment first anteriorly, then moving medially. The anterior part of the capsule is easily found by first identifying the patella tendon and then incising the capsule adjacent to the medial border of the patella tendon and continuing it medially until the medial collateral ligament is encountered. A curved forcep is then used to isolate the medial ligament from its external surface and by careful dissection medially, the tip of the forceps can be made to meet a curved retractor placed around the medial side approaching from the posterior part of the joint. With the tissues external to the medial collateral ligament protected, the remaining medial and posteromedial capsule can be divided.

Popliteal Neurovascular Structures

The popliteal artery and vein can be identified in the popliteal fossa through the lateral approach and followed up to the point where they enter the popliteal fossa through the hiatus in adductor magnus (Fig. 11.5D). The sciatic nerve can also be easily found and followed to its division into the posterior tibial and common peroneal branches. Distally, the vessels and nerves are carefully dissected as far distally as possible to allow retraction away from the proximal tibia, which will be required later during preparation of the proximal tibia for the tibial prosthesis.

With the proximal and distal femur detached, the femur with its attached adductors can be gently pulled laterally, while the soft tissue flap of the quadriceps and its overlying skin are retracted medially. The insertion of the adductor magnus into the adductor tubercle on the medial condyle is then found, carefully isolated, and then divided beginning distally and working proximally along the supracondylar ridge. Doing this the hiatus in the distal part of adductor magnus is easily found and the entry point of the femoral vessels from the adductor canal into the popliteal fossa identified.

Adductor Dissection

With the femur gently pulled laterally, division of the vastus medialis from the medial intermuscular septum is completed. The vessels are found and followed into the adductor canal. Carefully protecting the vessels, the adductor longus muscle is divided from its femoral attachment. This is then retracted medially and the course of the vessels proximally to the femoral triangle can be seen. The vessels lie on the adductor magnus muscle in the adductor canal. With a finger deep to the adductor magnus muscle beginning at its hiatus, the muscle insertion is divided from distal to proximal. The perforator branches of the profunda femoris vessels are directly under the adductor magnus muscle and care must be taken to identify, ligate, and divide them.

Approaching the proximal part of the dissection, the profunda femoris can be seen arising from the main trunk of the femoral vessels. If this branch can be preserved, then it should as it provides blood supply to the muscles of the posterior compartment of the thigh. The adductor brevis muscle is the last main muscle to be divided before the femur is delivered from the wound.

RECONSTRUCTION

The commonest total femoral prosthesis utilizes a distal rotating hinge mechanism and a proximal bipolar femoral head (Fig. 11.6A). When reconstructing a total femoral resection with a total femoral prosthesis, a number of important surgical considerations must be entertained.

- Special attention must be paid to reconstructing the hip capsule and reattaching the abductors to secure stability of the hip joint.
- Adequate tension should be imparted to the soft tissue to allow stability of the hip and knee joint and for the remaining muscle to function appropriately.
- The femoral prosthesis is rotationally unstable about its mechanical axis because of the rotating hinge mechanism distally and the bipolar head proximally. Points of soft tissue anchorage should be created to minimize uncontrolled rotation about its mechanical axis.

Capsular Reconstruction

A major aim of the capsulotomy is to preserve as much capsule as possible. A purse string type suture using nylon tape or nondissolvable suture should be passed around the periphery of the capsule to allow this to be drawn around the femoral neck to capture the femoral head. This can also be reinforced using the remnant sort hip muscles such as pectineus, the external rotators, and psoas, which can be sutured to the capsule.

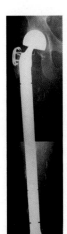
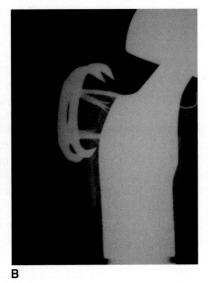
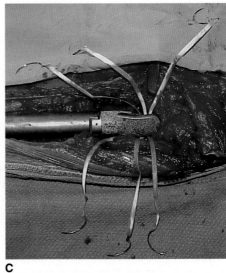

A   **B**   **C**

FIGURE 11.6

A: Anteroposterior radiograph of total femoral resection with bipolar femoral head and rotating knee replacement. **B:** Abductor reattachment with trochanteric grip and cables. Note fraying and rupture of cables. Failure to displace the trochanteric grip and greater trochanter indicates that the fragment of greater trochanter had united to the porous coating on the shoulder of the prosthesis prior to rupture of the encircling cables. **C:** If there is no greater trochanteric fragment to reattach to the prosthesis, the abductor tendon may be sutured to the prosthesis using nylon tape passed through holes in the prosthesis and threaded through the tendon of gluteus medius.

Abductor Reattachment

The abductors may be reattached to the prosthesis using a trochanteric grip and wire cables if a segment of greater trochanter remains (Fig. 11.6B). If a trochanteric osteotomy was not performed, a nylon tape can be woven through the muscle or tendon of gluteus medius and then passed through trochanteric holes that are usually found on the proximal parts of most tumor endoprostheses (Fig. 11.6C). This reattachment can be further reinforced by suturing the gluteus medius to the reconstructed vastus lateralis muscle.

Femoral Reattachment of Muscles

Reattaching the gluteus maximus tendon, the vastus lateralis muscle, and the adductor magnus tendon to the body of the endoprosthesis will assist in providing rotational stability to the entire construct. The shaft of the prosthesis may be tightly bound with nylon mesh that is held on with strong nylon tape or nondissolvable sutures. The gluteus tendon and other muscles can then be reattached to this sheath of mesh. The mesh provokes a fibrotic reaction, which strengthens the muscle and tendinous attachments over time.

Soft tissue Tension

The soft tissue tension is determined by the length of the construct. Overlengthening is common and nerve palsy may follow. Moreover, overlengthening may result in patellofemoral dysfunction and loss of range of stable motion. Patella subluxation may occur with overly tight soft tissue closure and this is a particular problem if excision of the biopsy tract has occurred. Lateral approaches are more susceptible to patella subluxation because of the built-in valgus of the knee and the ability of the femur to rotate laterally around its rotating hinge mechanism if there is a lateral pull from a tight lateral closure.

Deciding on the right combination of femoral and tibial component may not be simple because virtually all landmarks have been removed with the total femoral and proximal tibial resection. It is important to review the x-rays of the opposite knee to assess where the tip of the fibular sits in relation to the joint surface of the tibia. A tibial component should then be chosen that recapitulates the relationship of the tip of the fibular head to the joint surface as seen in the contralateral knee. Once the tibial component that achieves this is selected, the tension of the soft tissue can be adjusted by extending or shortening the body of the femoral prosthesis. This allows the joint line to be recreated as accurately as possible and for the patella to be placed as normally as possible in relation to the joint line. If the soft tissue tension is appropriate, the patella should sit over the proximal half of the anterior condyle of the distal femoral component. If the tissue tension is too tight, flexion will be restricted and during trialing of the component, the hinge prosthesis may rise out of the tibial component with flexion. Tissue tension that is too loose is easily noted by the laxity in the quadriceps mechanism.

Preparation of the Proximal Tibia

For an intra-articular resection, the lower limit of the proximal tibial osteotomy is the tibial tuberosity. A cut that is too close may cause patella tendon irritation from the prosthesis. A cut that is too distal may result in a surface area on which to seat the tibial component that is too small for available implants. Careful planning must be undertaken prior to the tibial osteotomy being performed. The tibial osteotomy should be neutral to the mechanical axis because most distal femoral prostheses have a built-in valgus angle that may be overaccentuated if the incorrect osteotomy is made with subsequent derangement of patellofemoral and tibiofemoral tracking. The tibial component also needs to accommodate the stem of the rotating hinge design and a valgus or varus cut is likely to lead to impingement of the component against the tibial endosteum, which may cause malseating of the component or perforation of the tibial cortex.

COMPLICATIONS

- Hip dislocation is a common complication because of the loss of extensive soft tissue attachments. It is important that special attention be paid to stabilize the hip joint and to reattach as much soft tissue to the prosthesis as possible.
- Infection is a high risk because of the prolonged nature of many procedures. Preoperative antibiotic prophylaxis, copious amounts of intraoperative lavage, and absolutely sterile techniques need to be employed. The dead space is likely to be enormous after this procedure and use of multiple wide bore drainage tubes is highly recommended.
- The rotatory movement of the rotating hinge mechanism combined with the instability of the total femur within the thigh and the ease at which soft tissue repairs may become unbalanced makes the patella prone to maltracking. Careful surgery with constant assessment of soft tissue tension when trialing a prosthesis and closing the defect or incision is required to minimize this complication.
- The common peroneal nerve is at particular risk of traction injury because it is bound to the neck of the fibular and uncontrolled movement of the limb may occur after femoral resection. There is the potential for greater susceptibility in patients undergoing chemotherapy because of the additional neurotoxic effect of chemotherapy on the nerves. Dissections should therefore be performed with care and constant vigilance be kept to ensure that the limb is not placed in an extreme position.
- Arterial injuries may occur particularly in the presence of large soft tissue components, which may distort normal anatomy. Vulnerable areas for injury include the division of the femoral artery to create its profunda branch, passage of the artery through the adductor hiatus where it may be tightly bound to the femur, where the anterior penetrating artery to the cruciates is given off, and also where the nerve divides into the anterior branch and passes through the interosseous space into the anterior compartment of the knee. Laceration, avulsion of branches, and development of intimal tears from traction may occur leading to an acutely ischemic limb.
- Venous compression or obstruction may lead to postoperative edema and the development of deep vein thrombosis. If this is suspected, vascular repair should be undertaken to avoid postoperative wound or limb problems.

POSTOPERATIVE MANAGEMENT

The limb should be wrapped in a soft spica made up of multiple rolls of cotton wool and crepe bandaging that extends from the foot to the groin. The purpose of this is to help obliterate the dead space to prevent hematoma collection. The bandage should be left on for about 5 days before the dressing is changed.

Drainage tubes are critical in such large surgery. They should remain in until drainage is at a minimum. They can be removed once flow drops to <10 mL/h for 4 consecutive hours. Drainage tubes should not be left in situ beyond 5 days because of the possibility of transmission of bacteria into the operative cavity. Intravenous antibiotics should be maintained until the drainage tubes are removed.

While in bed, the limb should be maintained in a position that prevents the femur or the tibia from flopping into external rotation. This is a typical position for the limb to adopt and may lead to peroneal nerve compression or dislocation of the hip. In rare situations, the entire femoral component may rotate 180 degrees about its mechanical axis without dislocating. This can be missed on inspection as the foot still points forward and there is no shortening. This complication is identified when the limb is seen to hyperextend but does not have flexion. Placing an extension splint firmly around the soft spica and placing the limb in a U-shaped supporting pillow will ensure that no abnormal rotation of the limb occurs.

Sutures or staples should be left in position for a minimum of 2 weeks. Oral antibiotics may be prescribed until the sutures or staples are removed.

Maintaining stability of the entire limb is essential when the patient starts to mobilize. A removable abduction hip brace with a flexion range from 0 to 90 degrees and a hinged extension to include the knee should be applied to help maintain stability when weight bearing.

A closely supervised program of rehabilitation should be prescribed because of the complex joint mechanics after such an operation. Graduated weight bearing and strengthening exercise should be undertaken between crutches until full weight bearing and adequate strength is recovered. During rehabilitation the hip knee brace should be applied. Patients should be forewarned of the prolonged nature of rehabilitation.

RESULTS

Prosthetic Survivorship

One of the first total femoral resection and prosthetic reconstructions was reported in 1965 (4). Since then, the benefits of this uncommon technique have seen an increase in its popularity. In the absence of septic or oncologic complications, the survival of total femoral prostheses is dependent on the fixation of the device at the hip and the knee. The in-built restraint to activity is likely a positive factor in prosthetic survival, which sees good short to medium-term survival (5–11). The favorable survival of these devices can also be attributed ironically to the poor survival of patients with extensive malignancy requiring total femoral resection who perish before their prostheses have an opportunity to fail (8,12). In this regard, total femoral replacement may offer patients with known limits in survival, for example, 2 to 5 years, the benefits of early weight bearing, and a functional limb without the encumberance that may follow biologic reconstructions or the psychosocial traumas of amputation. Long-term survival between 10 and 35 years has also been reported although this is not common. It does demonstrate that total femoral replacement may be an acceptable alternative in carefully selected patients (13,14).

Function

The function after total femoral replacement is dependent on the stability of the hip and knee joints and the remaining musculature that powers the limb. Early mobilization and weight bearing are features of total femoral replacement (15). Normal function, however, is the exception rather than the rule and patients should be counseled on their expectations of postoperative function (9,14). Despite this, in certain cases good function may occur (7). By contrast, others have demonstrated that loss of knee extension may impair the function of the total femoral replacement (3). An unstable knee as with total extensor mechanism resection or femoral nerve palsy may collapse during weight bearing because the lower limb relies on a strong hip and knee extension to maintain rigid during weight bearing. In this regard, techniques to arthrodese the knee have been recommended when reconstruction is being considered following total femoral resection that has also sacrificed the extensor mechanism (3). The complexity of total femoral replacement requires special attention to postoperative rehabilitation for maximal functional outcomes (16).

REFERENCES

1. Nicholson JT, Wieder HS Jr. Total resection of femur with turn-up plasty of tibia and prosthetic replacement of hip joint. *Ann Surg*. 1956;144:271–276.
2. McDonald DJ, Scott SM, Eckardt JJ. Tibial turn-up for long distal femoral bone loss. *Clin Orthop Relat Res*. 2001; 383:214–220.
3. Capanna R, Ruggieri P, Biagini R, et al. Subtotal and total femoral resection: an alternative to total femoral prosthetic replacement. *Int Orthop*. 1986;10:121–126.
4. Buchman, J. Total femur and knee joint replacement with a vitallium endoprosthesis. *Bull Hosp Joint Dis*. 1965;26:21–34.
5. Huang GK, Cao MJ. Prosthetic replacement using titanium-based alloy artificial total femur incorporating its total hip and total knee joints with plasma-sprayed ceramic coating. *Chin Med J (Engl)*. 1991;104:252–255.
6. Morris HG, Capanna R, Campanacci D, et al. Modular endoprosthetic replacement after total resection of the femur for malignant tumour. *Int Orthop*. 1994;18:90–95.
7. Faisham WI, Zulmi W, Halim AS. Modular endoprosthetic replacement after total femur resection for malignant bone tumor. *Med J Malaysia*. 2005;60(Suppl C):45–48.
8. Mankin HJ, Hornicek FJ, Harris M. Total femur replacement procedures in tumor treatment. *Clin Orthop Relat Res*. 2005;438:60–64.
9. Marcove RC, Lewis MM, Rosen G, et al. Total femur and total knee replacement. A preliminary report. *Clin Orthop Relat Res*. 1977;126:147–152.
10. Weigert M, Bonnemann D. Total replacement of the femur and its adjacent joints. *Arch Orthop Trauma Surg*. 1979;94:245–248.
11. Steinbrink K, Engelbrecht E, Fenelon GC. The total femoral prosthesis. A preliminary report. *J Bone Joint Surg Br*. 1982;64:305–312.

12. Jeon DG, Kim MS, Cho WH, et al. Clinical outcome of osteosarcoma with primary total femoral resection. *Clin Orthop Relat Res.* 2007;457:176–182.

13. Present DA, Kuschner SH. Total femur replacement. A case report with 35-year follow-up study. *Clin Orthop Relat Res.* 1990;251:166–167.

14. Nakamura S, Kusuzaki K, Murata H, et al. More than 10 years of follow-up of two patients after total femur replacement for malignant bone tumor. *Int Orthop.* 2000;24:176–178.

15. Katznelson A, Nerubay J. Total femur replacement in sarcoma of the distal end of the femur. *Acta Orthop Scand.* 1980;51:845–851.

16. Katrak P, O'Connor B, Woodgate I. Rehabilitation after total femur replacement: a report of 2 cases. *Arch Phys Med Rehabil.* 2003;84:1080–1084.

12 Allograft Prosthesis Composite Replacement for Bone Tumors of the Proximal Femur

George C. Babis, Vasileios I. Sakellariou, and Franklin H. Sim

Limb salvage has become the standard method of treatment of aggressive benign tumors and most bone malignancies (1) such as osteosarcoma, Ewing sarcomas, malignant fibrous histiocytomas, giant cell tumors, and metastatic bone lesions. Limb salvage requires en bloc resection of the involved bone with adequate margins, followed by reconstruction (1).

Allograft prosthesis composites have been used since the late 1980s in orthopaedic oncology (2—5). The main advantage, comparing to resection megaprosthesis, is the effective reattachment of the tendons of the hip abductors and iliopsoas muscles, thereby preventing dislocation and allowing better function (6). Additionally, incorporation and fusion of the allograft to the host bone decreases the possibility of resorption of the host bone around the proximal part of the prosthetic stem due to stress shielding (6). The allograft provides a dry virgin lattice for good cementing, but it does not need to be fixed to the distal part of the host femur with cement; hence, it does not compromise following revisions (7). Comparing to structural osteoarticular allografts, the main advantage is that joint deterioration and collapse that can be encountered with allograft cartilage is avoided (8). Subsequently, the biological capabilities of the allograft are combined with predictability and modularity of an implant.

The main disadvantages of segmental placement with allograft prosthesis composite are the technical difficulties and their cost. The long period of time that is necessary for healing at the graft-host junction and the potential for the transmission for disease are also major disadvantages. In addition to transmission of HIV, which has attracted the greatest attention, the possible transmission of hepatitis and other viral agents should be considered (9,10).

Besides, the biological characteristics of the allograft bone may lead to nonunion, resorption, or even fracture of the graft. Loosening of an allograft-prosthesis composite is not less problematic than loosening of a proximal femoral replacement. Allograft antigenicity and immune rejection, even yet unclear (11), may be related to incidents of resorption (9,12,13).

INDICATIONS

The precise indications for use of allograft composite vary from center to center, but essentially it is preferred in the following:

- For younger patients with a longer life expectancy
- When substantial portions of the periacetabular muscles and tendons can be spared
- When it is not planned to use radiation therapy, which can interfere with bone healing
- Also used in cases of short resections (<12 cm, mainly in treating benign tumors) because some modular resection prostheses have a minimal length of 12 cm (6).

SURGICAL TECHNIQUE

Preoperative Planning

A thorough oncological assessment is necessary before proceeding to this reconstructive procedure. Classification and staging of the tumor should be known. Life expectancy is a parameter that may alter the decision for the kind of reconstructive procedure. As previously referred, patients with short life expectancy should be better treated with proximal femoral replacement rather than an allograft reconstruction for which a long period of non–weight bearing is demanded. Technically, plain x-rays of the pelvis and the femur are essential to determine the level of resection, possible limb length discrepancy, as well as the size of the allograft to be used. Magnetic resonance images could also be helpful for the specification of the anatomical margins of the tumor.

The hip joint should be carefully examined preoperatively assessing the abductors sufficiency and the limb length. The patient should be informed for the potential of postoperative limb length discrepancy. If an elongation of more than 4 cm is expected, electrophysiology monitoring of the femoral and sciatic nerves could be beneficial.

A longer allograft than that templated should be available. The diameter of the allograft should preferably be matching with that of the host femur. As the allograft is usually underreamed and cemented to the stem, the medullary canal of the allograft should be equal to or slightly larger than the femoral canal of the host femur. The stem is templated according to the diameter of the host femoral canal. Cementless press fit fixation is preferred preserving host bone stock for future revisions. The femoral stem should be planned to bypass the allograft and the femoral isthmus. If that is not possible, additional screws and plates should be placed to stabilize allograft-host junction. Generally, we try to insert as less screws as possible as screw holes weaken the allograft and act as stress raisers, leading to allograft fractures. Intraoperative alterations of the initial templating are not rare, and allograft-host fixation alternatives should be scheduled and be available during surgery. Long strut grafts and cables or circlage wires should be available to be placed at the allograft-host junction. Dall-Milles cables or wires should be available for the trochanteric reattachment to the allograft. Templating of megaprosthesis should also be done, as intraoperative fracture of the only size matching allograft is possible.

ANESTHESIA AND PATIENT POSITIONING

Regional epidural anesthesia is generally preferred for the potential of postoperative pain control. The group of anesthesiologists should be aware of the duration of this procedure, which has a mean time of 4 hours and may exceed 6 hours, as well as the amount of blood loss, which has a mean value of 2,000 mL and sometimes may exceed 5,000 mL (14). Unfortunately, blood conservation techniques, such as intraoperative cell saving and postoperative autologous blood transfusion, should be avoided due to the risk of spreading the initial malignant disease.

The patient is positioned in a true lateral position with the affected hip uppermost. It is important that bony prominences of the legs and pelvis are protected with pads under the lateral malleolus and knee of the bottom leg and a pillow between the knees. The limb should be draped leaving free room for movement during the operation. The drapes should leave uncovered the lateral aspect of the femur and the knee as the incision may be extended distally.

ALLOGRAFT CHARACTERISTICS AND PREPARATION

Frozen structural allografts primarily possess the osteoconductive, and not the osteoinductive, property of bone grafts (7). They are biologically inert and therefore function as implants. Fresh allograft bone evokes an immune response in the host that may result in resorption of the graft or in a marked delay in the incorporation of the graft.

Deep-freezing and freeze-drying at −70°C have a shelf life of 5 years (15) and decrease the immunogenicity of allograft bone. These methods allow for long-term preservation and storage of allograft bone. Freeze-dried bone is weaker in bending and torsion than fresh-frozen bone (16–18), but it has the advantage of being less antigenic (19). The American Association of Tissue Banks have set standards in order to reduce the risk of diseases transmission (20,21). The risk of transmission of the human immunodeficiency virus is thought to be less than one in one million (20,21). Irradiation of the graft further reduces this risk (22), but radiation may weaken the allograft bone (23).

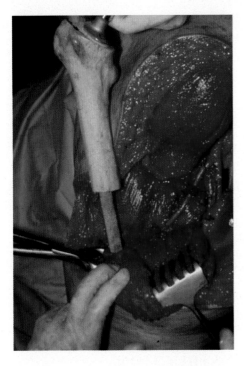

FIGURE 12.1

Intraoperative image, showing the trial reduction of the implant in the host femur and into the acetabulum, in order to assess the appropriate length of the graft.

At the time of reconstruction, the allograft is unwrapped, specimens are obtained from it for culture, and it is then placed in a warm antibiotic-containing solution. To reduce operative time, the graft is prepared on a separate table by part of the surgical team. The length of the bone resection is templated and measured before operation. An allograft that is longer than needed is ordered to allow for any intraoperative variations. The approximate length of the graft required is assessed by a trial reduction (Fig. 12.1) of the implant in the host femur and into the acetabulum. Hip stability and any preoperative limb-length discrepancy are taken into account in determining the length of the allograft.

The allograft is cleaned of soft tissue and then is reamed and broached (Fig. 12.2) until a good fit for the implant is achieved while allowing for a cement mantle of at least 2 mm around the stem. The graft does not have to be excessively reamed while still having a cement mantle of at least 2 mm.

A long-stem modular femoral prosthesis offering distal fixation is used. The femoral stem must be long enough to reach the distal femoral diaphyseal-metaphyseal junction, or else to achieve at least 6 cm of

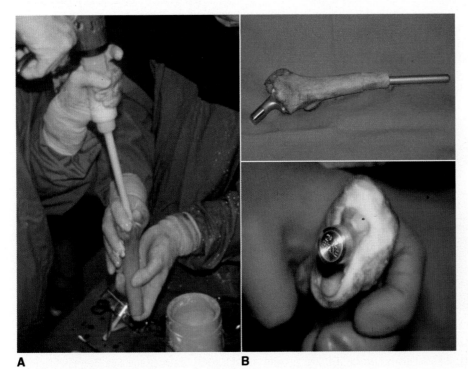

A   **B**

FIGURE 12.2

A: At a back table, the allograft is reamed and broached. **B:** Cement is pressurized into the graft. The stem is then inserted in the correct anteversion. Great care is taken to ensure that the cement is recessed around the allograft-host junction to allow host-bone contact.

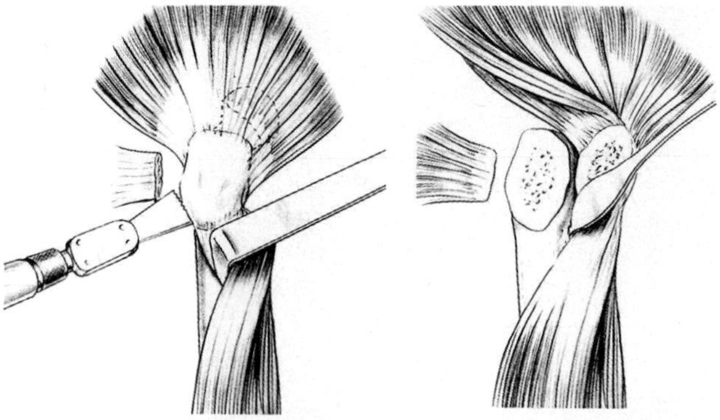

FIGURE 12.3

A sliding osteotomy of the greater trochanter is usually done because it is more stable than a transverse osteotomy and is associated with a lower risk of trochanteric migration. (Courtesy Langlais F, et al. Trochanteric slide osteotomy in revision total hip arthroplasty for loosening. *J Bone Joint Surg* [*Br*] 2003;85-B:510–516.)

prosthesis-shaft contact bypassing the allograft-host junction (6). Trial reduction of the prosthesis-allograft composite is done, and a transverse, oblique or step-cut osteotomy of approximately 2 by 3 cm is marked and made, according to the surgeon's preferences and allograft-host femoral canal matching. Adjustments are usually needed for correct anteversion and length. On the back table, the graft canal is cleaned and dried, and cement is pressurized into the graft. The stem is then inserted in the correct anteversion (see Fig. 12.2). Great care is taken to ensure that the cement is recessed around the allograft-host junction to allow host-bone contact. The composite is then inserted into the host stem, and the hip is reduced. Finally, wires or cables are passed around the lesser trochanter of the allograft for later attachment to the greater trochanter of the host.

SURGICAL TECHNIQUE OF RECONSTRUCTION

We mostly use the lateral approach (Hardinge) or the posterolateral approach (Moore). Oncological principles should be followed first. Open incision biopsy tracts should be excised. En bloc resection of the tumor should be done without compromising other compartments. Rising of large muscle flaps should be avoided. Reconstruction procedure should not interfere with meticulous en bloc tumor resection. In all cases, samples for biopsies and cultures should be obtained and quick biopsy and Gram stain results should be known before proceeding to reconstruction.

Substantial portions of the periacetabular muscles and tendons should be spared, if possible, so to be later reattached to the allograft. A sliding osteotomy of the greater trochanter is usually done because it is more stable than a transverse osteotomy and is associated with a lower risk of trochanteric migration (Fig. 12.3). The trochanteric osteotomy offers a better exposure of the hip joint, as well as a bony fragment for reattachment of the abductors to the graft. After the trochanteric osteotomy is done, the abductors and the vastus lateralis muscles are slightly displaced anteriorly, so that the anterolateral aspect of the femur is exposed to perform the femoral osteotomy. Care is taken not to strip any residual bone of its soft tissue completely, as it later is used as a vascularized autogenous graft if it is not included into the tumor mass. Before performing the resection osteotomy of the proximal femur, a Steinmann pin is inserted into the iliac crest and the distance to a reference point on the distal femur is used to determine the leg length and rotation of the host femur, as well as the length of the allograft. Then, the femur is osteotomized and excised.

There are several techniques to do a femoral osteotomy (Fig. 12.4). *A transverse osteotomy* (Fig. 12.4A) is the easiest to do but it does not provide adequate rotational stability. Fixation with one (anterolateral) or

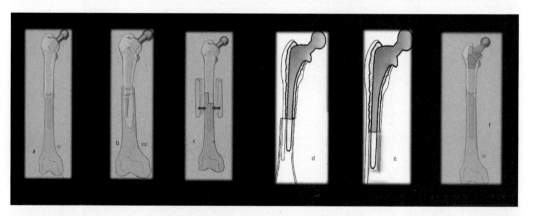

FIGURE 12.4

Options of femoral osteotomy and junction of allograft–host bone fixation. **A:** Transverse. **B:** Intussuception. **C:** Step cut. **D:** Intramedullary step cut. **E:** Step cut with lateral cortical extension and side sleeve junction. **F:** Oblique osteotomy.

usually two plates (one lateral and one anterior) is often needed for a stable construct. This results in developing many screw holes, which act as stress risers that weaken the allograft and potentially lead to allograft fracture. *Telescoping* the graft inside the host femoral canal or reversely the host femur into the allograft-prosthesis composite *(intussuception technique)* (Fig. 12.4B) is an option to obtain rotational stability and rigid fixation at the allograft-host junction. The medullary canal of the host femur has to be trimmed in order to better slide and grip inside the allograft and vice versa.

Otherwise, a *step-cut osteotomy* can be done (Fig. 12.4C), which is stable regarding rotation at the allograft-host femoral junction and develops a large allograft-host contact surface for allograft incorporation. *Step-cut osteotomy* is though technically demanding and can lead to rotational malalignment (24). A transverse osteotomy, which extends just through the lateral half of the femur, must be done carefully with an oscillating saw, with the medial aspect of the femur left intact. Then a midline anterior longitudinal femoral split (2 to 3 cm long) is carried out, and finally a new transverse osteotomy to the medial aspect of the femur is done and the proximal femur is excised. Then a spike of bone, about 2 cm in width and 2 to 3 cm in length on the medial side, remains attached to the healthy distal part of the femur, which has the shape of a step. Accordingly, the allograft is shaped with a reverse step cut and finally the allograft and the host femur match together as the key into the keyhole. This technique has several modifications. A long step cut 8 to 10 cm in length can be done to the allograft only, whereas the host femur has a typical transverse osteotomy. This step cut leaves a lateral cortical extension distally. If the inner diameter of the distal femur is larger than the inner diameter of the allograft, the allograft prosthesis component is inserted intramedullary into the distal host bone (Fig. 12.4D). Both the distal long stem and lateral allograft cortical extension are press fit into the distal host bone (25). Alternatively and most commonly, the inner diameter of the distal femur is smaller than the inner diameter of the allograft, and a lateral side-sleeve junction is developed, improving rotational stability (Fig. 12.4E). Finally, another type of femoral osteotomy is the *oblique,* which can be done orienting the oscillating saw from the lateral-distal to the medial-proximal aspect of the femur. *Oblique osteotomy* (Fig. 12.4F) combines the advantages of an easy technique providing also rotational stability.

After the femoral osteotomy is done and the proximal femur is resected, the acetabulum is reconstructed. This can be done with either a cemented or a cementless cup depending on the bone stock and the oncologic status of the patient. If the risk of postoperative instability is high, consideration should be given to the use of a constrained liner (26,27). Alternatively, a bipolar implant can be used, which provides good immediate stability and minimizes the socket failure (28).

The next step is to prepare the medullary canal of the host femur. A guide wire is inserted into the distal part of the host femur, and the canal is gently reamed. Excessive reaming of the distal femur should be avoided as it results in very tight distal fit and distraction at the host-allograft junction, which increases the risk of nonunion. Modular long stems with distal fixation are now available and preferred as they offer adequate stability. Press fit is considered to be safe when there is at least 6 cm of prosthesis-shaft contact bypassing the allograft-host junction (Fig. 12.5) (6). The use of cement distally should be preferably avoided as host femoral bone stock is compromised in case of a future revision.

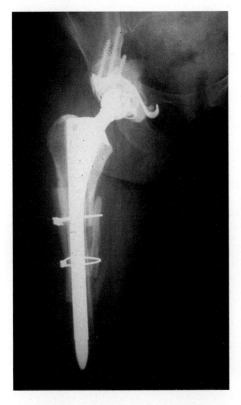

FIGURE 12.5

Press fit is considered to be safe when there is at least 6 cm of prosthesis-shaft contact bypassing the allograft-host junction.

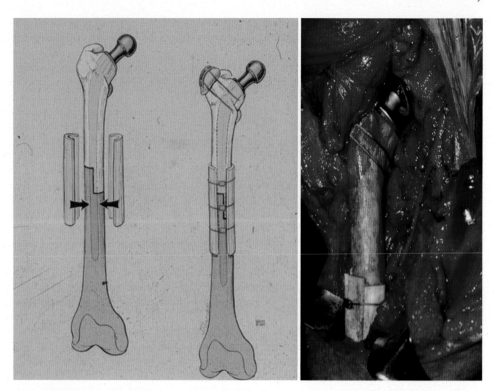

FIGURE 12.6

Use of strut grafts for additional rotational stability and assistance of allograft-host fusion.

The approximate length of the graft required is assessed by a trial reduction of the implant in the host femur into the acetabulum. Stability and any preoperative limb-length discrepancy are taken into account in determining the allograft length. The allograft-prosthesis composite, which has been already prepared at a back table as described to the previous section, is then inserted into the host femur, and the hip is reduced.

The allograft-host femur junction is secured firstly with two or more circlage wires. Thereinafter, two strut grafts are placed at each side of the junction and reinforced by circlage wires or cables (Fig. 12.6). The strut grafts offer additional rotational stability and assist allograft-host fusion (29). If the stem does not bypass the allograft host junction or if optimal stability is not achieved, double plates or combination of strut graft and plate may be attempted (29–32), with the disadvantages though referred above regarding creation of screw holes inside the allograft (30,33). If the stem bypasses the junction, but there is not primary stability, then cementing of both the prosthesis into the allograft and the allograft into the host may be tried (9,34).

The abductor mechanism with the greater trochanter or the remnants thereof are attached directly to its anatomic position to the allograft using Dall-Milles cables or wires in most cases to provide stable fixation, which enhances fusion and lessens the possibility of trochaneric migration. Alternatively, the abductors may be indirectly sutured to the fascia lata (Fig. 12.7). The final step of the reconstruction consists of reattachment of the

FIGURE 12.7

The abductor mechanism with the greater trochanter or the remnants thereof is attached directly to its anatomic position to the allograft using Dall-Milles cables or wires in most cases. Otherwise, it may be indirectly sutured to the fascia lata.

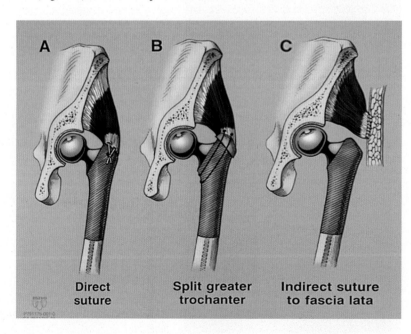

A   B   C

Direct suture   Split greater trochanter   Indirect suture to fascia lata

host tendons to the tendinous insertions of the allograft. Attachments of the soft tissue to the allograft through drill holes in the allograft should be avoided. This method has shown an unacceptable prevalence of failure. It is postulated that an increased vascular response leads to accelerated resorption of the allograft. Tendon to tendon repair is recommended and provides solid healing (35).

REHABILITATION

Unprotected weight bearing is prohibited until there is evidence of radiographic allograft-host union. This usually takes between 3 and 6 months but in some cases up to 2 years. For some time during this period, external stabilization of the hip may be necessary if the joint is unstable. The abductors should be protected either by avoiding active abduction of the hip or with the use of long spica cast in order to assist union of the greater trochanter and stabilization of the soft tissue for 6 to 12 weeks (36).

COMPLICATIONS

All reconstructions that are done after a major resection of an osseous tumor have a higher risk of complications than does the usual orthopedic reconstruction procedure, and allografts are not an exception. The reconstructive orthopedic surgeon should be aware of this difficult procedure with a wide range of potential intraoperative and postoperative complications that may have to deal with.

Allograft-host bone junction nonunion, postoperative infection, periprosthetic fracture, hip dislocation, and aseptic loosening of the femoral component are the most significant. The incidence of these complications varies according to the literature (37–41): nonunion of the allograft–host bone junction in 4.7% to 20% of cases, trochanteric nonunion in 25% to 27%, postoperative infection in 3.3% to 8%, periprosthetic fracture in 2% to 5%, hip dislocation is seen in 3.1% to 54%, and aseptic loosening in 1% to 3%.

Of 718 allograft procedures in the study by Mankin et al. (42), 156 failed. 85% of the failures were due to infection, local recurrence of the tumor, or fracture of the allograft. Most failures occurred during the first 3 years, with the greatest incidence during the first year after implantation. Despite these failures, the rate of amputation, including amputations associated with tumor-related complications, was only 7%, and 75% of the limbs were saved after an allograft failure.

Nonunion of the allograft-host junction is a major complication leading to almost definite failure of reconstruction (Fig. 12.8). Generally, achievement of good contact at the osteotomy line during insertion of the allograft prosthesis composite is difficult. Distal press fit fixation even desired is sometimes complicated with poor contact or even allograft–host bone diastasis. This is why usually a stem of smaller diameter is preferred in favor of wide allograft-host contact.

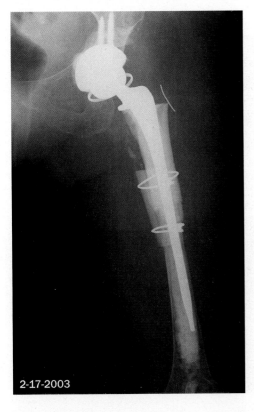

2-17-2003

FIGURE 12.8

Radiographic image showing nonunion at the junction of the allograft with the host femur 1 year postoperatively.

Many factors are associated with an increased risk of nonunion. Infection should always be ruled out as a possible cause. Chemotherapy strongly influences the outcome. In a review of 945 patients, Hornicek et al. (43) found that patients who were managed with chemotherapy had a higher rate of nonunion (27%) than those who were not managed with chemotherapy (11%). In a series of 112 patients with osteosarcoma who were treated with both preoperative and postoperative chemotherapy, Donati et al. (44) reported that the rate of nonunion was 49%, with regard to fixation.

Nonunion by itself has an adverse effect on the outcome. This negative impact is much greater when the nonunion is associated with either infection or fracture (43). A nonunion should be treated with autologous iliac bone, and the fixation should be revised if it is not rigid. Patients requiring three or more subsequent operations are more likely to have an allograft failure (43). In the series described by Hornicek et al. (43), despite aggressive treatment, 30% of the patients with a nonunion eventually had removal of the allograft or the extremity.

In certain cases, a vascularized fibular graft may be necessary to achieve healing of the junction. Efforts should be made to minimize the risk of nonunion, especially in patients with predisposing factors. The surgeon should maximize allograft–host bone contact and achieve rigid and stable fixation. Primary use of cancellous autograft at the junctions, although questioned by some (45), can be used. The use of osteoinductive material should be investigated as a possible means of reducing the prevalence of this complication.

Graft fracture remains a late risk due to the increased porosity of the allograft bone as cortical repair progresses. Most fractures (70%) occur in the first 3 years following allograft implantation (46). Berrey et al. (46) described three fracture types: type I, which is rapid dissolution of the graft, possibly related to a rejection process; type II, a fracture through the shaft; and type III, collapse or involvement of the articular surface, which is not applied to allograft prosthesis composites. Most type-II fractures originate from a screw hole within the allograft (Fig. 12.9).

Fractures are significantly more frequent in allografts that had been irradiated before implantation (47). Chemotherapy alone is not a risk factor for allograft fracture (33,48). Combination of chemotherapy and plate fixation is strongly associated with an increased risk of fracture (33). Nonunion has been reported to be an associated risk factor (46,48).

The management of type-II fractures is controversial. Minimally displaced fractures can heal with closed treatment, and this approach can be attempted. Repeat internal fixation and use of an autogenous graft from the iliac crest is infrequently successful but may be worth trying if the graft is otherwise excellent. If the first open reduction fails, graft replacement is recommended, since the rate of success with repeat reduction and grafting is extremely low (46). A vascularized fibular graft or replacement of the allograft with a new one might be indicated.

Deep infection is a disastrous complication of reconstruction with allograft prosthesis composites. It is seen in 12% to 15% of cases (49,50) and is the leading cause of failure of the allograft 10;75% of the infections were diagnosed within the first 4 months after implantation (49). A single organism, most frequently Staphylococcus epidermidis, was found to be the cause in the majority of the cases (49).

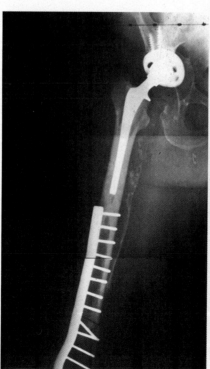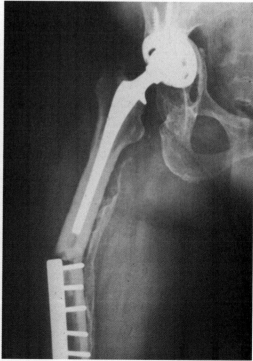

FIGURE 12.9

Type-II fractures originated from a screw hole within the allograft.

Local wound problems were the most critical factor associated with an increased risk of infection (49,50). Many of them were related to the fact that these reconstructions are frequently performed after resection of a malignant or aggressive benign lesion. Increased removal of bone and soft tissue, multiple operations, chemotherapy or radiation, skin slough, postoperative hematoma, and wound drainage are involved in this process (49,50). Preoperative contamination of an allograft has occurred but is rare (51). Management of the infected allograft is difficult. Rarely will a patient have a superficial wound infection that does not involve the allograft. A two-stage revision procedure is always performed; the allograft prosthesis composite is removed, followed be meticulous débridement. A cement spacer impregnated with antibiotics is used to retain leg length and prevent soft tissue contractures. After a 6-week intravenous and a total of 3 to 6 months of oral antibiotic administration, the second stage of reimplantation is decided, only after infection has been ruled out. Alternatively, a Girdlestone procedure may be followed. Limb salvage is possible in the majority of patients with an allograft infection, but approximately one third eventually need an amputation (49).

Hip dislocation can be attributed to suboptimal positioning of the acetabular component, use of small femoral heads, impingement, failure of offset restoration, and hip soft tissue balancing with abductors insufficiency. Reorientation of the acetabular component, use of femoral heads with larger diameter, when indicated use of constrain liner, removal of bone prominences or anterior capsule reducing the risk of impingement, and reattachment of the abductors either directly to the allograft or indirectly to the fascia lata are some options of dealing with the problem of dislocation. Postoperative cast immobilization in abduction for 3 to 6 weeks is helpful. Trochanteric nonunion and escape even usual (~20% in the literature (37,40,41) are not related to similar rates of clinical expression of abductors deficiency.

Leg length discrepancy <4 cm is managed conservatively with shoe raisers. If it exceeds 4 cm, revision may be considered due to the risk of permanent neurological deficits (sciatic nerve palsy most common) and progressive wear of the insert.

CONCLUSIONS/KEY POINTS

The technique of reconstruction of massive proximal femoral bone loss with an allograft-implant composite is a demanding procedure and requires meticulous surgical technique.

- Material selection and specification of the indications is of paramount importance.
- Oncological principles should never be disregarded.
- Preoperative planning and decision of the technique to be followed are important as different sizes of allografts suit for each technique.
- Intraoperative alterations should be scheduled.
- Cooperation of two surgical groups is essential.
- A stable allograft-host junction is essential for success.
- Preferably the allograft should be slightly oversized and underreamed.
- Cement fixation of the stem in the allograft should always be done.
- Stems with distal fixation should be used. They should bypass the allograft-host junction and offer a press fit fixation for at least 6 cm at the femoral shaft. Undersize of the stem is preferred in order to achieve good allograft-host contact at the junction.
- Step-cut osteotomy provides rotational stability but is technically demanding. Intussusception is often the preferred technique by present authors.
- Strut grafts enhance rotational stability.
- Fixation with screws and plates is sometimes needed. Screw holes inside the allograft should be as less as possible, as they act as stress raisers leading to allograft fracture even 2 to 3 years post surgery.
- Soft tissue reattachment is important for a good functional outcome.
- Complications are not uncommon, but they are usually managed without needing to amputate the limb. Nonunion, fracture, and infection are the most common complications and usually require surgical management.
- Although there is a high complication rate, it is a biologic reconstruction comparing to megaprostheses.
- It should be a limb salvage procedure of choice in cases with good life expectancy.

REFERENCES

1. Gitelis S. Limb salvage for appendicular tumors. *Curr Opin Orthop.* 1991;2:811–816.
2. Gitelis S, Piasecky P. Allograft prosthetic composite arthroplasty for osteosarcoma and other aggressive bone tumors. *Clin Orthop.* 1991;270:197–201.
3. Jofe MH, Gebhardt MC, Tomford WW, et al. Reconstruction for defects of the proximal part of the femur using allograft arthroplasty. *J Bone Joint Surg.* 1988;70A:507–516.
4. Johnson ME, Mankin HJ. Reconstructions after resection of tumor involving the proximal femur. *Orthop Clin North Am.* 1991;22:87–103.
5. Zehr RJ, Enneking WF, Scarborough MT. Allograftprosthesis composite versus megaprosthesis in proximal femoral reconstruction. *Clin Orthop.* 1996;322:207–223.

6. Donati D, Giacomini S, Gozzi E, et al. Proximal femur reconstruction by an allograft prosthesis composite. *Clin Orthop.* 2002;394:192–200.

7. Haddad FS, Garbuz DS, Masri BA, et al. Instructional course lectures, the american academy of orthopaedic surgeons—femoral bone loss in patients managed with revision hip replacement: results of circumferential allograft replacement. *J Bone Joint Surg Am.* 1999;81:420–436.

8. Dion N, Sim FH. The use of allografts in orthopaedic surgery—part I: the use of allografts in musculoskeletal oncology. *J Bone Joint Surg Am.* 2002;84:644–654.

9. Masri BA, Spangehl MJ, Duncan CP, et al. Proximal femoral allografts in revision total hip arthroplasty: a critical review. *J Bone and Joint Surg.* 1995;77-B (suppl III):306–307.

10. Nemzek JA, Arnoczky SP, Swenson CL. Retroviral transmission in bone allotransplantation. The effects of tissue processing. *Clin Orthop.* 1996;324:275–282.

11. Poitout DG, Lempidakis M, Loncle X, et al. Reconstructions massives du cotyle et du fémur proximal. *Chirurgie.* 1994–1995;120:254–263.

12. Hutchison CR, Mahomed N, Agnidis Z, et al. Proximal femoral allografts in revision hip arthroplasty—minimum five-year follow-up. *Orthop. Trans.* 1996;20:94.

13. Roberson JR. Proximal femoral bone loss after total hip arthroplasty. *Orthop Clin North Am.* 1992;23:291–302.

14. Gross AE, Blackley H, Wong P, et al. The use of allografts in orthopaedic surgery—part II: the role of allografts in revision arthroplasty of the hip. *J Bone Joint Surg Am.* 2002;84:655–667

15. Czitrom AA. Biology of bone grafting and principles of bone banking. In: Weinstein SL, ed. *The Pediatric Spine: Principles and Practice*, vol. 2. New York, NY: Raven Press; 1994:1285–1298.

16. Kang JS, Kim NH. The biomechanical properties of deep freezing and freeze drying bones and their biomechanical changes after in-vivo allograft. *Yonsei Med J.* 1995;36:332–335.

17. Pelker RR, Friedlaender GE, Markham TC. Biomechanical properties of bone allografts. *Clin Orthop.* 1983;174:54–57.

18. Pelker RR, Friedlaender GE. Biomechanical aspects of bone autografts and allografts. *Orthop Clin North Am.* 1987;18:235–239.

19. Friedlaender GE, Strong DM, Sell KW. Studies on the antigenicity of bone. I. Freeze-dried and deep-frozen bone allografts in rabbits. *J Bone Joint Surg.* 1976;58-A:854–858.

20. Buck BE, Malinin TI, Brown MD. Bone transplantation and human immunodeficiency virus. An estimate of risk of acquired immunodeficiency syndrome (AIDS). *Clin Orthop.* 1989;240:129–136.

21. Buck BE, Resnick L, Shah SM, et al. Human immunodeficiency virus cultured from bone. Implications for transplantation. *Clin Orthop.* 1990;251:249–253.

22. Fideler BM, Vangsness CT Jr, Moore T, et al. Effects of gamma irradiation on the human immunodeficiency virus. A study in frozen human bone-patellar ligament-bone grafts obtained from infected cadavera. *J Bone Joint Surg.* 1994;76-A:1032–1035.

23. Hamer AJ, Strachan JR, Black MM, et al. Biochemical properties of cortical allograft bone using a new method of bone strength measurement. A comparison of fresh, fresh-frozen and irradiated bone. *J Bone Joint Surg.* 1996;78-B(3):363–368.

24. Heijna MJ, Gitelis S. Allograft prosthetic composite replacement for bone tumors. *Semin Surg Oncol.* 1997;13:18–24.

25. MacLachlan CE, Ries MD. Intramedullary step-cut osteotomy for revision total hip arthroplsty with allograft-host bone size mismatch. *J Arthroplast.* 2007;22(5):657–662.

26. Goetz DD, Capello WN, Callaghan JJ, et al. Salvage of a recurrently dislocating total hip prosthesis with use of a constrained acetabular component. A retrospective analysis of fifty-six cases. *J Bone Joint Surg.* 1998;80-A:502–509.

27. Lombardi AV Jr, Mallory TH, Kraus TJ, et al. Preliminary report on the S-ROM constraining acetabular insert: a retrospective clinical experience. *Orthopedics.* 1991;14:297–303.

28. Curtiss PH Jr, Powell AE, Herndon CH. Immunological factors in homogenous-bone transplantation. III. The inability of homogenous rabbit bone to induce circulating antibodies in rabbits. *J Bone and Joint Surg.* 1959;41-A:1482–1488.

29. Chandler HP, Penenberg BL. *Bone Stock Deficiency in Total Hip Replacement: Classification and Management.* Thorofare, NJ: Slack; 1989.

30. Chandler H, Clark J, Murphy S, et al. Reconstruction of major segmental loss of the proximal femur in revision total hip arthroplasty. *Clin Orthop.* 1994;298:67–74.

31. Mankin HJ, Doppelt S, Tomford W. Clinical experience with allograft implantation. The first ten years. *Clin Orthop.* 1983;174:69–86.

32. Rosenberg A, Jacobs J. *Circumferential Proximal Femoral Allografting.* Boston, MA: Read at the Harvard Hip Course; 1998..

33. Thompson RC Jr, Pickvance EA, Garry D. Fractures in large-segment allografts. *J Bone Joint Surg.* 1993;75-A:1663–1673.

34. Head WC, Wagner RA, Emerson RH Jr, et al. Restoration of femoral bone stock in revision total hip arthroplasty. *Orthop Clin North Am.* 1993;24:697–703.

35. Enneking WF, Mindell ER. Observations on massive retrieved human allografts. *J Bone Joint Surg Am.* 1991;73:1123–1142.

36. Zmolek JC, Dorr LD. Revision total hip arthroplasty. The use of solid allograft. *J Arthroplasty.* 1993;8:361–370.

37. Blackley HRL, Davis AM, Hutchison CR, et al. Proximal femoral allografts for reconstruction of bone stock in revision arthroplasty of the hip. *J Bone Joint Surg [Am].* 2001;83:346–354.

38. Chandler H, Clark J, Murphy S, et al. Reconstruction of major segmental loss of the proximal femur in revision total hip arthroplasty. *Clin Orthop.* 1994;298:67–74.

39. Head WC, Berklacich FM, Malinin TI, et al. Proximal femoral allografts in revision total hip arthroplasty. *Clin Orthop.* 1987;225:22–36.

40. Gross AE, Hutchison CR. Proximal femoral allografts for reconstruction of bone stock in revision hip arthroplasty. *Orthopedics.* 1998;21:999–1001.

41. Haddad FS, Garbuz DS, Masri BA, et al. Structural proximal femoral allografts for failed total hip replacements: a minimum review of five years. *J Bone Joint Surg Br*. 2000;82(6):830–836.

42. Mankin HJ, Gebhardt MC, Jennings LC, et al. Long-term results of allograft replacement in the management of bone tumors. *Clin Orthop*. 1996;324:86–97.

43. Hornicek FJ, Gebhardt MC, Tomford WW, et al. Factors affecting nonunion of the allograft-host junction. *Clin Orthop*. 2001;382:87–98.

44. Donati D, Di Liddo M, Zavatta M, et al. Massive bone allograft reconstruction in high-grade osteosarcoma. *Clin Orthop*. 2000;377:186–194.

45. Vander Griend RA. The effect of internal fixation on the healing of large allografts. *J Bone Joint Surg Am*. 1994;76:657–663.

46. Berrey BH, Lord CF, Gebhardt MC, et al. Fractures of allografts. Frequency, treatment, and end-results. *J Bone Joint Surg Am*. 1990;72:825–833.

47. Lietman SA, Tomford WW, Gebhardt MC, et al. Complications of irradiated allografts in orthopaedic tumor surgery. *Clin Orthop*. 2000;375:214–217.

48. Sorger JL, Hornicek FJ, Zavatta M, et al. Allograft fractures revisited. *Clin Orthop*. 2001;382:66–74.

49. Lord CF, Gebhardt MC, Tomford WW, et al. Infection in bone allografts. Incidence, nature, and treatment. *J Bone Joint Surg Am*. 1988;70:369–376.

50. Dick HM, Strauch RJ. Infection of massive bone allografts. *Clin Orthop*. 1994;306:46–53.

51. Tomford WW, Starkweather RJ, Goldman MH. A study of the clinical incidence of infection in the use of banked allograft bone. *J Bone Joint Surg Am*. 1981;63:244–248.

13 Femoral Internal Fixation and Metastatic Bone Disease

Timothy A. Damron

Metastatic disease (including myeloma and lymphoma) involving the femur requires a different approach from that for primary bone disease. In most cases, resection for cure is not the goal; rather, palliation and maintaining function are the goals. In the femur, except for femoral neck fractures or extensive replacement of the proximal femur by tumor, internal fixation is usually indicated for metastatic bone involvement. Most cases warrant a third-generation "reconstruction" type of femoral nail to protect the entire femur, but for solitary lesions in the intertrochanteric region, some surgeons prefer the dynamic hip screw and cement. Unless otherwise indicated, this chapter focuses on the third-generation nail; where there are differences with the dynamic hip screw, those are noted in each section.

INDICATIONS

Third-Generation Intramedullary Reconstruction Nail

There are two main advantages of the intramedullary nail over a dynamic hip screw and side plate for metastatic disease in the femur. These include: 1.) Broadens range of anatomic locations covering much farther distal in the femur, and 2.) Provides prophylactic stabilization of nearly entire femur away from main lesion for smaller metastases that are either present and recognized, present but unrecognized, or potentially will develop elsewhere later in the disease course.

Indications for the femoral third-generation intramedullary reconstruction nail require consideration of four factors (Fig. 13.1). First, whether there is an actual or impending pathologic fracture; second, the specific location of the bone lesion in the proximal femur; and third, the underlying diagnosis, the latter of which relates to the fourth factor, expected survival. Locations that are acceptable for internal fixation of impending fractures are broader than those for actual pathologic fractures. *Diagnosis should be established by independent biopsy of the lesion, not by intramedullary reamings, and should precede any intramedullary instrumentation of the femur, including placing the guide rod.*

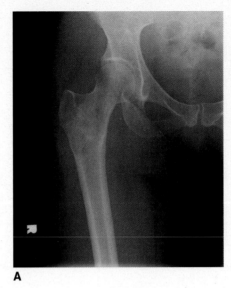
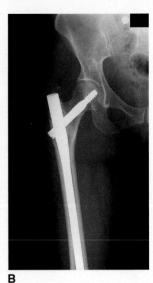

FIGURE 13.1

Indications for stabilization must consider four factors: impending versus actual fracture, location, diagnosis, and prognosis. **A:** In this case, the patient had pain recalcitrant to medical management and irradiation associated with this mixed lytic/blastic intertrochanteric lesion from breast carcinoma. The patient was felt to have an impending pathologic femur fracture. **B:** Due to the intact bone and relatively good prognosis, the patient was treated with a third-generation femoral reconstruction nail (Long Gamma Nail, Stryker) locked proximally and distally.

A　　　　　　　　　　　　　　　　　　　**B**

- *Location within the femur*
  - ○ Impending pathologic fractures
    - ❑ Femoral neck to distal femoral diaphysis
      - ● Rationale: If good bone stock remains in the femoral epiphysis to support the threaded portion of the reconstruction screw(s), an intramedullary reconstruction nail may still be utilized in this situation.
      - ● Key: Regardless of the location of the identifiable lesions, critically assess the remaining bone to ensure that adequate fixation is able to be achieved both proximal and distal to the lesion. Always have a backup plan.
  - ○ Displaced pathologic fractures
    - ❑ Intertrochanteric region to distal femoral diaphysis
    - ❑ Rationale: Once a fracture has occurred, the femoral neck is no longer a reasonable option for consideration of the reconstruction intramedullary nail.
    - ❑ Key: Adequate bone stock proximal and distal to the fracture is necessary to obtain secure fixation.
- *Established diagnosis*
  - ○ Independent biopsy of the bone lesion directly at site of lesion and/or fracture prior to instrumentation of the intramedullary canal with guide rod, reamers, or nail
    - ❑ Rationale: Unless the patient already has well-established terminal metastatic disease with previously biopsy-proven metastatic lesions in bone, a biopsy will exclude the possibility of a sarcoma, a condition that should not be treated in most cases by intramedullary nailing.
- *Adequate life expectancy to expect benefits to outweigh risks*
  - ○ Medically fit to survive procedure and perioperative period
    - ❑ Rationale: While the mortality risk of a percutaneously inserted intramedullary nail is relatively small, patients who are immediately preterminal due to medical issues related to their cancer are best referred for hospice if they are unable to be optimized preoperatively.
  - ○ Expected survival of 6 to 12 weeks minimum
    - ❑ Rationale: If patients are not expected to recover fully enough prior to their death to allow restoration of some function, the goals of the procedure are unlikely to be achieved.

Dynamic Hip Screw Device Indications

The anatomic location indicated for use of the dynamic hip screw device is much more limited than that of the third-generation femoral reconstruction nail because it covers a much more limited area of the bone. Weaknesses:

- More limited indications than third-generation reconstruction nail device
- Requires solid bone immediately adjacent to bone lesion for secure fixation, a situation which is rare, as the region of poor bone quality may often be underestimated by the imaging studies
- More prone to failure of internal fixation due to loss of secure purchase by screws in the bone
- Fails to address presence and/or development of more distal bone lesions

CONTRAINDICATIONS

Third-Generation Intramedullary Reconstruction Nail

Contraindications also involve the location of the tumor, the quality of the proximal and distal remaining femoral bone, and the patient's life expectancy (Table 13.1). All medical issues should be addressed preoperatively and optimized.

Dynamic Hip Screw Device Contraindications

In addition to those contraindications above, the dynamic hip screw device is contraindicated for the following pathologic fractures and lesions:

- Any anatomic site other than the intertrochanteric region
- Presence of additional lesions elsewhere in the femur away from the intertrochanteric region that may develop problems if they progress
- Inadequate proximal diaphyseal bone to provide secure screw fixation

TABLE 13.1   Contraindications and Alternative Surgical Options for Third-Generation Intramedullary Nail Fixation of the Femur

Category	Contraindication	Alternative Surgical Treatments
Location	Femoral neck fractures	Prosthetic hip endoprosthesis: hemiarthroplasty vs. total hip arthroplasty
	Distal femoral metaepiphysis lesions or fractures	1. Plate/screw fixation alone or supplementing reconstruction femoral nailing[a] 2. Distal femoral megaprosthesis total knee replacement
Bone Quality	Insufficient proximal femoral bone stock	1. Prosthetic hip endoprosthesis: hemiarthroplasty vs. total hip arthroplasty 2. Calcar replacement stem (hemi vs. total) 3. Proximal femoral megaprosthesis
	Insufficient distal femoral bone stock	1. Plate/screw fixation alone or supplementing reconstruction femoral nailing[a] 2. Distal femoral megaprosthesis total knee replacement
Life expectancy	<6 wk	Hospice care

[a]Retrograde nailing may be considered in this situation, but only with great caution, as it leaves the proximal femur unprotected (Fig. 13.2).

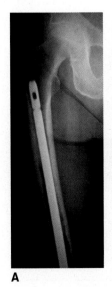 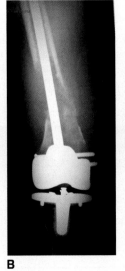 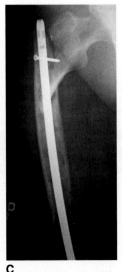

A   **B**   **C**

FIGURE 13.2

Retrograde femoral nails are not ideal for internal fixation of impending or actual pathologic femur fractures as they fail to adequately protect the proximal femur, a common site of bone metastases. This patient incurred a pathologic right distal femur fracture above a total knee arthroplasty. **A,B.** Biopsy showed metastatic carcinoma, and the patient underwent surgical stabilization utilizing a retrograde femoral intramedullary nail without bone cement supplementation. **C:** Subsequently, the patient developed a second pathologic fracture through the proximal femur just above the retrograde femoral nail in the region left unprotected by the original stabilization.

PREOPERATIVE PLANNING

- Confirm diagnosis
  - Preoperative metastatic workup to search for likely primary and identify extent of disease (if unknown)
    - Total skeleton bone scan
    - Computerized tomography of chest/abdomen/pelvis
  - Serum protein electrophoresis and urine protein electrophoresis to evaluate for multiple myeloma
  - Establish diagnosis of femoral lesion with tissue before proceeding with treatment (unless patient already has had tissue documentation of other bone metastases)
    - Preoperative needle biopsy
    - Intraoperative needle or open biopsy with frozen section
- Assess extent of bone defect and remaining bone, proximal and distal
  - Plain biplanar radiographs of entire femur
  - Consider MRI or CT to assess extent of defect
- Entertain alternative means of operative management
  - Consider alternatives if proximal (more likely) or distal bone proves inadequate to support fixation intraoperatively (Table 13.2)
    - Supplementation with bone cement
    - Proximal endoprosthetic device
  - Decide upon a backup plan and have implants available (see Table 13.2)
- Ensure all equipment will be available
  - Primary plan: third-generation femoral reconstruction nail (or dynamic hip screw) of choice with insertion equipment, flexible intramedullary reamers and guide rod(s), radiolucent fluoroscopy table or fracture table, and c-arm fluoroscopy
  - Backup plan(s): bone cement with insertion device of choice (Toomey syringe), third-generation intramedullary reconstruction nail (if primary plan involves dynamic hip screw device), endoprostheses, and associated insertion equipment (see Table 13.2)
- Consider preoperative embolization (Fig. 13.3)
  - Vascular malignancies: renal carcinoma, thyroid carcinoma, and myeloma
  - This is particularly important to consider for these techniques because whether the lesion is approached directly or indirectly (reaming through it), brisk bleeding may be encountered.

TECHNIQUE

Third-Generation Intramedullary Reconstruction Nail (Fig. 14.4A–P)

Positioning   A radiolucent table should be utilized. For impending fractures, a Jackson table or other equivalent vascular imaging table without metallic bars on the side that may impede fluoroscopic imaging is ideal (Fig. 13.4A and B). When traction is desired, as with displaced pathologic fractures, a fracture table is often preferable. In either case, the table should be chosen to minimize interference with intraoperative imaging. Typically, the patient is positioned supine with a bump under the operative hip (Fig. 13.4B). The ipsilateral arm should be secured over a pillow across the patient's chest to avoid interference during intramedullary instrumentation.

Landmarks
- Tip of greater trochanter. Adequate access to the region proximal to the tip is crucial, so attention must be paid to this when placing the bump under the hip during positioning and also during draping.
- Rotational landmarks: Anterior superior iliac spines, patella, and lateral femoral condyle should be assessed to ensure that postoperative rotation is optimal when dealing with displaced fractures.

TABLE 13.2 Reconstructive Alternatives to Internal Fixation Devices Based on Anatomic Region of Compromised Proximal Femoral Bone	
Anatomic Region with Compromised Bone (from Femoral Head Down to Designated Level)	**Reconstructive Alternative**
Base of femoral neck	Standard or long-stem cemented femoral stem
Inferior aspect of lesser trochanter	Calcar replacing cemented femoral stem
More distal	Proximal femoral replacement megaprosthesis

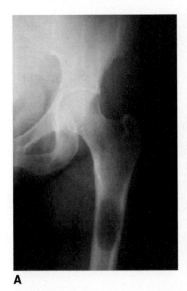
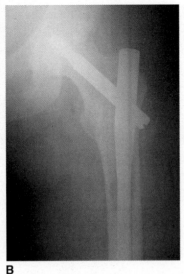

A   **B**

FIGURE 13.3

For metastatic lesions of the femur due to renal carcinoma, myeloma, or thyroid cancer, consideration should be given to preoperative embolization to minimize intraoperative bleeding. **A:** This patient with known metastatic thyroid cancer to the left femur subtrochanteric region with impending pathologic fracture had associated pain despite treatment with radioactive iodine. **B:** Considerable intraoperative bleeding was encountered during placement of this locked third-generation reconstruction nail (Long Gamma Nail, Stryker).

Surgical incision

- To establish diagnosis. If a biopsy is to be done as part of the procedure, the approach should be from the lateral thigh directly at the site of the lesion, NOT through the intramedullary canal (Fig. 13.4C)! The frozen section diagnosis should be established unequivocally to be metastatic disease, myeloma, or lymphoma before proceeding to operative fixation. If there is a possibility that the diagnosis represents sarcoma, the procedure should be aborted until a definitive diagnosis is rendered on permanent sections.
- For third-generation intramedullary nail insertion through the tip of the greater trochanter
  - Depending upon the size of the patient, the incision may vary from 2 to 6 cm.
  - Begin the incision at the center (anterior-posterior) of the tip of the greater trochanter and extend *proximally*.

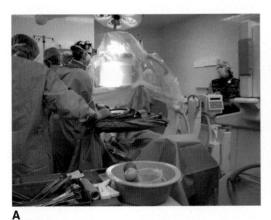
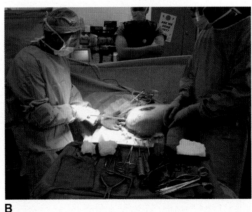

A   **B**

FIGURE 13.4

A: A typical intraoperative setup for femoral trochanteric nailing of an impending fracture is shown here. The patient is positioned on a radiolucent Jackson table to facilitate intraoperative imaging, the surgeon and assistants are on the operative side (patient's right in this case), the fluoroscopy c-arm unit is coming in from the patient's contralateral side (patient's left in this case) to minimize interference with the use of instruments by the surgeon, and the viewing screen at the foot of the bed where it is unobstructed by other personnel or equipment. **B:** When there is no fracture, a fracture table is unnecessary, as in this case of an impending pathologic fracture. In a supine position with a bump under the operative hip to facilitate access to the trochanteric region, the operative limb may be easily manipulated to allow exposure to the lateral biopsy/curettage site (the larger midshaft incision in this case) as well as to the tip of the trochanter, as shown here for insertion of instruments and the implant into the femoral canal. The operative limb is adducted and internally rotated to bring the tip of the greater trochanter more anterior. In much the same manner, the limb can also be easily manipulated to obtain both anteroposterior and frog-lateral x-ray views with the fluoroscopy unit. This obviates the cumbersome and time-consuming rotation of the fluoro unit much of the time.

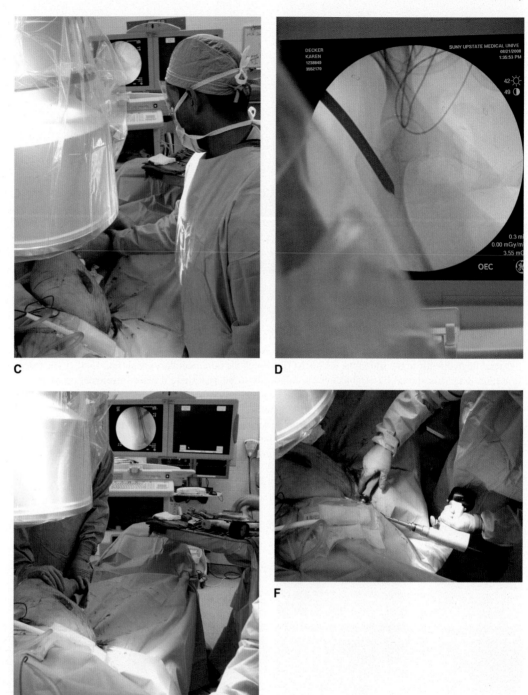

C   D

E   F

FIGURE 13.4 (*Continued*)

C: From the surgeon's viewpoint, the viewing screen should be positioned so that it can be easily visualized while manipulating the leg and instruments alike. **D:** Here, the fluoroscopy unit viewing screen shows an awl for a trochanteric nail being inserted through the tip of the greater trochanter. **E:** The intramedullary ball-tipped guide rod has now been inserted through the awl and passed into the distal femur. At this point, the length of the nail may be determined based upon the amount of exposed guide rod using a measurement tool. **F:** Viewed from above, the surgeon is utilizing a battery-powered reamer driver and flexible reamers inserted over the ball-tipped guide rod and through a soft tissue protector in the small proximal incision in order to prepare the canal. For reconstruction of trochanteric nail devices, overreaming of the distal shaft by 2 mm is recommended to allow some manipulation of the nail into the perfect position so that the proximal locking screw or screws are positioned well within the femoral neck and head. Overreaming by <2 mm serves no purpose and only makes it more difficult to manipulate the nail within the canal after it has been passed.

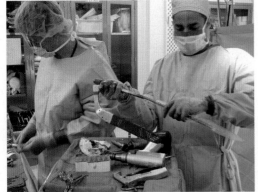

G

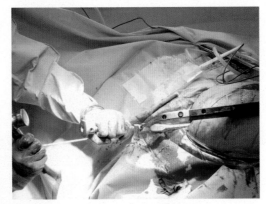

H

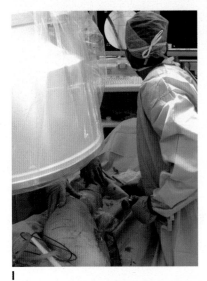

I

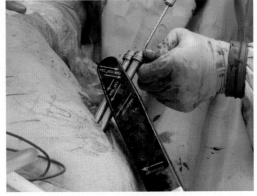

J

FIGURE 13.4 (*Continued*)

G: The intramedullary nail of appropriate length and diameter is assembled to an insertion device on the back table, taking care to make sure that the anterior bow position of the femur is reproduced. At this point, it is wise to confirm with the provided cannula for proximal screw insertion that the insertion handle is aligned well with the nail by inserting the cannula device through the appropriate slot(s) in the insertion handle and checking to make sure that the tip of the cannula contacts the center of the hole. **H:** Depending upon the type of nail, the device may be advanced by hand or with the insertion of the mallet on an impaction device. The latter is shown here. **I:** The position of the proximal interlocking hole relative to the femoral neck and head is crucial to evaluate fluoroscopically, as shown here. **J:** Proximal screws are placed through the nail and into the proximal femur by drilling and/or reaming through cannulae inserted into holes in the nail insertion handle, sometimes over partially threaded guided wires. **K:** Fluoroscopic visualization in two planes should be accomplished after drilling or placing the guide wire in order to confirm appropriate positioning within the femoral neck and head. Here, the drills for two proximal interlocking screws in a reconstruction type nail are advanced under fluoroscopic visualization.

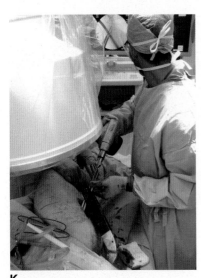

K

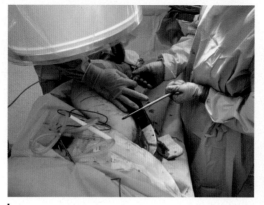

L

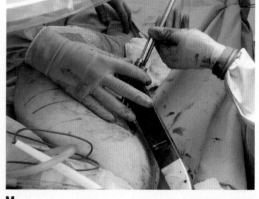

M

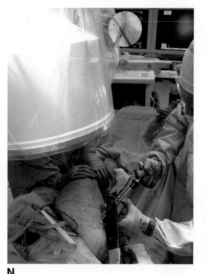

N

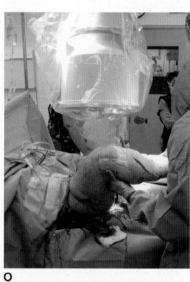

O

FIGURE 13.4 (*Continued*)

L to **N:** Interlocking screws are assembled to an insertion handle and then passed through the cannulae under fluoroscopic visualization into the proximal femur.
O: A good frog-lateral view of the inserted proximal femoral device assembly should be obtained in addition to the anteroposterior view in order to confirm adequate placement of the nail and screw(s). This photo illustrates how easily this is achieved in the supine position without the need to move the fluoroscopy unit, saving time and effort. **P:** In the supine position, distal interlocking screws are placed with the fluoroscopy c-arm unit in a cross-table lateral position perpendicular to the limb and parallel to the floor, the view magnified to cone down to the distal interlocking screw holes. The goal is to achieve "perfect circles" of the distal interlocking screw holes on the viewing monitor. This is facilitated by having the assistant focus on maintaining the desired position of the limb and providing counterresistance to the force of the surgeon as he drills and places the screws. Both anteroposterior and lateral views should be done after final distal interlocking screw insertion.

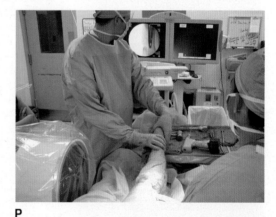

P

Surgical approach for biopsy. When the diagnosis has not been established, a lateral approach to the femur at the site of the lesion/fracture is preferred for open biopsy (Fig. 13.4B,C). However, particularly when there is substantial cortical breach or thinning to allow insertion of a needle, diagnostic tissue can be obtained simply by means of a Trucut core needle without the need to make an incision. The frozen section diagnosis should be established unequivocally to be metastatic disease, myeloma, or lymphoma before proceeding to operative fixation.

Surgical Approach for Device Insert

Third-generation reconstruction intramedullary nail. Carry the scalpel through skin, subcutaneous tissue, and iliotibial band/gluteal fascia directly down onto the tip of the greater trochanter from proximal to distal; turn the blade proximal and create at least a 2 to 3 cm area of fascial opening through which the operative finger can palpate the tip of the trochanter.

Canal Access and Preparation (Third-Generation Reconstruction Nail)

The trochanteric tip can be accessed quite easily and efficiently with a cannulated awl through which the ball-tipped intramedullary guide rod is inserted (Fig. 13.4D). Others may prefer to utilize a straight pin over which a rigid, large diameter (15 to 17 mm), proximal femoral reamer is passed to open the proximal bone before passing the longer guide rod into the distal femur. The danger in reaming the proximal femur with a large size reamer over a short pin is that slight errors in pin positioning may result in the cortex being inadvertently damaged before the surgeon recognizes it. Hence, this author prefers passage of the longer guide rod through the entire femur and checking it distally fluoroscopically in two planes to ensure it is appropriately seated in the femur before utilizing any reamers (Fig. 13.4E).

Once the guide rod is passed, this author does two things to expedite the remainder of the case.

1. On the drapes, mark the point at which the fully inserted guide rod tip is positioned. This provides a visual reference point to ensure that the rod has not backed out during reaming or removal of the reamers at each changeover. This also minimizes fluoroscopic exposure.
2. Measure for nail length. For the nail that the author utilizes most often, the only variable determined intra-operatively is the length (assuming the canal is reamable to 13 mm to allow the 11 mm nail to be inserted). Hence, measuring the length now allows the final nail to be selected, opened, and assembled to the insertion device while reaming is being completed, thus expediting the case.

Distal reaming for a reconstruction-type intramedullary femoral nail should be to 2 mm larger than the diameter of the nail (Fig. 13.1F). Proximal reaming must accommodate the larger proximal portion of the nail, and most systems provide a straight cannulated rigid reamer for this purpose.

Interlocking Screw Fixation

Proximal interlocking screw insertion utilizes an outrigger jig attached to the nail (Fig. 13.4G–O). Distal interlocking screw insertion is advisable in all cases and may be done by any one of a number of freehand techniques utilizing the appropriate size drill bit (Fig. 13.4P) (1). Both proximal and distal interlocking screw placement must be confirmed in two planes fluoroscopically (Fig. 13.4O and P).

Cement Supplementation

Bone cement may be needed in one of three situations (16).

1. Cement supplementation of proximal screw fixation. When proximal screw fixation is less than optimal, the screw may be removed and then reinserted after first injecting bone cement. However, care must be taken to avoid creating a cement arthrogram if either the k-wire or drill penetrated the subchondral bone during preparation for screw placement. When in doubt, injection of radiographic dye under pressure during fluoroscopic visualization should be considered first.
2. Cementation of biopsy or curetted defects by direct exposure. When the lesion or fracture has been approached directly for biopsy, the exposure provides an opportunity to supplement any defect in the bone with bone cement (Table 13.3). However, the immediate improvement in biomechanical stability must be weighed against the potential for impeding fracture healing in patients who have this potential.
3. Intramedullary supplementation of contained femoral defects. Defects may also be supplemented with bone cement introduced from the nail insertion site. However, as noted in Table 13.3, intramedullary cementation prior to nail placement is technically demanding. To make sure that the nail and proximal interlocking screws will be positioned expeditiously in the correct degree of anteversion and at the appropriate level in the femoral neck and head before the cement hardens and prevents repositioning of the nail, consideration should be given to inserting the nail and screw once and then removing it prior to introducing the cement if this technique is to be utilized. Furthermore, attention needs to be paid to potential extraosseous cement extrusion at sites of cortical disruption. Direct exposure of these sites may be required to avoid injury to vital structures.

Dynamic Hip Screw Device Technique

Positioning, anatomic landmarks, surgical approach for biopsy, and cementation considerations are the same as described previously for the third-generation intramedullary reconstruction nail. The unique aspects are described below.

Surgical Incision
- For dynamic hip screw devices
  - Begin the incision slightly posterior to midline at the level of the lesser trochanter and extend *distally* over 8 to 10 cm.

TABLE 13.3 Advantages and Disadvantages of Techniques of Direct Exposure Cementation

Technique for Direct Exposure Cementation	Advantages	Disadvantages
Cementation after nail placement	Technically easier Minimizes risk of malpositioned nail Easier extraction for complications (infection)	Less complete cementing
Cementation prior to nail placement	More complete cementing	Technically demanding Risks malpositioned nail due to premature cement hardening More difficult extraction for complications (infection) Potential cement extrusion at remote sites of cortical disruption

Surgical Approach for Device Insertion
- Dynamic hip screw device. A standard lateral approach to femur will suffice here.

Technique of Dynamic Hip Screw Fixation
- Curettage of lesion. Since cement supplementation of the dynamic hip screw device is almost always indicated in the situation of a pathologic fracture, a thorough curettage of the lesion is recommended. This should be accomplished through the fracture line or, in the situation of an impending fracture, through a lateral femoral defect at or above the site of planned dynamic screw insertion.
- Cementation of the defect. While 4.5 cortical screws may be placed through hardened cement, the large dynamic hip screw cannot. Hence two options exist for cement supplementation: cementing after placing the hip screw (± plate) and cementing prior to placement of hip screw and plate. Considerations are the same as those described in Table 13.3 for direct cementing during intramedullary reconstruction nail fixation. If the cement is going to be introduced prior to placement of the hip screw device before the cement hardens, preliminary trial placement of the plate and screws is advisable before the cement run. Alternatively, the hip screw alone (without plate) may be placed, then the cement introduced, and finally the plate applied while the cement is still doughy.
- Placement of the dynamic hip screw and side plate. In most instances, the goal here is to achieve an immediately rigid construct between the hip screw, plate, and bone cement. Hence, the biomechanics are different than those typically achieved in the fixation of a nonpathologic intertrochanteric fracture. Unless no bone cement is used and the fracture (if present) is expected to heal (in patients who are expected to live long enough to do so), the construct should not be dynamic at all. Hence, the locking screw should be tightened rigidly rather than loosely, as no sliding of the hip screw is expected.

PEARLS AND PITFALLS

- Regardless of the location of the identifiable lesions, critically assess the remaining bone to ensure that adequate fixation is able to be achieved both proximal and distal to the lesion. Always have a backup plan.
- Adequate bone stock proximal and distal to the fracture is necessary to obtain secure fixation.

POSTOPERATIVE MANAGEMENT

One of the goals of the procedure is to allow the patient to weight-bear as tolerated immediately postoperatively. Hence, if the construct is felt to be rigid, there is no reason to protect weight bearing postoperatively. Patients should be mobilized on the first postoperative day and advanced in physical therapy as they are able. Consideration should be given to perioperative antibiotic coverage, thromboembolic disease prophylaxis, and appropriate blood replacement. Irradiation of the entire instrumented region is advisable, as implant failures are significantly greater among patients who do not receive postoperative treatment (2).

COMPLICATIONS

In general, complications have diminished over time with the evolution of the reconstruction nails (8,11,17–19,21) (Table 13.4). Early use of second-generation reconstruction nails such as the Russell-Taylor nail was remarkable for

TABLE 13.4	Complications Reported with Femoral Intramedullary Nail Fixation of Actual and Impending Pathologic Fractures[a]			
Author	Year Published	Femoral Nails (N)	Fractures (F) vs. Impending (I)	Complications
Gibbons et al.	1995	43	43 F	0 implant failures 7 complications
Karachalios et al.	1993	14 R-T	14 F	0 mechanical failures
Piatek et al.	2003	22 LGN, recon, and locking	22 F	2 dislocations of nail 1 distal locking screw loosening 1 progressive tumor destruction
Samsani et al.	2003	39 LGN	11 F, 28 I	0 implant failures 14 minor technical, medical, or implant related complications
Wedin and Bauer	2005	22 Recon	22 F	3/22 (13.6%) failures
Weikert and Schwartz	1991	10 R-T	10 I	0 implant failures 0 complications

[a]Numerous other larger series exist but often include arthroplasty techniques and other anatomic sites (4–11).

technical difficulties in up to 63% (19/30), mostly due to nail insertion and placement of proximal interlocking screws (3). However, improved instrumentation and the shift to a trochanteric tip insertion site have coincided with less frequently reported difficulties. Distal interlocking screws are advisable even in prophylactic fixation cases to avoid proximal femoral fractures (1).

These patients need to be followed, however, because increasing failure rates with increasing time of survival postoperatively following femoral internal fixation techniques have been noted (10,12,13). In one series including 37 osteosynthesis procedures for the proximal femur, the 2-year reoperation rate after internal fixation was 35% (12). In another series of, the 5-year reoperation rate was 44% (13).

RESULTS

For the most part, good results can be expected (Table 13.5), but the results of femoral pathologic fracture fixation are not as good as that of the humerus (3,8,14,15,18–20). In fact, for proximal third femoral fractures in

TABLE 13.5	Results of Intramedullary Stabilization of Actual and Impending Pathologic Femur Fractures[a]			
Author	Year Published	Femoral Nails (N) and Type	Fractures (F) vs. Impending (I)	Results
Garnavos et al.	1999	30 R-T	30 F	No cancer patient returned to prefracture level of mobility
Karachalios et al.	1993	14 Recon	14 F	All patients free of pain and regained mobility
Mickelson and Bonfiglio	1982	2 Zickel	2 I	Successful stabilization with resection and Zickel nail, wire mesh, and cement reconstruction
Piatek et al.	2003	22 LGN, recon, and locking	22 F	63% able to walk at time of discharge
Samsani et al.	2003	39 LGN	11 F, 28 I	All patients achieved pain relief and improved mobility
Ward et al.	2003	89 Recon	20 F, 69 I	Satisfactory pain relief and functional preservation for most patients with impending fractures

[a]Numerous other larger series exist but often include arthroplasty techniques and other anatomic sites (4–11).

particular, a treatment controversy exists, as some authors have reported better results with arthroplasty than with internal fixation in lesions even farther distal than the femoral neck (2,10,12).

Comparing reconstruction nails to hip screws and glide-screw plates, the latter generally are reported to have higher complication rates (11,13). While early reports on the use of internal fixation techniques for proximal femoral pathologic fractures suggested less complications when bone cement was used to supplement internal fixation (6,13,14), more recent reports on third-generation reconstruction nails have not suggested such a difference (8).

REFERENCES

1. Chesser TJ, Kerr PS, Ward AJ. Pathological fracture after prophylactic reconstruction nailing of the femur. The need for distal locking. *Int Orthop*. 1996;20(3):190–191.
2. Wedin R, Bauer HC, Wersall P. Failures after operation for skeletal metastatic lesions of long bones. *Clin Orthop Relat Res*. 1999;(358):128–139.
3. Garnavos C, Peterman A, Howard PW. The treatment of difficult proximal femoral fractures with the Russell-Taylor reconstruction nail. *Injury*. 1999;30(6):407–415.
4. Bocchi L, Lazzeroni L, Maggi M. The surgical treatment of metastases in long bones. *Ital J Orthop Traumatol*. 1988;14(2):167–173.
5. Dutka J, Sosin P. Time of survival and quality of life of the patients operatively treated due to pathological fractures due to bone metastases. *Ortop Traumatol Rehabil*. 2003;5(3):276–283.
6. Habermann ET, Sachs R, Stern RE, et al. The pathology and treatment of metastatic disease of the femur. *Clin Orthop Relat Res*. 1982;(169):70–82.
7. Katzer A, Meenen NM, Grabbe F, et al. Surgery of skeletal metastases. *Arch Orthop Trauma Surg*. 2002;122(5):251–258. Epub 2001 Dec 4.
8. Piatek S, Westphal T, Bischoff J, et al. Intramedullary stabilisation of metastatic fractures of long bones. *Zentralbl Chir*. 2003;128(2):131–138.
9. Sosin P, Dutka J. Clinical and radiographic evaluation of mechanical sufficiency of the operative treatment of pathological fractures in bone metastases. *Ortop Traumatol Rehabil*. 2003;5(3):290–296.
10. Wedin R. Surgical treatment for pathologic fracture. *Acta Orthop Scand Suppl*. 2001;72(302):2p., 1–29.
11. Wedin R, Bauer HC, Rutqvist LE. Surgical treatment for skeletal breast cancer metastases: a population-based study of 641 patients. *Cancer*. 2001;92(2):257–262.
12. Wedin R, Bauer HC. Surgical treatment of skeletal metastatic lesions of the proximal femur: endoprosthesis or reconstruction nail? *J Bone Joint Surg Br*. 2005;87(12):1653–1657.
13. Yazawa Y, Frassica FJ, Chao EY, et al. Metastatic bone disease. A study of the surgical treatment of 166 pathologic humeral and femoral fractures. *Clin Orthop Relat Res*. 1990;(251):213–219.
14. Mickelson MR, Bonfiglio M. Resection and Zickel device fixation for metastatic tumor. *Clin Orthop Relat Res*. 1982; 164:261–264.
15. Dijstra S, Wiggers T, van Geel BN, et al. Impending and actual fractures in patients with bone metastases of the long bones. A retrospective study of 233 surgically treated fractures. *Eur J Surg*. 1994;160(10):535–542.
16. Dutka J, Sosin P, Libura M. Internal fixation with bone cement in reconstruction of bone defects due to bone metaseses. *Ortop Traumatol Rehabil*. 2006;8(6):620–626.
17. Gibbons CL, Gregg-Smith SJ, Carrell TW, et al. Use of the Russell-Taylor reconstruction nail in femoral shaft fractures. *Injury*. 1995;26(6):389–392.
18. Karachalios T, Atkins RM, Sarangi PP, et al. Reconstruction nailing for pathological subtrochanteric fractures with coexisting femoral shaft metastases. *J Bone Joint Surg Br*. 1993;75(1):119–122.
19. Samsani SR, Panikkar V, Georgiannos D, et al. Subtrochanteric metastatic lesions treated with the long gamma nail. *Int Orthop*. 2003;27(5):298–302. Epub 2003 Jun 11.
20. Ward WG, Holsenbeck S, Dorey FJ, et al. Metastatic disease of the femur: surgical treatment. *Clin Orthop Relat Res*. 2003;415(Suppl):S230–S244.
21. Weikert DR, Schwartz HS. Intramedullary nailing for impending pathological subtrochanteric fractures. *J Bone Joint Surg Br*. 1991;73(4):668–670.

14 General Considerations

Peter F. M. Choong

Complex reconstructive surgery is now commonplace for the knee as limb sparing surgery replaces amputation as the preferred technique for managing malignancies of the knee (1,2). Many of these techniques are also being extended to nonmalignant conditions (1,3–7) where significant bone loss and instability are dominant features such as with marked condylar bone defects associated with multiple revisions of a knee joint replacement or significant loss of bone integrity associated with periprosthetic fractures and also malunited or ununited fractures around the knee. The primary aim of reconstructive surgery is to achieve a stable mobile joint.

INDICATIONS

Primary Malignancies

The knee is the commonest site for the development of osteosarcoma. Over the last two decades, there has been a shift in surgical philosophy from amputation to limb sparing surgery (2,8). Much of this shift has been attributed to advances in imaging, chemotherapy, prostheses, and surgical techniques. Moreover, it has been shown that function is superior with limb salvage surgery (9) while patient survival is not affected by limb sparing surgery and the risk of local recurrence after limb sparing surgery is extremely low (10). A number of studies have also indicated the cost effectiveness of limb sparing surgery as compared to amputation (11,12).

Most osteosarcomas develop in the metaphysis of the femur (Fig. 14.1A,B). These tumors are often associated with a large soft tissue component that grows through the cortical bone of the metaphysis and extends proximally and distally from the metaphysis through the intramedullary bone (Fig. 14.1C,D). When developing in the immature skeleton, a metaphyseal osteosarcoma often meets resistance at the growth plate. Penetration of this structure is often a late event and may be regarded as a suitable margin if there is nonconclusive evidence of growth plate invasion (13). Invasion of the synovium in the supracondylar region is uncommon, and imaging frequently shows the pushing rather than the invasive characteristic of osteosarcoma as it

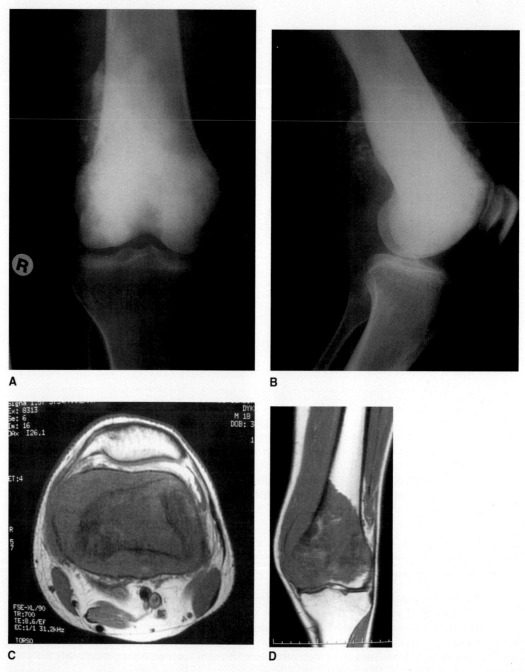

FIGURE 14.1

A: Anteroposterior radiograph of distal femoral osteosarcoma. Note the mixed sclerotic character of the tumor within the distal metaphysis and the extraosseous subperiosteal reaction. **B:** Lateral radiograph of distal femoral osteosarcoma. Excellent example of anterior and posterior cortical subperiosteal reaction. **C:** T1-weighted axial MRI clearly demonstrating the outline of the distal femoral cortex being overrun by the extraosseous extension of tumor. This sequence clearly demonstrates the anatomy of the popliteal fossa with clear delineation of the tumor capsule and the popliteal vessels and nerves, which lie well away from the tumor.
D: T1-weighted coronal MRI of the knee demonstrating the excellent marrow imaging using this modality, which permits accurate planning of surgical margins.

abuts the synovium. Invasion of the knee joint proper is also an uncommon occurrence (13) but may arise in the presence of pathologic fracture, cruciate ligament invasion, poor biopsy technique, and capsular invasion at the collateral ligaments. The surgical management of distal femoral osteosarcomas will depend on whether there is tumor within the joint or not. If there has been no breach of the joint capsule, then an intra-articular resection of the distal femur is preferred. A more complex extra-articular resection is indicated if invasion of the joint has occurred.

The size, shape, and direction of protrusion of the extraosseous soft tissue component will determine the nature of the soft tissue dissection, the structures that can be preserved, and those that will require sacrifice. The confluence of neurovascular structures in the popliteal fossa makes planning of surgical margins critical in the presence of a large posteriorly directed soft tissue component.

Metastatic Malignancies

The commonest malignant tumor of bone is a metastasis from carcinoma. Although the femur is a common site for metastasis, distal femoral metastases are less common than proximal femoral metastases. Metastases are usually from breast, lung, thyroid, kidney, and prostate primary tumors. Gastrointestinal tract tumors uncommonly target bone. Condylar metastases are easily treated by resection and megaprosthetic reconstruction (14,15). Extraosseous soft tissue components are uncommon except for renal metastases, and consequently, sacrifice of soft tissue attachments can be avoided and bone margins need not be extensive.

Isolated lesions are uncommon but may occur in relation to thyroid and renal metastases. Occasionally, late presentation of breast carcinoma metastases many years after the treatment of the primary may present as a solitary lesion. In all these cases, en bloc resection may be attempted with locally curative intent. More often, however, disease arises in multiple sites within a single bone and progression of disease is to be expected. In planning surgical management, protection of the whole bone should be sought in anticipation of further development of disease. Long stemmed cemented intramedullary fixation is preferred as a method for protecting the femoral diaphysis.

Nonneoplastic Conditions

Multiple revisions of joint replacement may lead to significant loss of distal femoral bone stock causing elevation of the joint line, loss of condylar offset, and disappearance of the epicondyles. Under such circumstances, reconstruction with standard prostheses or even those that include prosthetic augments or posterior stabilized designs may not be sufficient to provide adequate collateral stability or return a stable kinematic range of flexion and extension. Megaprosthestic reconstruction with a rotating hinge mechanism provides a unique opportunity for correcting the bone loss and instability in a single device (3–5,7).

Poorly united or nonunion of supracondylar or condylar fractures can provide complex challenges for reconstruction (Fig. 14.2A,B). Frequently, patients present with the late effects of their malunited or ununited fractures such as gross coronal plane malalignment, loss of range of motion, and pain of degenerative disease. In contrast to failed revision joint replacement, abnormalities of union are more frequently associated with fixed deformities and contractures. Surgical solutions to this include combinations of resection of sufficient bone and prosthetic implantation to allow correction of the deformity and soft tissue releases to correct the restriction of movement (Fig. 14.2C,D). Correction of chronic deformity always carries the risk of nerve and vascular injury.

CONTRAINDICATIONS TO LIMB SPARING SURGERY

Infection

Infection may not only threaten the success of knee surgery, but may also lead to amputation if it becomes uncontrolled. Major reconstructive surgery must not be undertaken in the setting of infection unless it is being performed as part of a staged approach to the management of acute/chronically infected joint prostheses.

Skeletally Immature Patients

Mobile reconstruction following resection of osteosarcoma of the distal femur in patients with open growth plates may lead to the development of significant limb length inequality. Predicted inequality may be reduced by surgically restricting growth in the contralateral limb by epiphysiodesis. However, the potential for ongoing growth in the contralateral limb may be so great that interrupting this may result in unacceptable stunting of overall height. In principle, the younger the patient, the greater is the potential for limb length discrepancy. If the anticipated inequality is substantial, then reconstruction is contraindicated and amputation should be considered. Matching leg lengths through modification of amputation limb prostheses may be easier to achieve

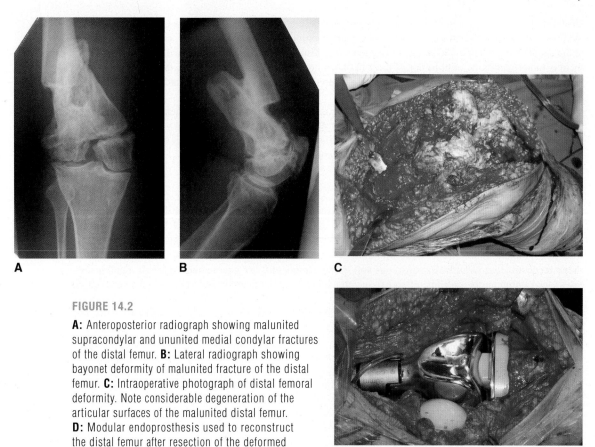

FIGURE 14.2

A: Anteroposterior radiograph showing malunited supracondylar and ununited medial condylar fractures of the distal femur. **B:** Lateral radiograph showing bayonet deformity of malunited fracture of the distal femur. **C:** Intraoperative photograph of distal femoral deformity. Note considerable degeneration of the articular surfaces of the malunited distal femur. **D:** Modular endoprosthesis used to reconstruct the distal femur after resection of the deformed distal femur.

than compensating for gross discrepancies in knee and ankle joint line heights. Alternatives to conventional above knee amputations include rotation plasty and telescopic prostheses. While the success of the former procedure is well described, telescopic prostheses remain experimental without significant clinical experience to mandate their use.

Poor Response to Chemotherapy

A good response to chemotherapy is often manifested by a reduction in symptoms and size of the metaphyseal lesion. Histologic examination usually demonstrates the presence of a fibrous rind around the tumor, which facilitates the development of sound oncologic margins. This is particularly important when the popliteal neurovascular structures are immediately adjacent to the extraosseous soft tissue component and require dissection from the fibrous rind. If the response to chemotherapy is poor, and it can be anticipated that the margins will be unsatisfactory, then the risk of local recurrence may be unacceptably high. Under this circumstance, limb sparing surgery may be contraindicated and amputation may be preferred. Being able to predict response to treatment and visualize the surgical margins preoperatively allows the team to appropriately counsel the patient and caregivers about amputation and its merits over limb sparing surgery before the procedure.

Involvement of the Popliteal Neurovascular Structures

Amputation should be strongly considered when both neural and vascular structures are involved at the level of the knee. Involvement of the vessels without neural, however, is not necessarily a contraindication to limb sparing surgery. Reconstruction of the vascular tree is possible and a viable and functioning lower limb may be expected. Involvement of only the neural structures, however, may result in a profound sensory and motor deficit below the level of the knee and amputation may be preferable to preservation of an insensate and immobile foot. Anecdotal reports of patient acceptance after tumor resection that includes the sciatic nerve now make limb sparing surgery less of an absolute contraindication when neural involvement is evident.

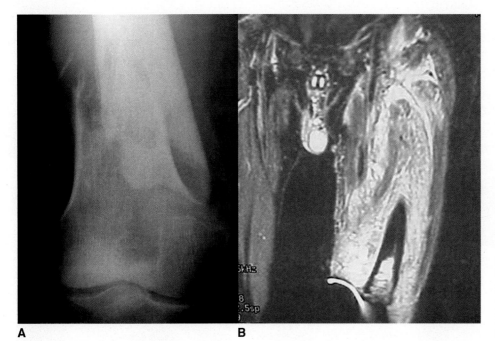

A   B

FIGURE 14.3

Radiograph of a pathologic fracture through a distal femoral central chondrosarcoma. Note the intense soft tissue edema, which is clearly demonstrated on MRI following the fracture. Soft tissue edema and hematoma may extend all the way proximally to the hip capsule, potentially complicating any plans for limb sparing surgery.

Pathologic Fractures

Pathologic fractures can be associated with extensive hematomas and posttraumatic inflammation, which is known to cause significant contamination of adjacent tissue planes with tumor (Fig. 14.3A,B). The risk of local recurrence under such a circumstance may be unacceptably high and amputation is an absolute indication if widespread contamination occurs. Low energy fractures such as that which may occur at the articular surface of a significantly weakened bone may only result in intra-articular contamination, which does not preclude limb sparing surgery via an extra-articular approach. Should limb preserving surgery be chosen over amputation in the setting of pathologic fracture, the patient should be protected from further disruption of the hematoma by immobilization (e.g., skeletal traction, spanning external fixation) and administered neoadjuvant chemotherapy. A response to chemotherapy after 10 to 12 weeks is usually accompanied by ossification and healing of the fracture, which serves to stabilize the fracture site sufficiently to allow safe manipulation of the limb during surgery. The patient must accept that the risk of local recurrence is higher with attempted limb sparing surgery after fracture.

INVESTIGATIONS

Plain Radiographs

Plain radiographs of the knee extending proximally sufficiently to visualize the whole extent of the tumor is mandatory. Composite images should be discouraged, but rather the whole tumor and its relationship to the entire knee should be visible on the single radiograph. High-quality images should be obtained, which allow scrutiny of the cortical destruction, periosteal reaction, and new bone formation in the case of primary malignancy (Fig. 14.4A,B). In the case of metastatic disease, radiographs of the entire femur should be obtained where possible to ensure that metastatic deposits at the limits of the prosthesis are accounted. If present, appropriate steps must be taken to ensure that these are treated appropriately at the time of surgery. 1:1 magnification should be obtained to permit appropriate templating of the distal femur, proximal tibia, and the intramedullary canal to select a stem of appropriate diameter and length. This may be particularly important in situations where abnormally large or small sizes of implants are required as these may not be present on the standard inventory of equipment and prostheses and may have to be especially requested.

The nature of the primary or secondary bone tumor will determine the appropriate surgical approach and reconstruction. The relative existence of lytic and sclerotic lesions in metastatic disease will also be a factor in determining the appropriate management of metastatic disease of the femur. It should be noted that radiographs on their own may not be sufficient to account for all malignant disease in a bone because the loss of 30% or more of bone is required before a lytic lesion becomes obvious on plain radiographs.

Radiographs are also important for assessing malunion and nonunion of the femur or its condyles. Long leg weight-bearing standing anteroposterior radiographs are valuable for assessing the mechanical alignment of the limb, the extent of the coronal or sagittal deformity, and the level at which the deformity is occurring.

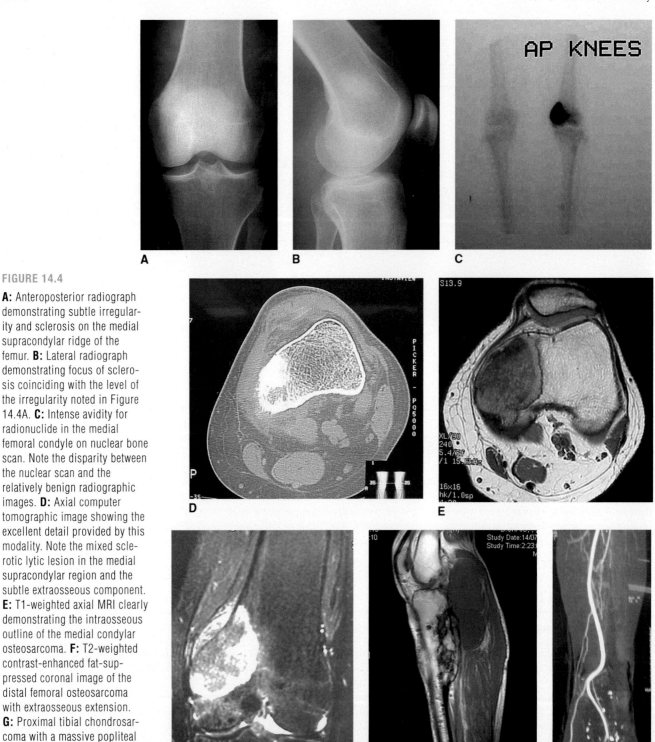

FIGURE 14.4

A: Anteroposterior radiograph demonstrating subtle irregularity and sclerosis on the medial supracondylar ridge of the femur. **B:** Lateral radiograph demonstrating focus of sclerosis coinciding with the level of the irregularity noted in Figure 14.4A. **C:** Intense avidity for radionuclide in the medial femoral condyle on nuclear bone scan. Note the disparity between the nuclear scan and the relatively benign radiographic images. **D:** Axial computer tomographic image showing the excellent detail provided by this modality. Note the mixed sclerotic lytic lesion in the medial supracondylar region and the subtle extraosseous component. **E:** T1-weighted axial MRI clearly demonstrating the intraosseous outline of the medial condylar osteosarcoma. **F:** T2-weighted contrast-enhanced fat-suppressed coronal image of the distal femoral osteosarcoma with extraosseous extension. **G:** Proximal tibial chondrosarcoma with a massive popliteal soft tissue component. **H:** Computer tomographic angiogram to assess compression by the popliteal chondrosarcoma.

Nuclear Scintigraphy

Nuclear scintigraphy with bone targeting tracers is an excellent modality for identifying areas of increased bone turnover (Fig. 14.4C) that may represent malignancy, prosthetic loosening, and periprosthetic fracture or nonunion. Unlike plain radiography, which requires at least 30% of bone loss to clearly identify a bone abnormality, scintigraphy may detect subtle increases in bone activity. More recently, co-registration of nuclear scans with multislice computed tomography (CT) has facilitated greater specificity and accuracy in the interpretation of results. Nuclear tracers such as thallium and glucose-6-phosphate that can detect metabolic activity may also be useful for identifying areas of increased metabolic activity. This is pertinent when assessing the nature of a malignancy because areas of increased metabolic activity may be targeted for biopsy, or the changes in tracer avidity between prechemotherapy/radiotherapy and postchemotherapy/radiotherapy may be important for determining response to treatment. Response to treatment can have significant bearing on the choice of surgical margin when planning resection of a malignant tumor.

Computed Tomography

CT is an excellent modality for delineating cortical and trabecular bone (Fig. 14.4D). Thus, CT has an important role in identifying bone loss of any cause including fracture, tumor, or periprosthetic lysis. Multiplanar and three-dimensional reconstructions may be invaluable for providing spatial information when planning reconstruction. Loss of extensive areas of cortical bone may require selection of bulk allografts or alternately segmental megaprostheses for reconstruction. Image degradation is encountered when CT scans are performed through metallic devices. The ability of sophisticated CT software to subtract the prosthetic image or suppress the metal artifact of existing prosthesis allows better delineation of periprosthetic lysis. Long leg alignment views may also be obtained to delineate the extent of malalignment in the setting of previous trauma or failed joint replacement. Appropriately configured CT scans are also useful for identifying the anatomic landmarks such as the femoral epicondyles and the relationship of these to existing prostheses if revision surgery, which includes correction of rotational deformity, is being planned.

Magnetic Resonance Imaging

Magnetic resonance imaging (MRI) provides unsurpassed soft tissue contrast allowing excellent delineation between different tissues (Fig. 14.4E,F). This modality is particularly useful for tumors of the knee as the close proximity of the popliteal neurovascular structures to any soft tissue component requires careful scrutiny and assessment. The confined space of the popliteal fossa and the need to ensure a safe plane of dissection between the neurovascular structures and the tumor mass mandate high-quality images in three planes. The intra-articular extension of tumors of the knee may occur through the suprapatellar pouch, cruciate ligaments, subarticular bone, and the collateral ligaments. These areas are particularly well visualized and an effusion indicating joint involvement is easily identified on MRI scans.

Angiography

Angiography may be indicated when involvement of the popliteal artery or its bifurcation into posterior and anterior tibial arteries is suspected. This is relevant when dealing with tumors that have a large soft tissue component (Fig. 14.4G,H). Tumors that extend superiorly may complicate the superficial femoral artery as it courses along the adductor canal or emerges through the hiatus in adductor magnus. Identifying any such eventuality preoperatively allows appropriate evasive action to be undertaken during surgery while sparing injury to either the vessels or the tumor capsule. CT angiography or MR angiography has now revolutionized the visualization of the vascular tree and in most circumstances has supplanted standard angiography for this purpose.

Angiography is imperative when dealing with large metastatic bone lesions. Metastases such as renal, thyroid, and myeloma, which are characterized by hypervascularity, may require preoperative embolization to minimize potentially life-threatening intraoperative hemorrhage. Conventional angiography by percutaneous puncture and catheterization of the vascular tree is the preferred route when embolization is being considered. It is also important to conduct surgery within 36 hours of embolization as there is a high risk of revascularization of the tumor after this time. The size, number, and extent of the vascular lesions within a bone may be important when deciding on whether resectional surgery or excisional curettage will be employed and also the type of implant to be used in any reconstruction.

ANATOMIC CONSIDERATIONS

Knee Joint

The important consideration regarding the knee joint is whether it is directly involved or has the potential to be involved in the tumor. The major areas where entry into the knee joint may occur include the suprapatellar pouch, the cruciate ligaments, the articular surface, and the collateral ligaments. Signal abnormalities on MRI scans in the sentinel areas described above should also alert the surgeon to the possibility of intra-articular extension of tumor. Not withstanding this, invasion of the knee joint is uncommon and may be heralded by the presence of an effusion.

The greatest vulnerability of the knee joint to tumor involvement comes from inadvertent transgression of the capsule during biopsy. The wide extent of the capsule beyond the articular margins of the knee joint makes it vulnerable to errant placement of a biopsy site. The capsule is thinnest at the suprapatellar pouch, which may also extend a significant distance proximal to the superior pole of the patellar and bulges medially and laterally to create the paracondylar gutters. Biopsy of a metaphyseal tumor will need careful consideration of all imaging to select the safest approach, which avoids the joint capsule. CT guided biopsy is preferred as this permits an excellent view of the anatomy, including an effusion if one exists.

Adductor Canal

The adductor canal passes proximally from the adductor hiatus in the adductor magnus muscle to the tip of the femoral triangle. The superficial femoral artery and vein course through the canal accompanied by the saphenous nerve and motor branch to vastus medialis obliquus. Where the adductor canal approaches the hiatus in adductor magnus, the vessels are tightly held together by a thickened fascia. Tumors with a large soft tissue component may abut strongly through the vastus medialis or the adductor magnus muscles against this fascia, increasing the tension in the fascia and flattening the adductor canal and its contents. Should this occur, very careful dissection is required when opening the adductor canal to avoid lacerating the vessels or the capsule of the adjacent tumor. The adductor magnus muscle attaches to the adductor tubercle on the medial condyle of the femur via a stout tendinous insertion. Division of this may release the pressure created by a large tumor as it presses against the adductor canal. Injury to the vein in the canal is a real risk and blunt dissection is recommended as the vessels have to be released from the canal and the hiatus through which they pass into the popliteal fossa, so that they may be swept away and protected when continuing with the dissection of the tumor in the popliteal fossa. If the vessels remain tethered to the hiatus, injury may occur or the dissection is made more difficult by being unable to move these structures aside as they are dissected away from the popliteal extension of the tumor.

Popliteal Vessels and Nerves

The neurovascular structures may be accessed either from the medial or lateral side of the popliteal fossa. However, because of their anatomic disposition, the vessels are best approached from the medial side of the knee and the nerves from the lateral side of the knee.

The tibial and peroneal branches of the sciatic nerve run distally closely applied to each other within a thin areolar fascia as they enter the popliteal fossa. As they pass through the popliteal fossa, the common peroneal branch passes laterally to emerge under the biceps tendon as it courses over the lateral head of gastrocnemius. The nerve is easily found by sharp dissection just above the tendon of biceps approximately 4 inches above its insertion into the fibular head. Here there is an interval between the ridge of fascia lata that inserts into the Gerde tubercle and the biceps tendon. Splitting this interval allows access into the popliteal fossa from the lateral side. The nerve often sits parallel and next to the belly of the biceps. The tendon of biceps can then be carefully divided and retracted backward to expose the popliteal fossa and the popliteal nerve in its bed.

The popliteal vessels are best exposed from the medial side. Here the upper border of the conjoint tendons of sartorius, gracilis, and semitendinosus are separated from the medial intermuscular septum and vastus medialis and retracted posteriorly. Dividing the distal attachment into the pes anserinus allows greater displacement of the muscles. The medial head of gastrocnemius is then exposed and can be divided from its femoral attachment, finally revealing the contents of the popliteal fossa from the medial side. The popliteal artery and the vein beneath it can then be seen passing distally through the fossa. There are many branches that arise from the popliteal vessels that pass into the vastus medialis and the profunda femoris network. These have to be carefully ligated and divided to free the popliteal vessels. A branch to the posterior cruciate ligament that passes straight forward to the notch of the femur may be substantial and must be sought with caution. In the case of a large posteriorly protruding tumor, this branch may tether the artery and vein to the femur, making its release difficult. It may also be accidentally avulsed, causing significant hemorrhage.

PATIENT POSITIONING

Patients should be prepared for a total knee replacement with a tourniquet applied about the upper thigh, a lateral knee support, and a foot rest to maintain the knee in flexion. In an obese lower limb or in a procedure requiring a long operative incision, the tourniquet may hinder exposure and may need to be discarded. Inflation of the tourniquet will depend on surgeon choice. Inflation may be reserved for the time just prior to cementation, for the dissection of the tumor, or only as a standby precaution if required. Most procedures are longer than a total knee replacement, so maintaining a tourniquet inflated throughout the entire duration of the procedure is not recommended.

INCISION

The choice of incision will depend on a number of factors including the site of the biopsy, the presence of an asymmetric soft tissue component of the tumor, or surgeon preference. A lateral thigh incision that curves across the lower knee below the tibial tuberosity may be preferred because of the preservation of the vascular supply of the anterior thigh skin, which arrives from the medial side (Fig. 14.5A). A disadvantage of this

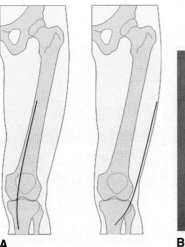

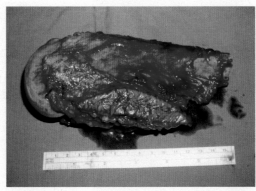

A   **B**

FIGURE 14.5

A: Incisions commonly used for tumors of the distal femur. **B:** Biopsies are usually performed through a medial or lateral approach. Biopsy tracks may be excised en bloc with the tumor via medial or lateral incisions.

incision is the large flap that is created, which may cause some difficulty when trying to dissect around the medial side of the knee. A slightly curved midline skin incision, which is an extension of a standard approach to the knee joint, provides good exposure to either side of the knee (Fig. 14.5A). The disadvantage is the potential for the incision over the knee cap to be under stress as the knee flexes and extends. Curving the incision to either side of the patella provides some relief from this stress.

Incisions should be performed to include the biopsy tract (Fig. 14.5B,C). Even the removal of a small ellipse of skin may be sufficient to subject the wound edge to unwanted tension. If excessive wound tension is anticipated, then muscle flap closure should be considered and the skin defect closed with split skin grafts. Occasionally, simultaneous medial and lateral incisions are required in very large tumors. Care should be taken to ensure that the strip of skin between the incisions is not so narrow as to lead to ischemic necrosis.

Closure of the wound usually requires suture of the deep fascia. If the patella is particularly mobile, it is possible to create an imbalance in the soft tissue tension during closure to displace the patella medially or laterally. The extensor mechanism is often partially defunctioned after surgery and patella maltracking may easily occur. Suturing the wound with the knee in flexion helps identify if excessive tension is being applied with closure.

COMPLICATIONS

- The peroneal branch of the sciatic nerve is particularly vulnerable to traction injuries because it is firmly held in place by the fascia lata at the fibular neck as it melds with the deep fascia of the lower leg and also the deep and superficial branches of the nerve soon after it enters the lower leg. Resection of the distal femur allows significant movement of the proximal femur. Thus, uncontrolled movements between the thigh and lower leg must be avoided once the distal femur is excised to protect the nerve against injury.
- The popliteal artery may be traumatized during its dissection in the popliteal fossa. This may cause the artery to go into spasm and, if significant enough, may lead to distal ischemia. Additionally, spasm in the artery may be a prelude for the development of arterial thrombosis, which may prolong ischemia or cause distal emboli with subsequent digital infarction. Careful handling of the artery should always be practiced, and vasodilators should be available if arterial spasm is severe. If thrombosis is suspected, an on-table angiogram should be performed and embolectomy undertaken if possible.
- Compartment syndrome is an important complication of distal femoral resection. The discomfort and pain of surgery must be assessed regularly to avoid missing a compartment syndrome. The cause of a compartment syndrome can usually be directly linked to the dissection of the popliteal artery and therefore, may begin anytime during or after surgery. The use of an epidural anesthetic may mask the symptoms of compartment syndrome. Frequent postoperative neurovascular observations are advised following this procedure regardless of what type of anesthetic is used. In general, the pain of compartment syndrome is very severe and this condition should be suspected if the standard postoperative pain is not easily resolved with standard levels of analgesia. Compartment syndrome is a clinical diagnosis and urgent fasciotomies should be considered if compartment syndrome is suspected. Compartment pressure monitoring may not be reliable and may give a false sense of security.
- Wound closure may be a problem if skin excision is included in the resection. This is particularly problematic if the reconstruction leaves the prosthesis exposed. Viable and healthy soft tissue cover is mandatory for

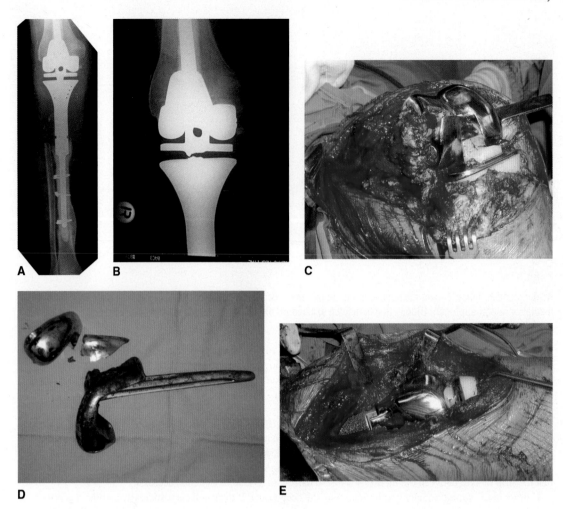

FIGURE 14.6

A: An 18-year-old man with a proximal tibial rotating hinge prosthesis for a knee osteosarcoma. He had previously fractured the stem of his tibial component requiring a revision of the proximal tibial component. Later, he developed a periprosthetic fracture at the level of the tip of his tibial prosthesis stem. **B:** The same patient presented 2 years later with an unstable knee and radiograph demonstrated a fracture through the rotating hinge component of his prosthesis. This was revised to a new rotating hinge component. **C:** Twelve months after the fracture of the axis of his joint, he represented with a clicking in his knee. At operation, a fracture of the lateral femoral condyle was noted. The femoral component was revised to a similar component. **D:** Two years after the fracture of his prosthetic femoral condyle, the patient represented with further clicking in his knee, and had catastrophic fracture of the femoral component treated by revision to a distal femoral tumor endoprosthesis (Fig. 14.6E).

prosthetic implant. Vulnerable sites include the medial and lateral aspects of the proximal tibia. Mobilization of the gastrocnemius muscle and its transposition over the prosthesis is an excellent solution for gaining soft tissue cover. The external surface of the gastrocnemius flap can then be skin grafted.

- Lateral patella subluxation or dislocation is a risk with distal femoral resections. An approach from the lateral side may result in a tight repair during closure, which may tether the patella laterally such that with flexion the patella dislocates laterally. This may be compounded by the use of a rotating hinge prosthesis that permits the leg to rotate laterally on the hinge mechanism, which increases the Q angle and further exacerbates patella maltracking. This should be avoided at all costs with appropriate positioning of the implants, repair of the arthrotomy without lateral tethering of the patella, and protection against uncontrolled and persistent external rotation of the lower leg in relation to the knee.
- Fracture of the prosthesis is an uncommon complication and may occur in particularly active individuals (Fig. 14.6A–E). The modularity of the megaprostheses allows salvage of limb salvage.

REFERENCES

1. Shin DS, Choong PF, Chao EY, et al. Large tumor endoprostheses and extracortical bone-bridging: 28 patients followed 10–20 years *Acta Orthop Scand*. 2000;71:305–311.
2. Choong PF, Sim FH. Limb-sparing surgery for bone tumors: new developments *Semin Surg Oncol*. 1997;13:64–69.

3. Harrison RJ Jr, Thacker MM, Pitcher JD, et al. Distal femur replacement is useful in complex total knee arthroplasty revisions *Clin Orthop Relat Res.* 2006;446:113–120.

4. Haspl M, Jelic M, Pecina M. Arthroplasty in treating knee osteoarthritis and proximal tibia stress fracture *Acta Chir Orthop Traumatol Cech.* 2003;70:303–305.

5. Wang J, Temple HT, Pitcher JD, et al. Salvage of failed massive allograft reconstruction with endoprosthesis *Clin Orthop Relat Res.* 2006;443:296–301.

6. Stumpf UC, Eberhardt C, Kurth AA. Orthopaedic limb salvage with a mega prosthesis in a patient with haemophilia A and inhibitors—a case report *Haemophilia.* 2007;13:435–439.

7. Whittaker JP, Dharmarajan R, Toms AD. The management of bone loss in revision total knee replacement *J Bone Joint Surg Br.* 2008;90:981–987.

8. DiCaprio MR. Friedlaender GE. Malignant bone tumors: limb sparing versus amputation *J Am Acad Orthop Surg.* 2003;11:25–37.

9. Aksnes LH, Bauer HC, Jebsen NL, et al. Limb-sparing surgery preserves more function than amputation: a Scandinavian sarcoma group study of 118 patients *J Bone Joint Surg Br.* 2008;90:786–794.

10. Sluga M, Windhager R, Lang S, et al. Local and systemic control after ablative and limb sparing surgery in patients with osteosarcoma *Clin Orthop Relat Res.* 1999;358:120–127.

11. Grimer RJ, Carter SR, Pynsent PB. The cost-effectiveness of limb salvage for bone tumors *J Bone Joint Surg Br.* 1997;79:558–561.

12. Wafa H, Grimer RJ. Surgical options and outcomes in bone sarcoma *Expert Rev Anticancer Ther.* 2006;6:239–248.

13. Quan GM, Slavin JL, Schlicht SM, et al. Osteosarcoma near joints: assessment and implications *J Surg Oncol.* 2005;91:159–166.

14. Orlic D, Smerdelj M, Kolundzic R, et al. Lower limb salvage surgery: modular endoprosthesis in bone tumour treatment *Int Orthop.* 2006;30:458–464.

15. Sanjay BK, Moreau PG. Limb salvage surgery in bone tumor with modular endoprosthesis *Int Orthop.* 1999;23:41–46.

15 Megaprosthesis of the Knee for Non-Neoplastic Conditions

Bryan D. Springer

The primary use for megaprostheses about the knee has been for reconstruction of the distal femur and proximal tibia after resection of a neoplasm (1–4). Complex primary and revision total knee arthroplasty (TKA) in patients with massive bone loss, ligamentous instability, or both is a significant challenge. Prosthetic knee design with articular constraint often is needed and hinged knee implant may be required in complex situations (5–7).

Previous fixed hinge designs have been associated with high failure rates because of increased transmission of stress to the bone-cement interface (Figs. 15.1 and 15.2) (8). With the advent of a rotating hinge design, the rotational freedom allows for dissipation of stresses from the bone-cement interface and a more anatomically matched prosthesis (9–11). The purpose of this chapter is to evaluate the current indication, surgical techniques, and results of a megaprosthesis of the knee in nonneoplastic conditions.

INDICATIONS

Megaprosthetic replacement of the knee is utilized as a salvage procedure for complex primary or revision TKA. The use of a megaprosthetic component in primary and revision knee surgery is relatively uncommon. Reports in the literature range form 0.14% to 13% of all revision knees (12, 13).

The ideal candidate for the use of a megaprosthesis is an elderly, low-demand patient with extensive distal femoral or proximal tibial bone loss. These patients may benefit substantially from early mobilization. Cemented megaprosthetic replacement allows for immediate weight bearing and transfers as early as postoperative day 1. Specific indications include

- Limb salvage following periarticular tumor resection
- Severe bony deficiency with associated collateral ligament disruption
- Extensor mechanism disruption
- Significant flexion and extension gap mismatch
- Acute treatment of supracondylar femur fractures with substantial bone loss in elderly patients
- Treatment of periprosthetic fractures about the knee with associated severe bone loss and/or poor bone quality (osteoporosis) in low-demand patients (Fig. 15.3)
- Salvage of previous nonunion/malunion of periprosthetic fracture about the knee (Fig. 15.4)

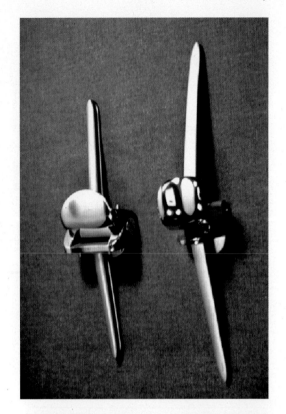

FIGURE 15.1

Early hinge designs were fixed hinges that only allowed motion in flexion and extension.

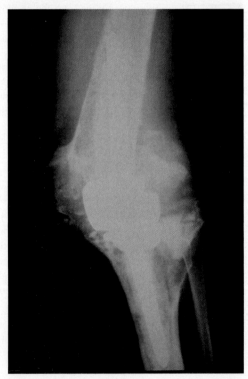

FIGURE 15.2

Due to high prosthetic constraint of early hinge designs, loosening was a common mode of failure.

CONTRAINDICATIONS

Contraindications for the use of megaprosthetic replacement in TKA include

- Patients medically unfit to undergo surgery
- Active infection of the limb
- Poor soft tissue coverage
- Higher demand patients in whom the limb can be reconstructed with allograft or standard primary or revision components

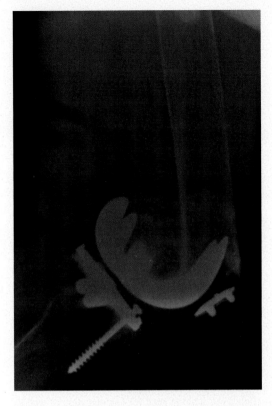

FIGURE 15.3

Distal femoral periprosthetic fracture above a TKA. The bone is of poor quality (osteoporotic) and there is little remaining host bone to allow for distal fixation.

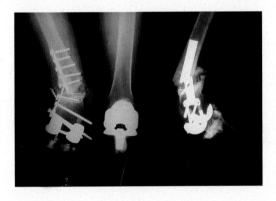

FIGURE 15.4

Nonunion/malunion of a supracondylar periprosthetic femur fracture.

PREOPERATIVE PREPARATION

As with any primary or revision TKA, preoperative planning is essential.

Imaging

Appropriate radiographs should include a standing anterior-posterior view, lateral view and merchant view. Each of these x-rays should be evaluated to assess bone loss and quality of remaining host bone. In addition, a long leg hip to ankle view may be utilized to asses the overall mechanical alignment of the extremity and to asses for other hardware that may interfere with placement of a long stemmed hinged TKA (e.g., total hip arthroplasty above a TKA).

Preoperative examination should include

- Examination of skin for color, temperature changes and effusion that would indicate infection
- Evaluation of old incisions
- Vascular and neurologic status of the limb
- Range of motion
- Collateral ligament stability
- Function of the extensor mechanism
- Recurvatum deformity

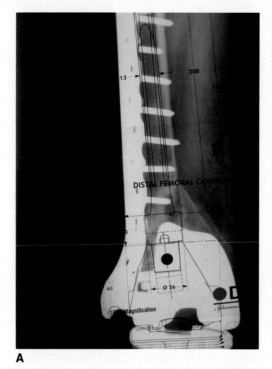
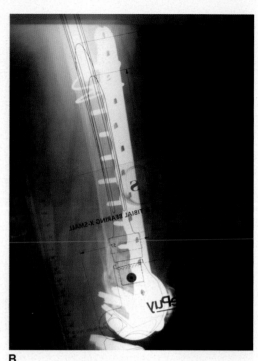

A   **B**

FIGURE 15.5

A,B: Preoperative templating to determine length of distal femoral resection as well as length and diameter of intramedullary stems is a crucial part of preoperative planning.

Templating of both the femoral and tibial components are mandatory. In addition to estimating the size of the components, templating is utilized to estimate bone resection levels and the need for augmentation as well as the length, position, and size of intramedullary stems (Figs. 15.5 A,B).

TECHNIQUE

Position and Draping

Patients should be placed supine on the operative table and all bony prominences well padded. A nonsterile tourniquet can be placed proximally on the upper thigh. The positioning should allow for free mobility of the operative limb throughout the full range of flexion and extension. A leg positioner should be used to allow the knee to flex and rest at 90 degrees and to assist in femoral and tibial preparation. In cases where large resections of the distal femur or proximal tibia are required, the entire extremity to include the groin and pelvis should be prepared and draped free.

Incision and Exposure

The approach to the knee is determined by the previous surgical incisions and the condition of the soft tissue around the knee. Whenever possible, prior incision should be utilized. When multiple incisions are present, use the most laterally based incision. Any flaps that are created should be full thickness to avoid compromise of the blood supply to the skin. Standard medial parapatellar approach or extensile exposures may be required. Once exposed, removal of the failed tibial and femoral components should proceed, preserving as much of the remaining bone as possible. Remove all cement and debris and debride all bony surface down to good quality bone.

Tibial Preparation

Prepare the tibial canal and establish a proximal tibial supportive bony platform perpendicular to the mechanical axis.

- The tibial surface may be cut utilizing extramedullary or intramedullary instrumentation (Fig. 15.6).
- The tibial canal is prepared by reaming to the appropriate size and depth based on preoperative templating or until cortical contact is made (Fig. 15.7).
- Determine the appropriate depth of the tibial resection. The purpose of this cut is to obtain a flat, supportive bony platform. It may be unnecessary to cup below all defects as these may be filled in with bone graft or augmented.
- Cut the proximal tibial using the preferred instrumentation. Determine the need for block or wedge augmentation and make the appropriate bony cuts on the tibia. The tibial baseplate can then be sized. A trial tibial component with the appropriate length stem trial and augments can then be inserted (Fig. 15.8).

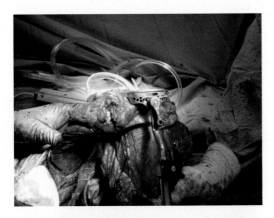

FIGURE 15.6

Tibia can be cut using either intramedullary or extramedullvary (shown here) alignment guides perpendicular to the mechanical axis of the tibia.

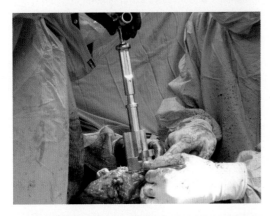

FIGURE 15.7

The intramedullary canal of the tibial is prepared with the appropriate reamers.

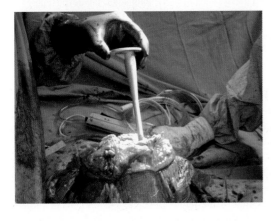

FIGURE 15.8

The trial tibial implant can be placed to ensure a stable tibial platform.

Distal Femoral Resection

The rotation of the femoral component is critical to achieving proper flexion gap symmetry and patellofemoral mechanics. In the revision setting, however, many of the key bony landmarks used to determine femoral component rotation such as the epicondylar axis, posterior condylar axis and trochlear grove are absent or damaged (Fig. 15.9). Prior to diaphyseal resection it is imperative to mark the rotation of the deepest section of the trochlear groove on the remaining diaphyseal segment. This will allow for correct femoral prosthesis rotational alignment (Fig. 15.10).

The length of the femur to be resected is measured with calipers and matched with the sizes of available implants for the particular implant system being utilized. This is confirmed with the preoperative templating plan. The femur is then osteotomized perpendicular to the long axis.

Femoral Canal Preparation

- Identify and progressively ream the femoral canal to the appropriate size based on preoperative templating or until cortical contact is made. Avoid eccentric reaming of the femoral shaft.
- The canal should be reamed to 2 mm over the anticipated stem diameter based on preoperative templating to allow for adequate cement mantle.
- If a bowed femoral stem is to be utilized, the femoral canal should be flexibly reamed.

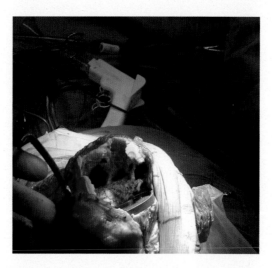

FIGURE 15.9

In patients with massive distal femoral bone loss, bony landmarks used to determine femoral component rotation are often absent.

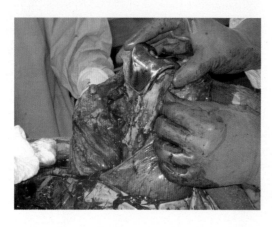

FIGURE 15.10

In the absence of bony landmarks, the deepest part of the trochlear groove should be marked on the diaphysis prior to distal femoral resection to allow for proper femoral component rotation.

BALANCE THE KNEE IN FLEXION

- Keeping in mind that a hinged TKA is often indicated to treat a significant flexion/extension gap mismatch (>10 mm), an attempt should be made to maximize stability in flexion.

BALANCE THE KNEE IN EXTENSION

- Extension gap stability is achieved by distal augmentation of the femur (loose extension gap) or further resection of the distal femur (tight extension gap). Most hinge system will allow a certain degree of hyperextension. This is usually limited with an extension stop bumper. It is important to limit any hyperextension so as to avoid stress on the bumper that could result in implant breakage.

Perform a Trial Reduction and intraoperative Radiographic Evaluation.

- When reasonable gap balance is achieved, assemble the trial component with the appropriate stem length and diameter.

With the appropriate trial in place, the knee should be taken through a range of motion to ensure proper stability and patellar tracking. Particular attention should be paid to patellofemoral tracking, one of the most common complications associated with hinged TKA. If patellar tracking is inappropriate, femoral component rotation must be evaluated and adjusted accordingly. The femur can be flexed to 90 degrees and the femoral component rotated so it is parallel to the cut tibial surface. The hinged components will substitute for coronal and sagittal plan imbalance. Intraoperative radiographs with trial components are recommended to ensure appropriate alignment of the extremity, restoration of joint line and position of stems within the intramedullary canal of the femur (Figs. 15.11.A,B) .

Assembly and Insertion of Real Components

If intraoperative trialing and radiographs confirms appropriate alignment, stability and patellofemoral tracking, the real implants should be opened. Meticulous care and attention should be paid to assembly of the real components. The operating surgeon or an experienced assistant should assemble the real components on the

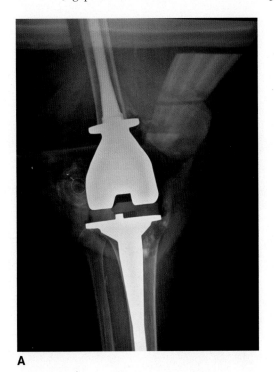

A

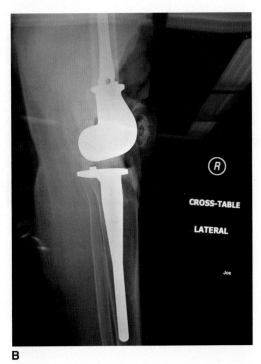

B

FIGURE 15.11

A,B: Intraoperative radiographs with the trial components in place are used to determine overall alignment and placement of the components.

back table. Ensure the appropriate stem length, diameter, and offset match the intraoperative trials. If necessary, insert the real components provisionally into the bone to ensure proper fit.

The femoral and tibial canals should be copiously lavaged and dried. The distal diaphyseal bone of the femur and tibia should be restricted with a canal plug if cemented stems are to be used. The tibial and femoral components should be cemented separately under separate mixing conditions allowing for the cement to fully cure before proceeding to cementing the next component.

Once all components have been cemented, the linked polyethylene is assembled. Care should be taken to ensure proper assembly of the linking mechanism (Figs. 15.12 A–D and 15.13 A–C). Stability and patellar tracking should again be assessed, ensuring proper patellofemoral tracking.

Each rotating hinge system that is available has a different mechanism of linked constraint between the femoral and the tibial component. It is important for the surgeon to be familiar with the system being used to ensure proper assembly.

PEARLS AND PITFALLS

- If a large exposure is required, a sterile tourniquet should be utilized in order to allow exposure to the proximal aspect of the thigh, groin and pelvis.
- In patients with severe distal femoral, proximal tibial bone loss or resection of the distal femur or proximal tibial may be required. As such, familiarity with the distal femoral and popliteal space anatomy is important to avoid damage to the superficial femoral artery during distal femoral resection; the popliteal artery and sciatic nerve during posterior dissection; and the tibial artery, tibial nerve, and peroneal nerve during proximal tibial dissection and resection.
- Because hinged TKA is often used in a salvage situation, most patients have had multiple previous incisions. Large exposures and bony resection may often compromise the already tenuous soft tissue envelope. Consultation with a plastic surgeon preoperatively to assess the need for soft tissue coverage at the time of the procedure may be warranted in some cases.
- Ensure the tibial reamers remain in line with the shaft of the tibia when reaming. Retained cement, sclerotic bone, or tibial deformity may influence reamer position and lead to cortical perforation.
- In patients with substantial proximal bony deficiency, a long stem cemented or cementless tibial stem may be required for fixation. In patients with metaphyseal or diaphyseal deformity, an offset stem may be required to obtain appropriate alignment in the intramedullary canal.

POSTOPERATIVE MANAGEMENT

- Suction drainage should be utilized and left in place until drainage is <30 mL in 8 hours.
- Standard postoperative antibiotics are administered for 24 hours.

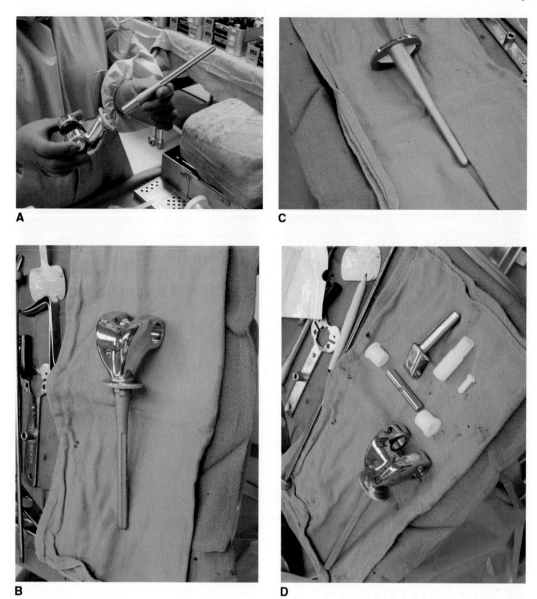

FIGURE 15.12

A–D: The real components should be assembled on the back table by the surgeon or someone familiar with the system to ensure proper assembly.

- Meticulous care should be taken with regards to the soft tissue envelope. Often times large exposure and lengthy surgical time can lead to soft tissue healing issues.
- Institution of physical therapy can be started when soft tissue envelope allows and progressed as tolerated.
- In general patients are allowed to weight bear as tolerated with an assistive device until quadriceps strength is adequate to allow for transfer to a cane.

COMPLICATIONS (SEE RESULTS)

Common complications following hinged TKA include

- Wound complications
- Patellofemoral complications
- Deep periprosthetic infection
- Hardware failure most commonly of axle/bushings

RESULTS

The largest experience with the rotating hinge design has been for the reconstruction of the distal femur and proximal tibia after resection of a neoplasm (1–4). Frequently, en bloc resection of the distal femur or proximal tibia or both is required to obtain adequate margins in tumor surgery. The development of custom implants and modularity has allowed for increased success of limb salvage in patients with musculoskeletal oncologic

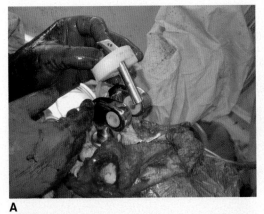

A

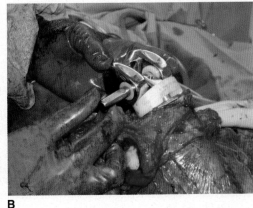

B

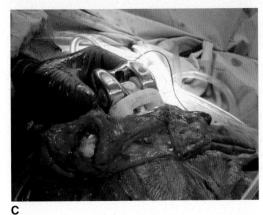

C

FIGURE 15.13

A–C: Once the real components have been assembled, care should be taken to assemble the axle, bushing, and yoke of the hinged prosthesis appropriately.

diseases. Likewise, patients with massive bone loss or ligamentous instability or both with nonneoplastic disorders may require a linked articulated implant to maintain skeletal continuity. Modular and segmental replacement allow for maintenance of motion and functional restoration. Alternative options include reconstruction with a large segmental allograft, arthrodesis, or amputation. With advent of newer prosthetic design, hinged TKA is being used with increasing frequency in revision TKA (14–16).

Although long-term results for the proximal femoral replacement for nonneoplastic disease have been reported, due to the rarity with which megaprosthetic replacement is required in TKA the literature is devoid of large outcomes series.

Springer et al reported on 25 patients using the modular segmental kinematic rotating hinge prosthesis for nonneoplastic limb salvage (17). The indications included nonunion of supracondylar periprosthetic femur fractures, severe bone loss and ligamentous instability, acute periprosthetic fracture, and fracture of a previous hinge prosthesis. The average age of the patients was 72 years. At a mean follow-up of 58 months, both Knee Society knee and functional scores improved. There were eight complications (31%) with the most common being infection. The patients in this study had significant resolution of pain and improvement in motion, functional outcome, and overall satisfaction. The authors concluded, however, that because of high complication and infection rates, the rotating hinge prosthesis should be reserved as a final salvage option.

Utting and Newman used a customized hinged knee replacement for the salvage of limb threatening situations in elderly patients (18). Indications included periprosthetic fracture, massive osteolysis/bone loss and reimplantation following deep infection. Twenty-five patients had mid to long term follow-up. Infection was the most common complication but no prosthesis had failed for aseptic complications.

Rosen et al reported on the use of segmental distal femoral replacement for the acute treatment of complex distal femur fractures in the elderly patients (19). Twenty-four patients (average age 76 years) were followed for an average of 11 months. Seventy-one percent resumed their prefracture level of ambulation. No significant surgical or medical complications were reported. Other smaller series have likewise reported improved pain relief and the ability for rapid mobilizations in this select group of elderly patients (20–22).

Megaprosthetic reconstruction of the knee for nonneoplastic conditions should be considered a salvage operation for the low demand elderly patient. New prosthetic designs have led to improved outcomes. While the majority of studies show a relatively high complication rate, this procedure allows for rapid mobilizations and restoration of function in this patient group. Meticulous preoperative planning and surgical technique are of paramount importance to ensure a successful outcome and minimize complications.

REFERENCES

1. Choong PF, Sim FH, Pritchard DJ, et al. Megaprostheses after resection of distal femoral tumors: a rotating hinge design in 30 patients followed for 2–7 years. *Acta Orthop Scand.* 1996;67:345–351.
2. Kawai A, Muschler GF, Lane JM, et al. Prosthetic knee replacement after resection of a malignant tumor of the distal part of the femur: medium to long-term results. *J Bone Joint Surg.* 1998;80A:636–647.
3. Shih LY, Sim FH, Pritchard DJ, et al. Segmental total knee arthroplasty after distal femoral resection for tumor. *Clin Orthop* 1993;292:269–281.
4. Frink SJ, Rutledge J, Lewis VO, et al. Favorable long-term results of prosthetic arthroplasty of the knee for distal femur neoplasms. *Clin Orthop.* 2005;438:65–70.
5. Cuckler JM. Revision total knee arthroplasty: How much constraint is necessary? *Orthopedics.* 1995;18:932–936.
6. Hartford JM, Goodman SB, Schurman DJ, et al. Complex primary and revision total knee arthroplasty using the condylar constrained prosthesis: an average 5-year follow-up. *J Arthroplasty.* 1998;13:380–387.
7. Karpinski MR, Grimer RJ. Hinged knee replacement in revision arthroplasty. *Clin Orthop.* 1987;220:185–191.
8. Jones EC, Insall JN, Inglis AE, et al. GUEPAR knee arthroplasty results and late complications. *Clin Orthop.* 1979;140:145–152.
9. Draganich LF, Whitehurst JB, Chou LS, et al. The effects of the rotating-hinge total knee replacement on gait and stair stepping. *J Arthroplasty.* 1999;14:743–755.
10. Kabo JM, Yang RS, Dorey FJ, et al. In vivo rotational stability of the kinematic rotating hinge knee prosthesis. *Clin Orthop.* 1997;336:166–176.
11. Kester MA, Cook SD, Harding AF, et al. An evaluation of the mechanical failure modalities of a rotating hinge knee prosthesis. *Clin Orthop.* 1988;228:156–163.
12. Springer BD, Sim FH, Hanssen AD, et al. The kinematic rotating hinge prosthesis for complex knee arthroplasty. *Clin Orthop.* 2001;392:181–187.
13. Barrack RL, Lyons TR, Ingraham RQ, et al. The use of a modular rotating hinge component in salvage revision total knee arthroplasty. *J Arthroplasty.* 2000;15:858–66.
14. Barrack RL. Evolution of the rotating hinge for complex total knee arthroplasty. *Clin Orthop.* 2001;392:292–299.
15. Barrack RL. Rise of the rotating hinge in revision total knee arthroplasty. *Orthopedics.* 2002;25:1020.
16. Jones RE, Barrack RL, Skedros J. Modular, mobile-bearing hinge total -knee arthroplasty. *Clin Orthop.* 2001;392:306–14.
17. Springer BD, Sim FH, Hanssen AD, et al. The modular segmental kinematic rotating hinge for nonneoplastic limb salvage. *Clin Orthop.* 2004;421:181–187.
18. Utting MR, Newman JH. Customised hinged knee replacements as a salvage procedure for failed total knee arthroplasty. *Knee.* 2004;11:475–479.
19. Rosen AL. Strauss E. Primary total knee arthroplasty for complex distal femur fractures in elderly patients. *Clin Orthop.* 2004;425:101–105.
20. Davila J, Malkani A, Paiso JM. Supracondylar distal femoral nonunions treated with a megaprosthesis in elderly patients: a report of two cases. *J Orthop Trauma.* 2001;15:574–578.
21. Freedman EL, Hak DJ, Johnson EE, et al. Total knee arthroplasty including a modular distal femoral component in elderly patients with acute fracture or nonunion. *J Orthop Trauma.* 1995;9: 231–237.
22. Harrison RJ Jr, Thacker MM, Pitcher JD, et al. Distal femur replacement is useful in complex total knee arthroplasty revisions. *Clin Orthop.* 2006;446:113–120.

16 Megaprosthesis of the Distal Femur

Kristy L. Weber

The distal femur is a common site for primary malignant bone tumors and, therefore, it frequently requires resection and reconstruction in an orthopedic oncology practice. In addition, patients who require multiple revision surgeries after a routine total knee replacement (TKR) for degenerative arthritis may end up with substantial bone loss, necessitating a resection of the distal femur. Therefore, this chapter is relevant to both orthopedic oncologists and revision knee surgeons alike. The examples provided are primarily from patients with bone tumors, but the technique section should apply to both situations. For more detail related to reconstruction for non-neoplastic conditions, see chapter 15. Although reconstructive options after resection of the distal femur include an osteoarticular allograft, allograft-prosthetic composite, and allograft arthrodesis, this chapter focuses on the use of a distal femoral megaprosthesis with rotational hinged knee replacement. The rationale for the modular rotational hinged knee design is that it provides stability in the anterior-posterior and varus-valgus planes while allowing rotation of the tibia on the femur. Theoretically, stress at the bone-cement interface is diffused by this rotational ability and decreases the risk of aseptic loosening. The goal of this type of reconstruction (as opposed to allograft or arthrodesis reconstruction) is to provide the patient a rigid, durable reconstruction that will allow immediate weight bearing (cemented stems).

INDICATIONS

The indications below do not distinguish between cemented and uncemented prosthetic designs. In general, the choice between these options is surgeon-dependent as both are reported in the literature with similar outcomes.

- Patients who require resection of the distal femur for aggressive benign or malignant primary bone tumors (Figs. 16.1 and 16.2)
- Patients who require resection of the distal femur for malignant soft tissue sarcomas that invade the bone
- Patients with extensive metastatic disease to the distal femur with destruction of the condyles and no good option for stable nonprosthetic fixation
- Patients with bony tumor recurrence or aseptic loosening of a distal femoral megaprosthesis
- Patients with severe distal femoral bone loss combined with ligamentous instability
- Patients with an acute periprosthetic femur fracture or nonunion that cannot be stabilized or healed with a stemmed revision prosthesis, allograft struts, or internal fixation
- Patients with a history of high dose radiation to the distal thigh or femur and a subsequent fracture (Fig. 16.3)
- Patients with failed fixation or nonunion of a distal femoral fracture (Fig. 16.4)
- Patients with severe osteoporosis and a complex supracondylar or intracondylar femur fracture

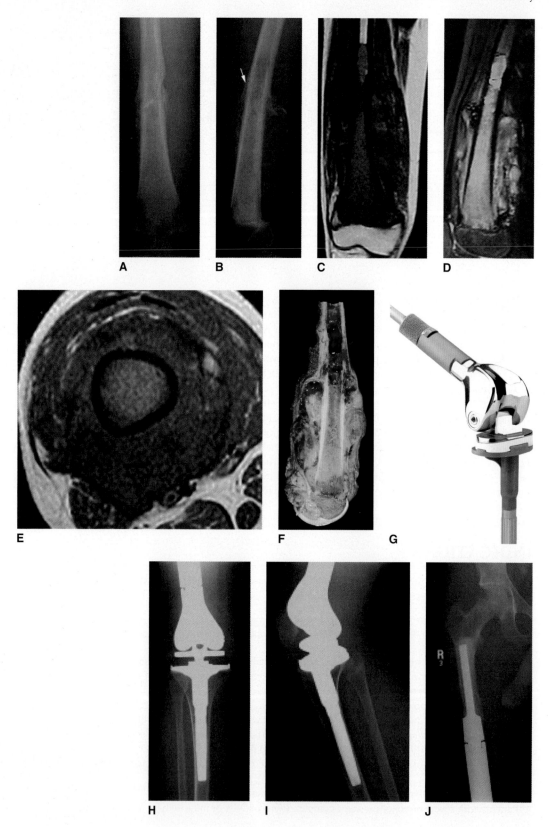

FIGURE 16.1

AP (**A**) and lateral (**B**) radiographs of the right mid-distal femur in a 15-year-old boy with an osteosarcoma after several months of neoadjuvant chemotherapy. Note the periosteal elevation and Codman's triangle at the proximal extent of the tumor (see *arrow*). Coronal T1-weighted (**C**), sagittal T2-weighted (**D**), and axial T1-weighted (**E**) MR images of the distal femur showing the extent of marrow involvement and proximity of the tumor to the posterior neurovascular structures. **F:** Lateral view of the gross specimen. **G:** Actual picture of the cemented prosthesis with a metal stemmed tibial component. AP (**H**) and lateral (**I**) radiographs of the cemented reconstruction. **J:** AP radiograph showing the small remaining segment of proximal femur with a cemented stem.

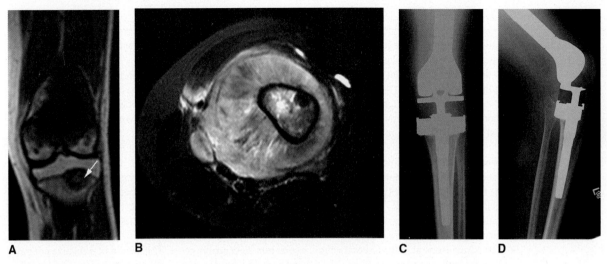

FIGURE 16.2

Coronal T1-weighted (**A**) and axial STIR (**B**) MR images of the left distal femur in a 16-year-old boy with metastatic osteosarcoma to the lungs and a skip metastasis in the ipsilateral proximal tibia (see arrow). AP (**C**) and lateral (**D**) postoperative radiographs show a cemented distal femoral prosthesis as well as an augmented proximal tibia after the skip metastasis was resected. This allowed his patellar tendon attachment to be maintained. A cemented metal stemmed tibial component was used.

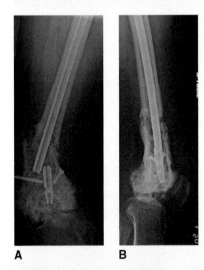

FIGURE 16.3

AP (**A**) and lateral (**B**) radiographs of the left distal femur in a 43-year-old man who was previously treated with radiation for a distal femoral lymphoma. He developed a late postradiation femur fracture treated with a locked intramedullary rod. Eventually it progressed to a nonunion with hardware failure. This clinical scenario would be an indication for a distal femoral prosthetic reconstruction.

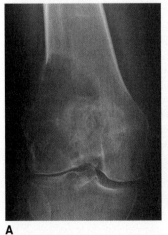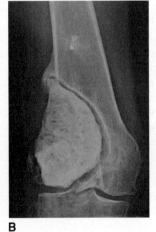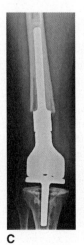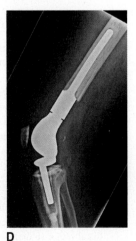

FIGURE 16.4

A: AP radiograph of the right distal femur in a 63-year-old woman with a giant cell tumor of the lateral femoral condyle. This was treated with curettage and cementation of the lesion. **B:** AP radiograph of the distal femur 16 months after surgery that shows an intercondylar fracture that has not healed and causes pain and disability. AP (**C**) and lateral (**D**) radiographs after salvage with a cemented distal femoral prosthesis.

CONTRAINDICATIONS

- Patients in whom an adequate surgical margin cannot be obtained with resection and reconstruction. In these cases, an amputation should be considered.
- Patients with significant comorbidities such that they would not survive the procedure (i.e., cardiac, pulmonary)
- Patients with an infected knee joint, history of knee infection or systemic sepsis (although there are options short of amputation to reimplant a megaprosthesis after clearing the infection with intravenous antibiotics and an antibiotic-impregnated cement spacer within the knee joint)
- Patients receiving chemotherapy who have not had a reasonable recovery of their absolute neutrophil count prior to surgery (author prefers ANC > 1,500)
- Patients whose malignant bone tumor or skip metastasis extends to within 130 mm of the proximal end of the femur as this does not allow stable fixation of the distal femoral stem. In this case a total femoral replacement can be considered.
- Patients whose distal femoral sarcoma has progressed while on chemotherapy. These patients are usually not candidates for limb salvage surgery.
- Tumor involvement of the femoral neurovascular bundle or sciatic nerve. This would be a relative contraindication as these structures can be resected and bypassed, but the overall function of the leg is decreased.
- Tumor involvement of the surrounding quadriceps to a significant degree that requires complete removal of the compartment is a relative contraindication. A free, innervated latissimus dorsi flap can be used in these situations to regain some knee extension.
- Patients who are extremely young, as the prosthesis is often custom-made and will require multiple revisions as well as limb/prosthetic lengthening. This is a relative contraindication. The author generally recommends rotationplasty or amputation to patients <10 years old as this is usually definitive surgery and requires no restriction from physical activities. The author acknowledges that there are expandable custom implants currently used in very young children for limb salvage procedures.

PREOPERATIVE PREPARATION

Patient Expectations

It is imperative to confirm the patient's understanding of the goals and likely outcomes of the surgery prior to the procedure. The surgery is being done to provide local control of a malignant bone tumor or to salvage a prior failed reconstruction and should be agreed upon by the patient and surgeon (and family for children <18 years of age) as the most appropriate procedure. The patient will be expected to work diligently in the postoperative period to regain knee motion and quadriceps strength in order to walk as normally as possible. This will require regular exercise and, often, formal physical therapy. Depending on whether a cemented or uncemented prosthetic design is used, the patient may be restricted initially from placing full weight on the extremity. The patient needs to be aware of the long-term outcomes of distal femoral reconstruction with a megaprosthesis, which include aseptic loosening. The surgeon may suggest restrictions on impact loading activities to maximize the lifespan of the prosthesis, and this may affect a patient's lifestyle or recreational activities.

History/Physical Examination

At the time of the preoperative consultation, an updated history and physical examination should be performed with careful attention to recent changes in signs and symptoms such as pain, neurologic status, fevers, fatigue, weight-bearing status, recent infection, and injury to the extremity. On physical examination, the entire extremity should be carefully assessed for knee passive and active range of motion, motor strength (especially quadriceps), deformity, sensation, leg length discrepancy, signs of an infected knee joint, abrasions to the extremity, ingrown toenails, or a rash. Prior incisions or open biopsy tracts should be documented, and it should be determined if this will influence the surgical approach. The author is not concerned about the presence of needle biopsy tracts and does not excise them during the procedure, but there are differing opinions on this point.

Radiographs

In the older, nononcologic patient, plain radiographs that include an appropriate amount of femur and tibia as well as a chest radiograph should be sufficient. Oncology patients should have new plain radiographs of the distal femur to include the knee and a postchemotherapy MRI scan to assess any change in tumor size. If the local tumor has progressed while on chemotherapy, the patient is likely no longer indicated for a limb salvage procedure. The MRI scan will also allow careful evaluation of the marrow extent of tumor so that the resection can be done with a clear margin. The status of the soft tissue and neurovascular bundle involvement is critical. If the tumor involves the neurovascular structures, an MR angiogram or standard angiogram may be warranted. Oncology patients should also be restaged for their overall disease with a new chest CT scan. Generally, these patients have already had a bone scan to identify skip metastasis if present. Skip metastases in the femur are usually incorporated into the resection.

Laboratory Tests

Patients should have laboratory tests prior to surgery that include a complete blood count, protime, prothrombin time (PT), electrolytes, and a type and screen/cross for blood products. The hemoglobin should be assessed to determine the potential need for packed red blood cells during the case. For oncology patients, the white cell count (including absolute neutrophil count) should be adequate to minimize the chance of postoperative infection. It is also important to check the calcium and magnesium as these can be low with chemotherapy. Adult patients for revision knee surgery with a megaprosthesis should have laboratory studies that are appropriate for their comorbidities (i.e., liver function tests, etc.). If there is any concern for infection in the native knee or prior knee reconstruction, a C-reactive protein, erythrocyte sedimentation rate, and joint aspiration should be performed.

Consultations

The anesthesia team should be consulted in advance to determine the method of anesthesia (regional, general, or combined). It is critical in oncology patients or nononcology patients with a significant valgus deformity at the knee to check the neurologic status of the limb postoperatively. For patients who have received Adriamycin, a preoperative echocardiogram may be requested by the anesthesia team. For patients over 50 years old, an ECG is often necessary. Additional preoperative clearance may be necessary from the Cardiology, Pulmonary, or General Medicine services as determined by the patient's medical condition. In the oncology patient, a Plastic Surgery consultation should be obtained if a large soft tissue defect or loss of the quadriceps/extensor mechanism is anticipated as part of the tumor resection.

Equipment Needs

Templating for the anticipated prosthesis and stems is done on the preoperative radiographs. It is important to determine whether the femoral canal can accept the minimum standard diameter stem (usually 11 mm). If not, smaller stems need to be available. The length of the remaining proximal femur after resection should be determined, as 130 mm is necessary for standard length femoral stems. Additional equipment may be needed as follows:

- Cemented versus uncemented femoral component
- Polyethylene versus metal stemmed tibial component
- Supplemental autograft or allograft (possible allograft struts for revision cases)
- Patellar resurfacing component (The author does not resurface the patella in young oncology patients, but reserves this for older patients with arthritis affecting the patellofemoral joint).
- Intraoperative fluoroscopy
- Doppler to assess vascular supply to foot
- Cement removal instruments for revision cases
- Hardware removal instruments if internal fixation is present
- Body exhaust system/hood (depending on surgeon preference)

TECHNIQUE

This technique is primarily geared toward placement of a cemented prosthesis (cemented femoral stem and polyethylene stemmed tibial component). When appropriate, alternative technical points related to uncemented designs are noted. The use of a polyethylene tibial component, as opposed to one with a metal baseplate and modular stems, requires that the polyethylene component be adequately supported by cortical bone around its periphery. In cases of poor quality proximal femoral bone in either primary or revision situations, an uncemented Compress system (Biomet, Inc.) may be indicated (1). This chapter is not focused on the placement or lengthening techniques for expandable prostheses in skeletally immature patients.

Setup

The patient is placed in the supine position on an operating table that can accommodate fluoroscopic views. Anesthesia is given. The author prefers that the patient not be paralyzed for the resection when close dissection is required around the neurovascular bundle. A urinary catheter is placed. The leg is prepped and draped in its entirety (including the foot) above the level of the anterior superior iliac spine to allow for placement of a sterile tourniquet if necessary. The author uses a sandbag taped across the operating table at the level of the knee to facilitate stabilizing the knee in an upright flexed position during the reconstruction. A blood transfusion may be necessary intraoperatively or postoperatively, especially if the patient has been on preoperative chemotherapy, so an appropriate type and cross should be confirmed.

Incision

Elevate the extremity and inflate the tourniquet. Standard incision options include anterior and lateral. However, the incision may need to be modified to accommodate open biopsy scars or prior knee incisions. Prior open biopsy incisions need to be removed by incorporation into the new incision so as to avoid potentially leaving residual viable tumor cells in the scar. The author finds the anterior incision to be the most versatile and easiest to use if the patient requires subsequent revision knee surgery. Start the incision proximal to the level of planned femoral resection and end just medial to the tibial tubercle. Protect the patellar tendon throughout the case, especially when the patella is everted laterally.

Resection

The finer points of tumor resection can be supplemented from other textbooks, as this book is focused on the reconstructive techniques. It is presumed that an intra-articular resection will be performed in the vast majority of cases. Briefly, the distal femur is dissected circumferentially to allow for a safe resection. The author cuts longitudinally along the rectus femoris tendon during the initial exposure, leaving a small medial cuff of the tendon to facilitate a tight extensor mechanism repair. The patella is everted laterally, and the joint and joint fluid are inspected. If there is extensive hemorrhage or soft tissue to suggest that the tumor has contaminated the knee joint, an extra-articular resection should be considered. The vastus intermedius is usually left covering the underlying bone tumor, although at times more of the quadriceps should be resected depending on the size, extent of soft tissue mass, and location of the tumor. The vastus medialis is retracted medially. The medial collateral ligament is transected just proximal to the medial meniscus. Medially, the origin of the gastrocnemius and insertion of the adductor muscles are released from the femur. This may be facilitated by flexing the knee. Care must be taken when dissecting along the adductor canal, as the femoral vessels are tethered close to the medial femur in this location. The femoral vein is the most medial structure at this level, and there may be multiple branches draining the tumor. These are ligated so that the main neurovascular bundle can be retracted posteriorly. The medial intermuscular septum separating the anterior and posterior compartments of the thigh is incised to allow dissection along the distal posterior femur into the popliteal fossa. Branches of the popliteal artery and vein leading to and from the femoral intercondylar notch are dissected and ligated, as the vessels are tethered to the femur in this location. The medial dissection continues proximal to the level of the planned bone transection (the author prefers to cut the femur at least 2 cm further than the most proximal location of disease noted on a preoperative T1-weighted MR image).

For the lateral dissection, the lateral quadriceps and majority of the rectus femoris muscles are retracted laterally along with the patella, which is everted when possible. The lateral patellofemoral ligaments are cut. The lateral collateral ligaments are transected just proximal to the lateral meniscus. The lateral intermuscular septum separating the anterior and posterior thigh compartments is identified and carefully dissected to allow entrance to the posterior compartment. The origin of the lateral head of the gastrocnemius muscle is released from the femur. Dissection continues proximal to the level of planned bone transection and circumferential subperiosteal dissection is done at this level. Mark the mid-anterior femoral cortex just proximal to the planned cut with an osteotome and marking pen for later rotational alignment during the reconstruction. Do this prior to cutting the cruciate ligaments or the true rotation may be disrupted. The author prefers to then cut the femur proximally with a power saw perpendicular to the femur while protecting the posterior soft tissues with a malleable retractor. Other surgeons may prefer to disarticulate the femur at the knee joint and transect the femur at the end of the dissection. At this time, a large curette is used to obtain a frozen section at the proximal femoral marrow margin. After the sample is removed, bone wax is placed over the end of the bone to prevent spillage of marrow contents. Bone wax is also placed on the end of the distal femoral segment to prevent spillage from the tumor side. A Kern or other large clamp is used to elevate the distal femoral fragment from its proximal end and the dissection continues posteriorly to free the remaining soft tissue attachments. Meanwhile the frozen section is being analyzed as opposed to sending the frozen section after the complete resection, which can cause a delay prior to reconstruction while the tourniquet is still inflated. The anterior cruciate ligament (ACL) is sharply divided from its tibial insertion. The posterior cruciate is divided either anteriorly or posteriorly. The posterior knee capsule is finally divided while protecting the popliteal vessels. At this point the specimen is removed from the operative table, and the resection length is carefully measured from the cut proximal end to the medial joint line. At the author's institution, the musculoskeletal pathologist immediately cuts the distal femoral specimen coronally with a table saw so that the gross distance from the cut femoral end to the visible tumor can be measured. Along with the frozen section results, the surgeon uses this information to determine whether additional bone needs to be resected to allow for an adequate margin.

For patients with nononcologic indications for distal femoral resection, the femur can often be subperiosteally dissected to maintain the majority of the quadriceps. The remaining steps are similar. If a standard, unstemmed knee prosthesis is in place, the femur can be transected just proximal to the femoral component. The standard prosthetic distal femoral segment is 65 mm in length added to a length of 10 to 40 mm depending on whether a porous coated body segment is included with the stem; so this should be taken into account when planning the resection length. Use of the cement removal or cementless revision instruments is required when removing a stemmed femoral prosthesis. Fluoroscopic guidance is used to minimize the possibility of penetrating the cortex during prosthesis or cement removal. A cortical window proximal to the end of the stemmed femoral component can facilitate its removal, although this requires that onlay strut grafts are cabled to the femur during the reconstruction or a longer stemmed revision is used to bypass this cortical defect and minimize a postoperative fracture. The author uses a sterile tourniquet unless the dissection extends too proximally in the thigh. It is ideal if the entire resection and reconstruction can be completed within a 2-hour tourniquet time. If not, the tourniquet should ideally stay inflated throughout the resection until the margins are clear. It can then be reinflated after being deflated for at least 30 minutes.

Prosthetic Reconstruction

The operative team changes gowns, gloves, instruments, light handles, suction, electrocautery, and superficial drapes when performing a prosthetic reconstruction after malignant tumor resection. For a prosthetic revision case or for indications of massive bone loss or fracture without malignancy, this step is not necessary. The wound is irrigated with pulsed lavage saline with or without antibiotics and hemostasis is obtained (Fig. 16.5).

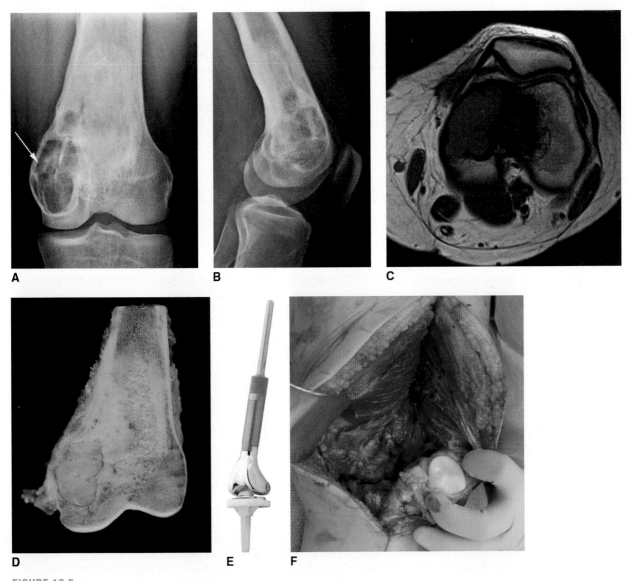

FIGURE 16.5

AP (**A**) and lateral (**B**) radiographs of an 18-year-old woman with a recurrent grade 1 fibrosarcoma of the left distal femur (see *arrow*). She was treated for a presumed benign tumor with curettage and bone grafting 1 year ago. **C:** T1-weighted axial MRI showing the endosteal cortical erosions from the tumor. There is minimal soft tissue extension medially. **D:** A coronal view of the gross resected specimen. **E:** An example of a distal femoral megaprosthesis with a polyethylene tibial component. **F:** View of the defect after tumor resection with the patella exposed showing no degenerative changes.

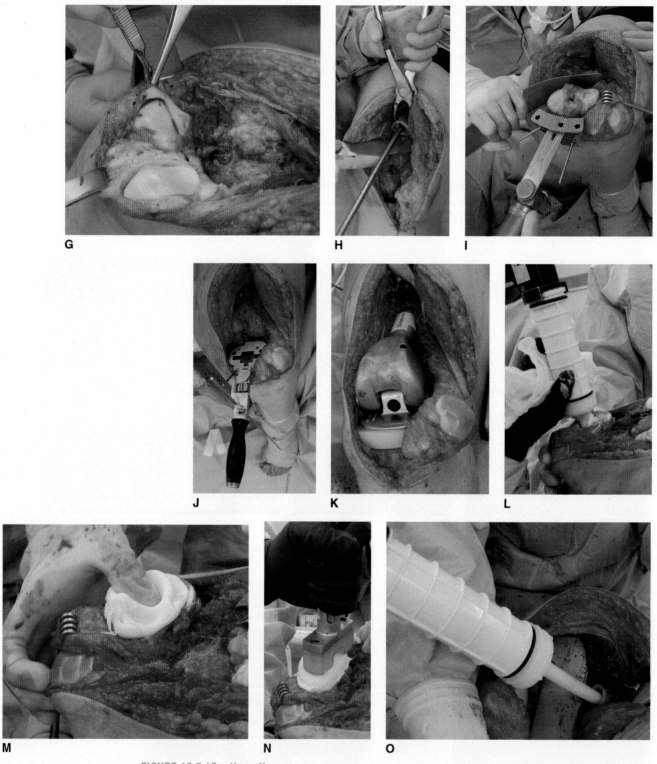

FIGURE 16.5 (*Continued*)

G: Sharp removal of the menisci from the tibial plateau. **H:** Flexible reaming of the proximal femur slightly further than the length of the prosthetic stem (for cemented stems). **I:** Making the tibial cut using the appropriate jigs. **J:** Using both an intramedullary and extramedullary alignment guide to judge rotation of the tibial tray. **K:** Placement of the trial prosthesis to assess length and tension on the neurovascular structures. **L:** Injection of cement into the tibia after the punches and keel have been used. No cement restrictor is necessary as a bone plug is created with the tibial punches. **M:** It is important to identify where the keel of the polyethylene tibial component will be placed within the cement to assure appropriate rotation. **N:** Placement of the real polyethylene component with excess cement removed. **O:** Injection of cement into the femur that was previously irrigated and dried.

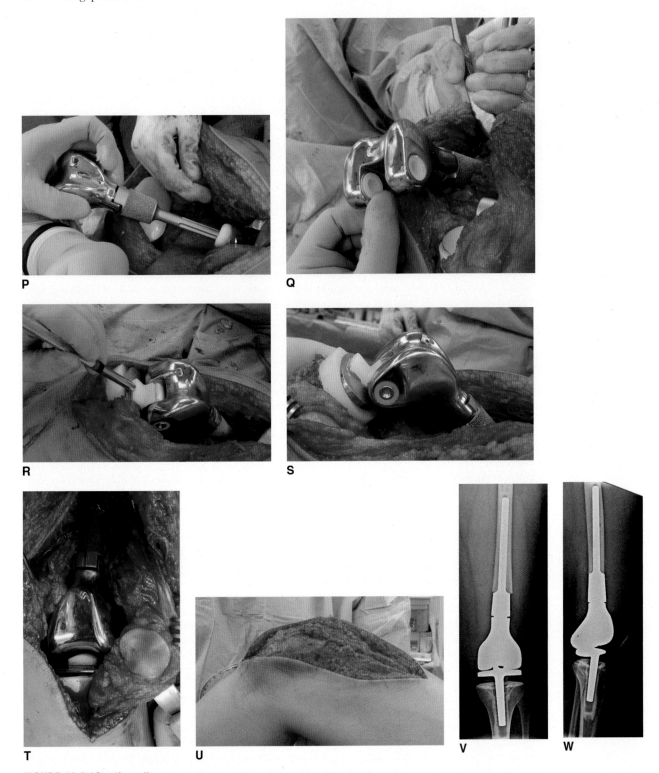

FIGURE 16.5 (*Continued*)

P: Placement of the real femoral prosthesis with attention to the appropriate rotation, which was marked earlier on the anterior femoral surface with an osteotome (see *arrow*) **Q:** Placement of the bushings within the femoral component. They are placed from the inner side of the prosthesis. After the femoral and tibial components are placed together, the metal axle locks them in place. **R:** Placement of the bumper to prevent hyperextension of the knee. **S:** Lateral view of the final reconstruction. **T:** AP view of the final reconstruction and patella. **U:** Testing the fascial repair to knee flexion of 90 degrees prior to final closure. AP (**V**) lateral (**W**) radiographs immediately postoperatively showing the cemented distal femoral prosthesis in good position.

The author starts with preparation of the femoral side. The bone wax is removed. For placement of a cemented femoral stem, a guide wire is placed into the femur and flexible reamers are used to enlarge the canal 2 mm larger than the planned femoral stem diameter. The largest diameter stem that does not require excessive removal of endosteal bone should be used (try to use a minimum of 11 mm [cemented] or *14 mm* [*uncemented*]). Reaming should extend several centimeters proximal to the length of the stem to allow for a cement restrictor. A standard femoral stem length is approximately 130 mm with additional lengths available up to over 200 mm. They are available in straight or curved versions with/without an attached porous-coated body segment. *For an uncemented femoral component, straight reamers are used with line-to-line reaming. For placement of a Compress uncemented stem, it requires implantation of an Anchor Plug with crossed pins and a Spindle at the prosthesis/bone interface to allow compression.* A planer reamer is used to prepare the distal end of the femur to fit perfectly with the taper of the real stem. Place the trial femoral stem in the canal at this point to be sure it fits well. The stem is removed, the femoral canal is packed to minimize blood loss, and attention is directed to preparation of the tibia.

The remaining menisci are sharply removed. The patellar tendon attachment on the tibia may need to be subperiosteally elevated to some degree to expose the anterior surface of the tibia. For revision cases, the tendon may be contracted and preclude full patellar eversion. The surgeon should be prepared to perform a tubercle osteotomy or lengthening of the extensor mechanism to achieve adequate exposure and facilitate placement of the revision components. A portion of the fat pad might be removed depending on surgeon preference. A drill is used to identify the tibial canal starting just anterior to the tibial insertion of the ACL. A T-handled canal finder is used to open the canal and assess the correct alignment (intramedullary). The author prefers to use both intramedullary and external alignment guides. The tibial cutting guide is placed and the surface is cut neutral to the tibial axis in all planes (i.e., no posterior slope) while protecting the posterior neurovascular structures with a malleable retractor. The patella is retracted carefully so as not to damage the cartilage surface in cases where it is not to be resurfaced. In cases of a malignant bone tumor, the tibial cartilage is often pristine, and the amount of bone removed should correlate with the thickness of polyethylene planned for the tibial component (usually 10 to 12 mm is removed). It is important to recreate the normal joint line for adequate patellar function. The trial tibial baseplate is placed on the tibial surface and aligned carefully with the longitudinal axis of the tibia. There should be no overhang of the tibial component when aligned in the correct rotation. If using an external alignment guide, the drop rod should align with the center of the ankle or second metatarsal. The baseplate is secured with pins, and the sequential tibial stem punches are used to prepare the bone for the polyethylene component. The trial tibial polyethylene component is placed along with the trial femoral component. The length of the entire trial reconstruction (from femoral body to bushings to polyethylene tibia) should equal the total bone resected from the femur and tibia. The femoral components are modular, so there are multiple segment length options. The author uses a porous coated body segment on the femoral stem if the resection length allows. Do not overlengthen the extremity in patients who have received preoperative chemotherapy, as there is a risk of peroneal or sciatic nerve palsy postoperatively from a stretch injury. Palpate the posterior neurovascular structures for tightness during knee extension and also check the distal pulses in the extremity. When placing an expandable prosthesis in a growing child, it is possible to safely lengthen the extremity approximately 1 cm. The femoral component should align with the rotational mark made on the anterior femoral cortex during the resection. Smooth flexion and extension of 110 to 120 degrees should be possible. If the patella does not track well, a lateral release can be performed. A lateral release is more often necessary in revision cases where the scarring is more extensive. If the patella requires resurfacing (for extensive degenerative changes or after removal of a prior patellar component), it can be cut freehand or by using the cutting guide. The tendency if cutting freehand is to take too much bone laterally and inferiorly. Use a caliper to determine whether the appropriate thickness of bone remains prior to placing the trial patellar component. In a revision situation, a metal tibial baseplate with modular stems may be used rather than a stemmed polyethylene component. In this scenario, straight handheld reamers are used during the initial tibial canal preparation and a cement restrictor may be used distal to the tip of the planned stem.

The femoral canal is now irrigated using a long-tipped pulse lavage system. For cemented stems, a cement restrictor is placed 1 to 2 cm beyond the planned stem length. Place the trial stem again to be sure the restrictor does not impede stem placement. The real femoral components are assembled on the back table. Pack the femoral canal while the cement is being mixed. The tibial canal and surface are also irrigated and packed, but generally no cement restrictor is necessary as the keel punches effectively create a "bone plug" distal to the planned end of the component. A cement gun is used with modern cementing technique. It is surgeon preference as to whether antibiotics are included within the cement for primary reconstruction scenarios. Antibiotics are commonly used in revision situations. The author cements the tibial polyethylene component (and patella if indicated) in one step. Pressure is maintained on the components until the cement is hard so that they do not rotate or "lift off" the bone. The femoral component is then cemented in the appropriate rotational alignment using a cement gun. Uncemented stems are placed using an impactor for a tight fit in the canal. The uncemented femoral stems have small antirotational fins on the prosthesis. Once the cement has hardened and all excess is removed, the tourniquet is released. The metal tibial rotating component, axle, and bumper (to prevent hyperextension of the knee) are placed, and the knee is flexed to at least 90 degrees with assessment of the neurovascular structures in full extension.

Closure

Hemostasis is obtained and irrigation is performed. Deep drains are placed to exit closely in line with the incision in tumor cases. A careful layered closure is performed with specific attention to the fascial repair around the patella, which should be reinforced with heavier suture. The repair should be tested with flexion of the knee to 90 degrees prior to closure of the subcutaneous layers. The author uses staples to close the skin as the incision crosses anteriorly over the knee. A sterile dressing is applied with care not to compress the peroneal nerve. The author places the leg in a continuous passive motion (CPM) before leaving the operating room. Calf high compression stockings and sequential compression devices are placed on both legs, and the patient is awakened and taken to the recovery room.

PEARLS AND PITFALLS

- Position the patient as distal as possible on the operating table in case fluoroscopy is necessary (for revision cases when cement needs to be removed from the femoral canal). Have the appropriate cement removal instruments available along with allograft struts and cables.
- Achieve an adequate margin even if it means resection of additional femoral bone.
- Maintain a soft tissue envelope around the distal femur if removing a malignant bone tumor.
- The adductors and gastrocnemius muscles do not need to be reattached after release from the femur.
- Mark the mid anterior cortex on the femur with an osteotome prior to transection to allow for appropriate rotation of the prosthetic component during reconstruction.
- Protect the femoral neurovascular bundle during the femoral and tibial cuts. There are usually branches of the artery and vein that course into the intercondylar notch and tether the vessels at this level.
- The operating team should change gowns, gloves, instruments, and superficial drapes after resection of a malignant bone tumor prior to prosthetic reconstruction to avoid contamination.
- Use a small curette to widen the medial and lateral flanges after using the tibial keel punches to allow enough space for the trial polyethylene component to fit easily.
- Be careful when initially extending the patient's knee after the trial implants are placed. Patients who receive preoperative chemotherapy are more sensitive to stretch on the peroneal nerve and may develop a temporary palsy if the limb is overlengthened.
- Consider cementing the tibial and femoral components separately to allow for excellent cement mantle without rushing. For young patients with malignant bone tumors, the author does not resurface the patella.
- Perform a lateral release if necessary for patellar tracking.
- Place the drains distal and closely in line with the incision for tumor cases.
- Reinforce the fascial repair around the patella during closure. Test this level of repair by flexing the knee 90 degrees before proceeding to the subcutaneous closure.
- If a CPM is to be used, the author advises placing it on the patient in the operating room and starting motion as soon as possible so the initial pain can be controlled in the recovery area prior to transfer to the inpatient unit.

POSTOPERATIVE MANAGEMENT

Medical Issues

Patients who receive neoadjuvant chemotherapy prior to the procedure may have a low hemoglobin. Even if the case is done with tourniquet control, there will likely be bleeding via the wound drains postoperatively (especially if the patient is using a CPM), and close monitoring of the blood count is necessary. Young patients can tolerate a lower hemoglobin than older patients, so symptoms of dizziness, headache, and orthostatic hypotension should be noted. In addition, patients previously receiving chemotherapy may need replacement of calcium or magnesium.

Postoperative antibiotics are given in accordance with documented protocols. However, there is some controversy as to whether immunocompromised cancer patients who have a large bone and soft tissue resection with reconstruction using a megaprosthesis should receive intravenous or oral antibiotics longer than what is mandated for routine procedures. This concern originates from the higher incidence of postoperative infection noted in these patients compared to patients who have a primary TKR for degenerative disease.

Pain Control/Neurologic Status

If the patient has general anesthesia, the postoperative pain is often controlled with narcotic medications via a PCA pump with later transition to oral medications. If the patient has a regional anesthetic (indwelling epidural, peripheral nerve blocks), it is important to establish a careful neurologic examination in the immediate postoperative period. The neurologic structures are sensitive to stretch especially in patients who receive neoadjuvant chemotherapy, and resection of large distal femoral tumors can result in a temporary peroneal or sciatic nerve palsy. If the patient has a regional anesthetic, the author prefers not to use a CPM postoperatively, as the patient may develop a peroneal palsy from direct pressure on the lateral calf by the CPM.

Rehabilitation

Patients who have had reconstruction with a cemented megaprosthesis can bear weight on the extremity on postoperative day 1. They will need assistive devices to ambulate until their quadriceps strength improves such that they can perform an unassisted straight leg raise. Patients with an uncemented stem often require protected weight bearing for 6 to 12 weeks. There are different views on whether to use a CPM postoperatively to assist with the knee range of motion. The author recommends a CPM for 3 to 5 days as an inpatient until the patient can achieve 90 degrees of passive knee motion in physical therapy. Many patients who have this procedure are young adolescents, and the author finds the CPM helpful when the patient's motivation to rehabilitate the knee is low. An ice pack is maintained on the distal thigh to decrease swelling and bleeding while in the CPM. The patient is sent home with an outpatient prescription for physical therapy to continue quadriceps strengthening, gait training, and knee range of motion.

COMPLICATIONS

The studies available for distal femoral prosthetic reconstruction usually include multiple variables as this is a relatively rare procedure. Thus, the complications are difficult to compare across series when both tumor and nontumor cases are included across multiple age groups with multiple types of stem fixation.

Infection

Prosthetic infections are often associated with severely immunocompromised patients, a prior history of prosthetic infection, or poor remaining soft tissue coverage of the prosthesis (Fig. 16.6). Schwartz et al. reported a 7% superficial infection rate, while deep infection ranges from 0% to 14.5% in major series (2–8).

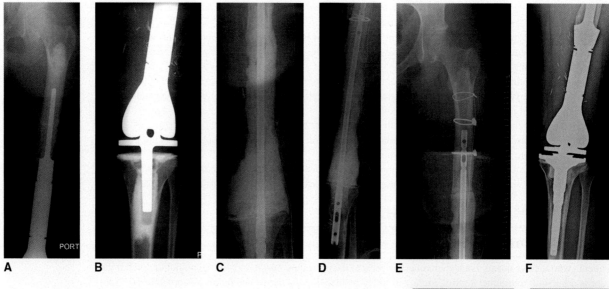

A   B   C   D   E   F

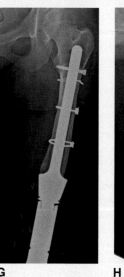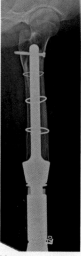

G   H

FIGURE 16.6

A,B: AP radiographs of the femur in an 18-year-old woman with an infected left distal femoral cemented prosthesis (methacillin-sensitive *Staphylococcus aureus*) after an initial irrigation and débridement. **C–E:** Radiographs of the femur after removal of the entire prosthesis and cement. A proximal femoral osteotomy was performed to remove all cement and cables were placed around the femur after a large cement spacer with antibiotics was inserted. **F–H:** Fifty-four months after reimplantation of a cemented distal femoral prosthesis with a healed femur and no signs of loosening or infection.

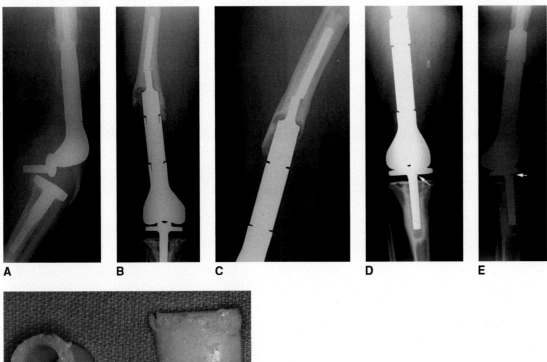

FIGURE 16.7

Examples of failed prostheses include (**A**) a dislocated tibial metal rotating component, (**B,C**) broken femoral stem, (**D,E**) broken tibial metal rotating component (see *arrows*), and (**F**) failed polyethylene bushing and bumper.

Hardware Failure

All parts of the metal and plastic prostheses are subject to failure (Fig. 16.7). There have been prosthetic improvements over time with addition of extramedullary porous coating, modular segments, and forged (vs. casted) metals. However, the metal femoral or tibial stems can fracture as documented in multiple series (5,6,8). Schwartz et al. (6) reported a 9% incidence of femoral stem fatigue fracture in the earlier custom-casted implants, and only a 1.2% incidence in the modular forged implants. Myers et al. (5) reported a 0.6% incidence of fracture in the fixed hinge implants versus 3.5% in the modular implants. The likelihood of bushing or axle failure is more common and does not always require revision of the prosthesis. Myers et al. (5) reported a 28% failure in the fixed hinge implants versus a 6% failure in the modular implants at a mean of 11 years after surgery (5). Schwartz et al. (6) reported a 11.8% bushing or axle failure at a mean 160-month follow-up.

Neurovascular Injury

This complication occurs in 0% to 12.5% of cases (4,6,9,10). Care must be taken not to overlengthen the extremity in patients undergoing chemotherapy. The highest incidence of this complication is found in skeletally immature patients who have expandable prostheses and subsequent lengthening procedures.

Periprosthetic Fracture

Tyler et al. (11) specifically evaluated 154 Compress uncemented prostheses and reported a 3.9% periprosthetic fracture rate. The osseointegrated surface was stable radiographically in all cases, and the limbs were salvaged with further surgery.

Local Recurrence/Amputation

The available series combine patients with benign, malignant, and metastatic tumors of the distal femur, but the overall local recurrence rate in recent series ranges from 0% to 7% (2–4,6,12). Amputation of the limb can be

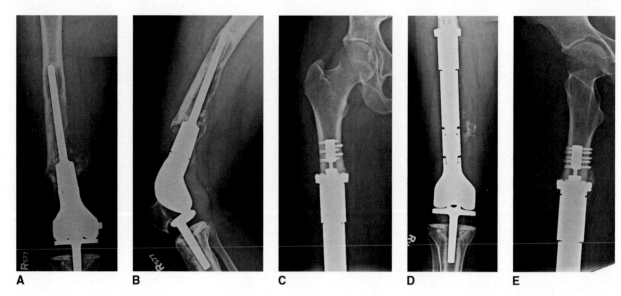

FIGURE 16.8

AP (**A**) and lateral (**B**) radiographs of the right distal femur in a 32-year-old woman 15 years after placement of a cemented distal femoral prosthesis for osteosarcoma. Note the extensive osteolysis and aseptic loosening. A workup for infection was negative. **C–E:** Radiographs 6 months after revision to a Compress uncemented prosthesis with new bone formation at the bone-prosthesis interface.

indicated due to tumor recurrence, deep infection, or repeated prosthetic failure and occurs in 3.6% to 17% of patients at long term follow-up (2,3,5).

RESULTS

The available literature documenting the results of prosthetic reconstruction after distal femoral resection is difficult to compare given the rarity of the procedure and numerous confounding variables. Most tumor-related articles do not separate patients on the basis of tumor grade, stage, or life expectancy. Many articles include multiple surgeons, cemented and uncemented stem designs, children and adults, and multiple anatomic areas in the series. Finally, "prosthetic survival" is not consistently defined.

Revision/Aseptic Loosening—Cemented Stems (Oncologic)

Aseptic loosening is the most common mode of failure for distal femoral prostheses over time (Fig. 16.8). The more recent cemented femoral stems are designed with a porous-coated body segment to allow for extracortical bone bridging (Fig. 16.9). Although it was initially thought this would allow transfer of stress from the

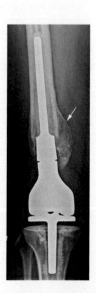

FIGURE 16.9

An AP radiograph of the distal femur in a 60-year-old man who is 5 years after resection of a chondrosarcoma and reconstruction with a cemented prosthesis. Note the extensive extracortical bone bridging along the porous coated body segment (see *arrow*).

prosthesis to the bone, it is now thought to isolate the joint and any metal or polyethylene debris from reaching the bone-cement junction. This is thought to decrease the risk of aseptic loosening. Two important recent series separated the results of older custom-cemented implants from the newer modular cemented implants (5,6). The first series is a retrospective study of 186 cemented distal femoral prostheses implanted after tumor resection. The grade and stage of tumor were documented with most cases being high-grade localized sarcomas. Using revision of the stemmed components as an endpoint, the overall series had a prosthetic survival of 77%, 58%, and 50% at 10, 20, and 25 years. At 15-year follow-up, the 101 older custom implants had a 52% survival compared to a 94% survival of the modular designs. Aseptic loosening occurred in only 3.5% of the modular stems. All cases of mechanical failure were able to be revised to new components. A functional evaluation could be performed in 160 patients with a mean Musculoskeletal Tumor Society (MSTS) score of 86.7% and a mean knee flexion of 110 degrees (6). The second series is a retrospective study of 335 distal femoral prostheses after tumor resection that were separated into 162 prostheses with a fixed hinged design and 173 with a modular rotating hinged design. The vast majority of the modular components had a hydroxyapatite collar. Overall revision for any cause occurred in 17% at 5 years, 33% at 10 years, and 58% at 20 years. Aseptic loosening occurred in 35% of the fixed hinged designs while there was none noted in the modular hinged designs with an HA collar at 10 years (5). Other series of cemented distal femoral prostheses report 5-year prosthetic survival of approximately 85% and 10-year survival from 55% to 79% (2,7,13). In recent series, the aseptic loosening rate ranges from 0% to 8.4% at mean follow-up of 52 to 90 months (2,4,7). One series presented an alternative of custom cross pin fixation of the cemented stems placed into short proximal femoral segments to decrease the incidence of aseptic loosening (14). Twenty patients were followed for more than 2 years and had no aseptic loosening at final follow-up.

Revision/Aseptic Loosening—Cemented Stems (Nononcologic)

The largest series of cemented distal femoral rotating hinged prostheses for nontumor primary or revision indications (severe bone loss with ligamentous instability, nonunion of a periprosthetic fracture, etc.) reports on 69 patients at 75-month follow-up. The average patient age was 72 years and there was a 32% complication rate with reoperation in 27% of cases. There was a 13% aseptic loosening rate, but only one patient required a revision for this finding. Overall, the knee range of motion and functional scores improved postoperatively, but the authors stated that this procedure should only be used as a final salvage option if a constrained condylar design is not possible (8).

Revision/Aseptic Loosening—Uncemented Stems (Oncologic)

Uncemented femoral stems gained popularity as an alternate option to decrease the rate of aseptic loosening. Capanna et al. (3) reported on an early series of 95 modular uncemented prostheses after tumor-related distal femoral resection at a mean of 52 months. There were no cases of aseptic loosening, but 42% of cases developed failure of the bushings at a mean of 64 months. There was a 6% incidence of femoral stem failure that was associated with the use of narrow stems. There was a 5% infection rate in primary cases and 6% in revision cases. Griffin et al. (15) also noted an increased risk of femoral stem failure as the stem diameter decreased. In 74 distal femoral uncemented prostheses, there was only a 2.7% incidence of aseptic loosening. The Compress uncemented prosthesis is an innovative concept that works on the principle of compression at the prosthesis-bone interface with the goal to increase bone mass and strength. It is often utilized in difficult revision cases when there is poor bone quality or a short segment of remaining proximal femur (see Fig. 16.8). One study evaluated the 5-year results of the Compress system with a standard uncemented femoral stem and found the functional results were similar and the prosthetic survival was 88% and 85%, respectively. The authors found that a femoral stem diameter of <13.5 mm was associated with aseptic loosening (1).

Patellar Complications with Distal Femoral Prosthetic Reconstruction

Several series have reported specific patellar complications after distal femoral prosthetic reconstruction (6,8,12). Schwab et al. (12) looked at this issue in 43 cases and found 63% had patellar complications with the most common being patella baja and patellar impingement. The authors stated that patellar impingement on the tibial polyethylene component is related to inaccurate restoration of the joint line.

Functional Results after Distal Femoral Prosthetic Reconstruction

Malo et al. (16) compared the overall functional results after reconstruction of the distal femur with 31 uncemented prostheses compared to 25 cemented hinged prostheses. Multiple functional scoring systems were used at a minimum of 1-year follow-up. The cemented design functional scores were significantly better on the MSTS 1993 and TESS scores. In another study, the function decreased in correlation with the amount of quadriceps that was resected (3).

Revision of Distal Femoral Prostheses

Few articles have reported on the results of revision of cemented or uncemented distal femoral prostheses (17,18). Hsu et al. reported 17 cemented Waldius fixed hinge prostheses and Mittermayer et al. reported a similar series of 15 uncemented Kotz prostheses that were revised with new components. The most common cause of the revision was aseptic loosening but the subsequently revised cases in both series had similar functional results as those of the primary reconstruction (17,18) (see Fig. 16.8).

Expandable Distal Femoral Prostheses

Finally, this chapter did not focus on the technical aspects of distal femoral expandable prostheses in skeletally immature patients but there are series available for review (9,10,19). Patients in this age group present a challenge to the orthopedic oncologist given the issues of leg length discrepancy and smaller femoral diameter. There is a higher complication rate when using the expandable prostheses related to failure of the prosthesis, the expansion mechanism, or nerve palsies. The options for lengthening include an open procedure with removal of the entire pseudocapsule around the prosthesis and replacement of a modular segment with a larger segment (10) (Fig. 16.10), coaxial lengthening by turning a screw in the distal end of the femoral prosthesis (9), or noninvasively by an external electromagnetic field (19) (Fig. 16.11).

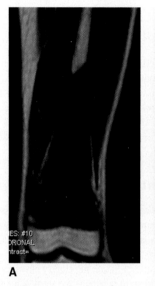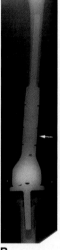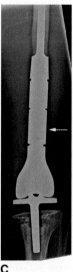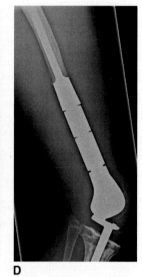

FIGURE 16.10

A: Coronal T1-weighted MR image of the left distal femur in a 12-year-old boy with osteosarcoma. **B:** AP radiograph after resection and reconstruction with a modular, cemented distal femoral prosthesis (*arrow* points to 30-mm segment). AP (**C**) and lateral (**D**) radiographs after an operative lengthening procedure where the 30 mm body segment was replaced with a 50 mm body segment (*arrow* points to 50-mm segment).

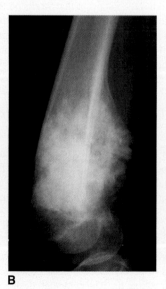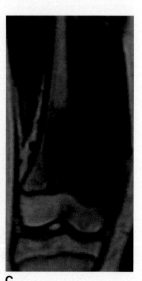

FIGURE 16.11

AP (**A**) and lateral (**B**) radiographs of the distal femur in a 10-year-old girl with osteosarcoma. **C:** T1-weighted coronal view shows the extent of the marrow involvement.

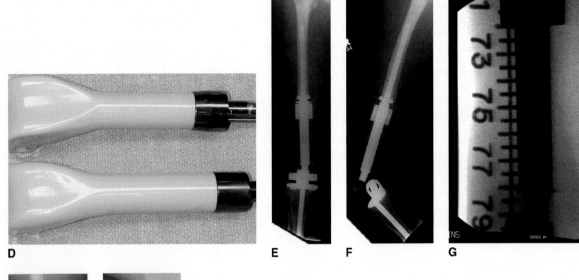

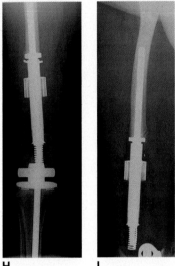

FIGURE 16.11 (*Continued*)

D: The Repiphysis expandable prosthesis was cemented to allow future noninvasive lengthening. AP (**E**) and lateral (**F**) postoperative views of the prosthesis. The body of the distal femoral component is radiolucent. **G:** Fluoroscopic view as the prosthesis lengthens while an external electromagnetic force is applied AP (**H**) and lateral (**I**) radiographs 1 year after the initial lengthening.

REFERENCES

1. Farfalli GL, Boland PJ, Morris CD, et al. Early equivalence of uncemented press-fit and Compress femoral fixation. *Clin Orthop Relat Res.* 2009;467:2792–2799.
2. Bickels J, Wittig JC, Kollender Y, et al. Distal femur resection with endoprosthetic reconstruction: a long-term followup study. *Clin Orthop Relat Res.* 2002;400:225–235.
3. Capanna R, Morris HG, Campanacci D, et al. Modular uncemented prosthetic reconstruction after resection of tumours of the distal femur. *J Bone Joint Surg.* 1994;76:178–186.
4. Frink SJ, Rutledge J, Lewis VO, et al. Favorable long-term results of prosthetic arthroplasty of the knee for distal femur neoplasms. *Clin Orthop Relat Res.* 2005;438:65–70.
5. Myers GJ, Abudu AT, Carter SR, et al. Endoprosthetic replacement of the distal femur for bone tumours: long-term results. *J Bone Joint Surg Br.* 2007;89:521–526.
6. Schwartz AJ, Kabo M, Eilber FC, et al. Cemented distal femoral endoprostheses for musculoskeletal tumor: improved survival of modular versus custom implants. *Clin Orthop Relat Res.* 2010;468:2198–2210.
7. Sharma S, Turcotte RE, Isler MH, et al. Cemented rotating-hinge endoprosthesis for limb salvage of distal femur tumors. *Clin Orthop Relat Res.* 2006;450:28–32.
8. Springer BD, Hanssen AD, Sim FH, et al. The kinematic rotating hinge prosthesis for complex knee arthroplasty. *Clin Orthop Relat Res.* 2001;392:283–91, 2001.
9. Arkader A, Viola DC, Morris CD, et al. Coaxial extendible knee equalizes limb length in children with osteogenic sarcoma. *Clin Orthop Relat Res.* 2007;459:60–65.
10. Eckardt JJ, Kabo JM, Kelley CM, et al. Expandable endoprosthesis reconstruction in skeletally immature patients with tumor. *Clin Orthop Relat Res.* 2000;373:51–61.

11. Tyler WK, Healey JH, Morris CD, et al. Compress periprosthetic fractures: interface stability and ease of revision. *Clin Orthop Relat Res.* 2009;467:2800–2806, 2009.

12. Schwab JH, Agarwal P, Boland PJ, et al. Patellar complications following distal femoral replacement after bone tumor resection. *J Bone Joint Surg.* 2006;88:2225–2230.

13. Biau D, Faure F, Katsahian S, et al. Survival of total knee replacement with megaprosthesis after bone tumor resection. *J Bone Joint Surg Am.* 2006;88:1285–1293.

14. Cannon CP, Eckardt JJ, Kabo JM, et al. Custom cross-pin fixation of 32 tumor endoprostheses stems. *Clin Orthop Relat Res.* 2003;417:285–292.

15. Griffin AM, Parsons JA, Davis AM, et al. Uncemented tumor endoprostheses at the knee: root causes of failure. *Clin Orthop Relat Res.* 2005;438:71–79.

16. Malo M, Davis AM, Wunder J, et al. Functional evaluation in distal femoral endoprosthetic replacement for bone sarcoma. *Clin Orthop Relat Res.* 2001;389:173–180.

17. Hsu RW, Sim FH, Chao EY. Reoperation results after segmental prosthetic replacement of bone and joint for limb salvage. *J Arthro.* 1999;14:519–526.

18. Mittermayer F, Windhager R, Dominkus M, et al. Revision of the Kotz type of tumour endoprosthesis for the lower limb. *J Bone Joint Surg.* 2002;84:401–406.

19. Gitelis S, Neel MD, Wilkins RM, et al. The use of a closed expandable prosthesis for pediatric sarcomas. *Chir Organi Mov.* 2003;88:327–333.

17 Distal Femur Osteoarticular Allograft

Luis A. Aponte-Tinao, German L. Farfalli, Miguel A. Ayerza, and D. Luis Muscolo

Distal femur osteoarticular allografts are utilized for reconstruction of the proximal side of the knee after tumor resection. Osteoarticular allografts do not sacrifice the side of the joint that is not compromise by the tumor and have the possibility of attaching soft-tissues. Reconstruction of the ligaments, tendons, and joint capsule must be meticulous and precise, since the longevity of these grafts is related in part to the stability of the joint. Care must be taken to avoid malalignment that will put greater stress on the allograft cartilage.

INDICATIONS

- The procedure is appropriate for the treatment of a massive osteoarticular defect after tumor resection or massive traumatic bone losses.
- The major neurovascular bundle must be free of tumor.

CONTRAINDICATIONS

- Patients in whom preoperative imaging studies demonstrate evidence of intra-articular compromise of the tumor.
- Inadequate host soft tissue to reconstruct the joint.
- Patients with cartilage degenerative disease of the proximal tibia.

PREOPERATIVE PREPARATION: ALLOGRAFT SELECTION

Fresh frozen allografts are obtained and stored according to a technique that has been previously described (1). Poor anatomical matching of both size and shape between the host defect and the graft can significantly alter joint kinematics and load distribution, leading to bone resorption or joint degeneration. To improve accuracy in size matching between the donor and the host, we developed measurable parameters based on CT scans of the distal femur. In the axial view of the distal femur, we measure the maximum total width and anteroposterior width of the medial and lateral condyles (Fig. 17.1), and the width of the intercondylar notch. The allograft is selected on the basis of a comparison of these measures with those of the donor.

TECHNIQUE

All operations are performed in a clean air enclosure with vertical airflow and usually with spinal anesthesia. The patient is placed on the operating table in the supine position. A sandbag is placed under the ipsilateral buttock. A long midline incision is made (Fig. 17.2), beginning in the middle part of the thigh, and a medial

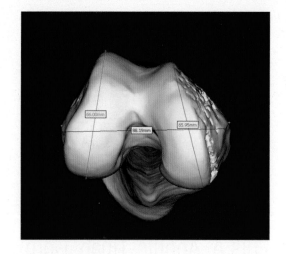

FIGURE 17.1

Axial view of a distal femur allograft CT scan prior to implantation that shows the measure of the maximum total width and the anteroposterior width of the medial and lateral condyles.

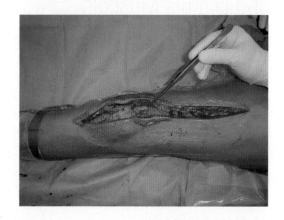

FIGURE 17.2

Intraoperative photograph that shows the long midline incision that is made beginning in the middle part of the thigh.

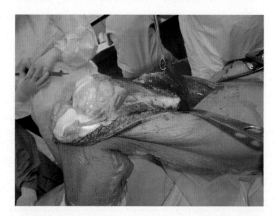

FIGURE 17.3

Intraoperative photograph showing wide exposure of the distal femur after medial parapatellar arthrotomy is performed.

parapatellar arthrotomy is performed with the eversion of the patella in a similar way as in a total knee replacement to enable a wide exposure of the distal part of the femur and the knee joint (Fig. 17.3). The biopsy track is left in continuity with the specimen. The cruciate and collateral ligaments are identified and sectioned near the femur insertion to ensure that there is enough host tissue to reconstruct these ligaments with the donor. The distal part of the femur is approached through the interval between the rectus femoris and the vastus medialis. If there is an extraosseous tumor component, a cuff of normal muscle must be excised. Femoral osteotomy is performed at the appropriate location as determined on the basis of the preoperative imaging studies. All remaining soft tissues at the level of the transection are cleared. After the posterior and medial structures have been protected and retracted, the osteotomy is performed perpendicular to the long axis of the femur. Following the osteotomy, the distal part of the femur is pulled forward in order to expose the soft-tissue attachments of the popliteal space. The popliteal artery is mobilized, and the geniculate vessels are ligated and transected. Both heads of the gastrocnemius are released, and the posterior capsule is sectioned near the femoral insertion. The distal femur is then passed off the operative field (Fig. 17.4).

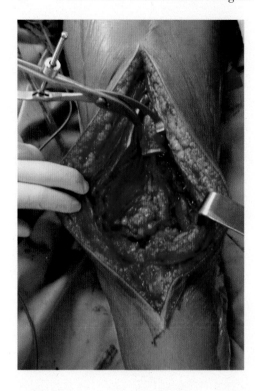

FIGURE 17.4

Intraoperative radiograph made after the distal femur is passed off the operative field, showing the osteoarticular defect.

Simultaneous with the tumor resection, the allograft specimen is prepared in the back table. The graft is taken out of the plastic packaging and placed directly in a warm normal saline solution. After being thawed, the donor bone is cut to the proper length and soft-tissue structures such as the cruciate ligaments, collateral ligaments, and posterior capsule are prepared for implantation. It is crucial for joint reconstruction to have adequate soft-tissue structures in order to repair them to correspondent host tissues.

After resection of the tumor, the distal femoral transplant is inspected to confirm that the size is appropriate and no degenerative changes are present (Fig. 17.5). In order to avoid varus-valgus malalignment between the graft and the recipient we placed both on the back table surface to compare angular valgus and osteotomy parallelism between the host and donor (Fig. 17.6). Then the insertion of an allograft segment tailored to fit the bone defect is performed. Fitting the osteotomy between the host and donor in close apposition is a crucial step. When cortical bone is avascular, as in the allograft side, long-lasting stability is required and under this situation absolute stability offers the best conditions and chances for healing. The diaphyseal osteotomy is stabilized by internal fixation with an anterior short plate (Fig. 17.7), and in order to minimize the risk of fracture an additional lateral condylar buttress plate is placed in order to covers the entire length of the allograft (Fig. 17.8). Once we have secured the allograft bone with the host the knee is flexed to allow joint reconstruction (Fig. 17.9). We repair posterior capsule suturing autologous capsular tissues to the capsular tissues provided by the allograft with two number-1 nonabsorbable sutures along the medial and lateral aspects from posterior to anterior (Fig. 17.10). After the posterior capsular tissues are secured, the posterior cruciate ligament is repaired suturing autologous cruciate tissues to the cruciate tissues provided by the allograft (Fig. 17.11). Finally, the anterior cruciate ligament, and the medial and lateral collateral ligaments are repaired as the posterior cruciate ligament (Figs. 17.12 and 17.13). The patella is reduced if it was not originally deattached suturing parapatellar ligaments. Two suction drains are inserted, and after lavage of the wound with saline solution, a meticulous suture repair of the quadriceps is required. A layered closure of the subcutaneous tissues and skin is then performed.

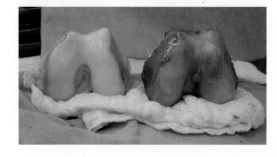

FIGURE 17.5

Intraoperative photograph after resection of the tumor that shows how the distal femoral transplant is inspected to confirm that the size is appropriate and no degenerative changes are present.

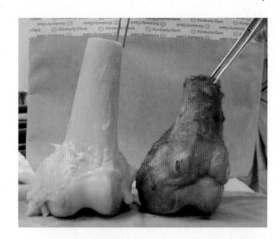

FIGURE 17.6

Intraoperative photograph that shows, in order to avoid varus-valgus malalignment, how the graft and the recipient are placed on the back table surface to compare anatomical axis.

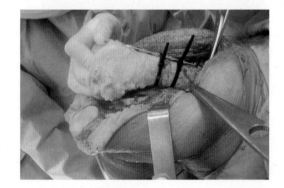

FIGURE 17.7

Intraoperative photograph of the graft and the recipient showing fitting of the diaphyseal osteotomy before compression is made with an anterior short plate.

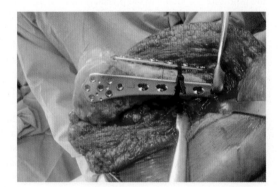

FIGURE 17.8

Intraoperative photograph showing the osteotomy between the host and donor in close apposition with adequate compression after internal fixation with the anterior short plate and how an additional lateral condylar buttress plate is placed in order to covers the entire length of the allograft.

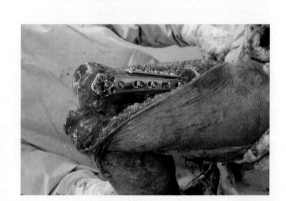

FIGURE 17.9

Intraoperative photograph made when the knee is flexed to allow joint reconstruction, after internal fixation of the osteotomy.

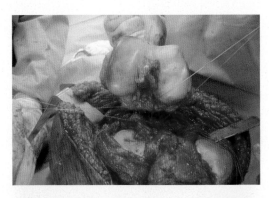

FIGURE 17.10

Intraoperative photograph made when the posterior capsule is repaired from posterior to anterior before the posterior cruciate is repaired.

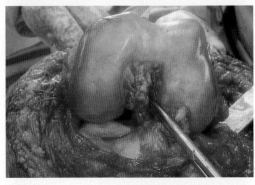

FIGURE 17.11

Intraoperative photograph made when the posterior cruciate ligament of the host is repaired with the corresponding allograft tissue.

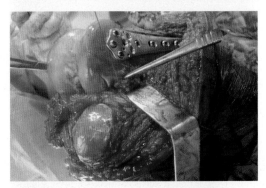

FIGURE 17.12

Intraoperative photograph when the posterolateral reconstruction is performed.

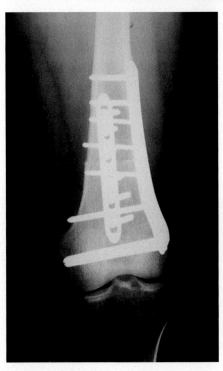

FIGURE 17.13

The radiographic control shows an adequate articular space and solid union of the osteotomy.

POSTOPERATIVE MANAGEMENT

After reconstruction, the knee is placed in full extension and secured with a knee immobilizer or locked hinged postoperative brace. After 2 days, the drains are removed and the wound is inspected. Ice or a cryotherapy device is used to help minimize postoperative swelling and discomfort. Postoperatively, a physical therapist instructed patients on brace use, crutched walking, and quadriceps contractions. The goals during the first week postoperative week are to minimize swelling and obtain passive complete extension. Passive flexion exercises are started 2 weeks postoperatively with the goal of obtaining at least 60 degrees of flexion. At 4 weeks postoperatively, active assisted knee motion is initiated until full active extension and 90 degrees of flexion are obtained. The patient is allowed partial weight bearing at 8 to 12 weeks, according to the stability obtained during the reconstructive procedure.

PEARLS AND PITFALLS

- The procedure is best performed by an orthopedic oncologic surgeon with experience in knee reconstructive surgery and sports-medicine surgery.
- All previous biopsy sites and all potentially contaminated tissues, including any needle biopsy tracks, should be removed en bloc.
- Poor anatomic matching of the size and shape between the host defect and the graft significantly alter joint kinematics and load distribution, leading to bone resorption or joint degeneration.
- Reconstruction of the ligaments and joint capsule must be meticulous and precise because the longevity of these grafts is related, in part, to the stability of the joint.
- Care must be taken to avoid malalignment that will put greater stress on the allograft cartilage.
- Uniform cortical contact, compression of the osteotomy gap, and rotational stability were noted to be better when internal fixation with plates and screws was used.
- To obtain a solid allograft construct, the internal fixation should span the entire length of the allograft.
- Locking compression plate is now used for the majority of our patients because we believe that it imparts greater mechanical stability to the reconstruction.

COMPLICATIONS

Although osteoarticular allografts are ideal material for biologic reconstruction of skeletal defects, biomechanically and biologically related complications including bone graft fractures and resorption, cartilage degeneration, joint instability, and delayed bone union or nonunion still occur (1–6). These biomechanically related complications can be grouped into two main categories, (a) related to geometric matching between the allograft and the host defect and (b) the stability achieved during surgery of the allograft-host bone and soft-tissue junction sites. Anatomical and dimensional matching of the articular surface, adequate joint stability obtained by host-donor soft-tissue repair, and joint alignment have been associated with minor degenerative changes at the articular surface. Clinicopathological studies performed in human retrieved allografts found earlier and more advanced degenerative changes in articular cartilage in specimens retrieved from patients with an unstable joint (2).

Poor anatomical matching of both size and shape between the host defect and the graft can significantly alter joint kinematics and load distribution, leading to bone resorption or joint degeneration. To improve accuracy in size matching between the donor and host, we developed measurable parameters based on CT scans of the distal femur (1). In the axial view of the distal femur, we measure the maximum total width and anteroposterior width of the medial and lateral condyles, and the width of the intercondylar notch. These measurements are available in our hospital based bone bank and allow appropriate selection of the graft to match the patient. Selection and placement of a graft not anatomically matching the size of the osteoarticular defect may alter joint kinematics and pressure distribution, which may in turn reduce the functional life of the graft.

Although allograft-host union may be related with a variety of biological factors involving immunology, tissue typing or graft preservation, a successful union mainly relies upon biomechanical factors. In allograft reconstruction there is a high stress at the osteotomy site between the host and allograft bone and if the graft is not protected with appropriate internal fixation, nonunion or fracture may result. Under these circumstances, if the graft is protected and a solid union is achieved, it may be able to support continuous mechanical loads. Chemotherapy is always a major concern when an allograft reconstruction is considered (7,8). The antiblastic toxicity of chemotherapeutic drugs is known to have an inhibitory effect on allograft union and repair in animals (7). Studies performed in human retrieved allografts seem to associate preoperative chemotherapy with retarded host-donor union (2). In a recent report (8) of 200 osteoarticular allografts that were analyzed (64 without chemotherapy and 126 with chemotherapy), nonunion rate was markedly increased in patients that received chemotherapy (32% vs. 12%), with no differences in infection or fracture rate. Excessive motion at the host-graft interface as a result of an inadequate fixation can inhibit bone union. Further, the biologic incorporation of a cortical allograft is a slow process of induction requiring creeping substitution. A stable host-graft interface with a high degree of contact and a rigid surgical construct may be particularly important to obtain an allograft long-term survival since the deleterious effect of chemotherapy seems to be a reversible process, and allograft healing may occur at the end of the chemotherapy period (7).

Reconstruction of the ligaments, tendons, and joint capsule must be meticulous and precise, since the longevity of these grafts is related in part to the stability of the joint. Care must be taken to avoid malalignment that will put greater stress on the allograft cartilage and may originate intra-articular fractures.

RESULTS

In a review (3) that reported 386 patients managed with an osteoarticular allograft, according to their grading system, excellent or good results for 73% of the patients when followed for more than 2 years. In other study (5) of 114 patients who were managed with an osteoarticular allograft of the distal femur or the proximal tibia, the authors reported that the 5-year survival rate for the grafts was 73% and the rate of limb preservation was 93%, with a mean radiographic score of 83%. One third of the patients had radiographic evidence of articular deterioration after 5 years. Other authors (4) reviewed the cases of 83 patients who were managed with a distal femoral osteoarticular allograft and followed for a minimum of 2 years. According to the grading system of Mankin et al., the results were good or excellent for 70% of the 53 patients managed without chemotherapy compared with only 53% of the 30 patients managed with chemotherapy. In a recent report (6), 80 osteoarticular distal femur allograft reconstructions were followed for a mean of 82 months. Overall allograft survival was 78% at both 5 and 10 years, and the rate of allograft survival without the need of a subsequent knee prosthesis resurfacing was 71% at both 5 and 10 years. Age, gender, the use of chemotherapy, or the percent of resected femur did not have statistically significant effect upon the overall allograft survival rates. Those patients who retained the original allograft had excellent functional and radiographic results.

REFERENCES

1. Muscolo DL, Ayerza M, Aponte-Tinao LA. Massive allograft used in orthopaedics oncology. *Orthop Clin North Am.* 2006;37:65–74.
2. Enneking WF, Campanacci DA. Retrieved human allografts. A clinicopathological study. *J Bone Joint Surg.* 2001;83A:971–986.
3. Mankin HJ, Gebhardt MC, Jennings LC, et al. Long-term results of allograft replacement in the management of bone tumors. *Clin Orthop.* 1996;324:86–97.
4. Mnaymneh W, Malinin TI, Lackman RD, et al. Massive distal femoral osteoarticular allografts after resection of bone tumors. *Clin Orthop.* 1994;303:103–115.
5. Muscolo DL, Ayerza MA, Aponte-Tinao LA. Survivorship and radiographic analysis of knee osteoarticular allografts. *Clin Orthop.* 2000;373:73–79.
6. Muscolo DL, Ayerza MA, Aponte-Tinao LA, et al. Use of distal femoral osteoarticular allografts in limb salvage surgery. *J Bone Joint Surg Am.* 2005;87:2449–2455.
7. Friedlander GE, Tross RB, Doganis AC, et al. Effects of chemotherapeutic agents on bone. Short-term methotrexate and doxorubicin (Adriamycin) treatment in a rat model. *J Bone Joint Surg.* 1984;66A:602–607.
8. Hazan EJ, Hornicek FJ, Tomford WW, et al. The effect of adjuvant chemotherapy on osteoarticular allografts. *Clin Orthop.* 2001;385:176–181.

18 Distal Femur Allograft Prosthetic Composite

D. Luis Muscolo, Miguel A. Ayerza, and Luis A. Aponte-Tinao

D istal femur osteoarticular allografts are utilized for reconstruction of the proximal side of the knee after tumor resection. Osteoarticular allografts do not sacrifice the side of the joint that is not compromise by the tumor and have the possibility of attaching soft-tissues. Reconstruction of the ligaments, tendons, and joint capsule must be meticulous and precise, since the longevity of these grafts is related in part to the stability of the joint. Care must be taken to avoid malalignment that will put greater stress on the allograft cartilage.

INDICATIONS

- The procedure is indicated for the treatment of massive osteoarticular defects after tumor resections or traumatic bone losses.
- The major neurovascular bundle must be free of tumor.
- Patient with degenerative arthritis or cartilage defects of the proximal tibia
- Inadequate host soft tissues to reconstruct and obtain a stable joint with an osteoarticular allograft
- Inadequate anatomical matching between the receptor and potential available donors

CONTRAINDICATIONS

- Patients in whom preoperative imaging studies demonstrate evidence of intra-articular compromise of the tumor
- Patients who received previous or will receive postoperatively high doses of radiotherapy
- Gross tissue deficiencies, particularly of the extensor mechanism, irreparable from soft tissues provided by the allograft

PREOPERATIVE PREPARATION: ALLOGRAFT SELECTION

Fresh-frozen allografts are obtained and stored according to a technique that has been previously described (1). In allograft prosthetic composite anatomical matching of both size and shape is not critical as in osteoarticular allograft. However, it is critical that the bone transplanted is the same as the resected (e.g., distal femur for distal femur) in order to reproduce as much normal biomechanical loading as possible at the construct.

TECHNIQUE

All operations are performed in a clean-air enclosure with vertical airflow and usually with spinal anesthesia. The patient is placed on the operating table in the supine position. A sandbag is placed under the ipsilateral buttock. A long midline incision is made, beginning in the middle part of the thigh, and a medial parapatellar arthrotomy is performed with the eversion of the patella in a similar way as in a total knee replacement to enable a wide exposure of the distal part of the femur and the knee joint (Figs. 18.1 and 18.2). The biopsy track is left in continuity with the specimen. The collateral ligaments are identified and, if they are not affected

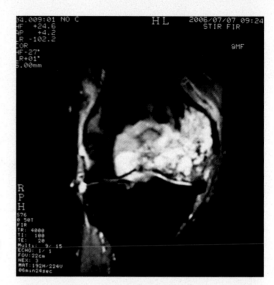

FIGURE 18.1

Coronal magnetic resonance image that illustrates the preoperative tumor growing assessment with extension to the medial collateral ligament.

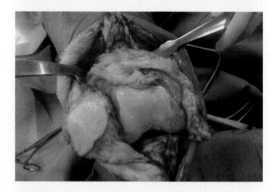

FIGURE 18.2

Intraoperative photograph showing wide exposure of the distal femur after a medial parapatellar arthrotomy is performed. Note degenerative arthritic compromising both distal femur and proximal tibia of the joint.

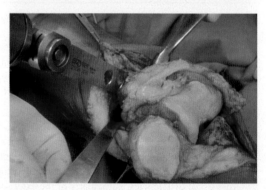

FIGURE 18.3

Intraoperative photograph made when the femoral osteotomy was performed.

by the tumor, sectioned near the femur insertion to ensure that there is enough host tissue to reconstruct these ligaments with the donor. The cruciate ligaments are resected with the specimen. The distal part of the femur is approached through the interval between the rectus femoris and the vastus medialis. If there is an extraosseous tumor component, a cuff of normal muscle must be excised. Femoral osteotomy is performed at the appropriate location as determined on the basis of the preoperative imaging studies. All remaining soft tissues at the level of the transection are cleared. After the posterior and medial structures have been protected and retracted, the osteotomy is performed perpendicular to the long axis of the femur (Fig. 18.3). Following the osteotomy, the distal part of the femur is pulled forward in order to expose the soft tissue attachments of the popliteal space. The popliteal artery is mobilized, and the geniculate vessels are ligated and transected. Boths heads of the gastrocnemius are released, and the posterior capsule is sectioned near the femoral insertion. The distal femur is then passed off the operative field (Fig. 18.4).

Simultaneous with the tumor resection, the allograft specimen is prepared in the back table. The graft is taken out of the plastic packaging and placed directly in a warm normal saline solution. After being thawed, the donor bone is cut to the proper length and soft tissue structures such as the collateral ligaments and posterior capsule are prepared for implantation. It is crucial for joint reconstruction to have these adequate soft tissue structures in order to repair them to correspondent host tissues. The femoral cuts are done in the back table in order to place the prosthesis in the allograft (Figs. 18.5 to 18.7). After the appropriate size of the prosthesis is

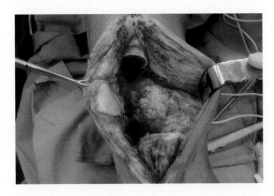

FIGURE 18.4

Intraoperative photograph made after the distal femur is passed off the operative field, showing the osteoarticular defect.

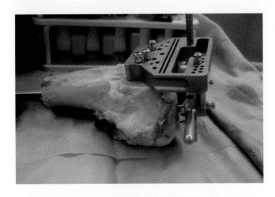

FIGURE 18.5

Intraoperative photograph after the anterior cut for the femoral prosthetic implantation is performed in the allograft.

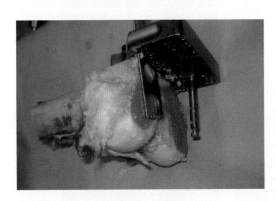

FIGURE 18.6

Intraoperative photograph after the distal cut of the femoral prosthetic implantation is performed.

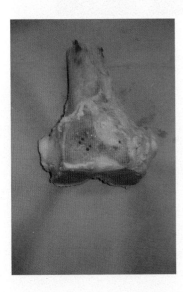

FIGURE 18.7

Intraoperative photograph showing the distal femur allograft previous to the intercondylar cuts.

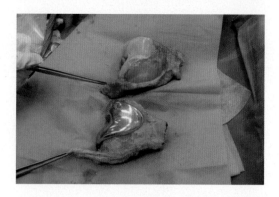

FIGURE 18.8

Intraoperative photograph showing the distal femur allograft with the femoral component. Note the medial collateral ligament that is long enough to allow soft tissue reconstruction, in order to substitute the original ligament potentially contaminated by the tumor and preserved in the resected specimen shown.

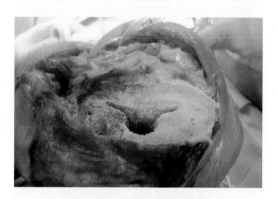

FIGURE 18.9

Intraoperative photograph after the proximal tibia cut is performed for tibial component as in a regular knee prosthetic reconstruction.

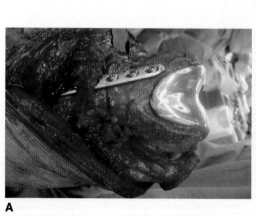

A

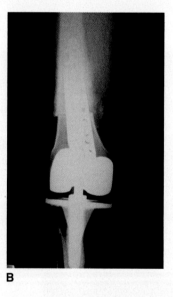

B

FIGURE 18.10

(A) Intraoperative photograph showing the osteotomy between the host and donor in close apposition with adequate compression after internal fixation. **(B)** Intraoperative xrays may be obtained to confirm alignment and position of reconstruction.

selected, it is cemented to the femoral allograft with a noncemented stem to avoid collapse of the metaphyseal bone (Fig. 18.8).

The tibial cuts are then performed (Fig. 18.9) and the tibial component is cemented. The diaphyseal osteotomy of the femur is stabilized by internal fixation with an anterior plate (Fig. 18.10). Once we have secured the allograft bone with the host, the knee is flexed to allow joint reconstruction. We use a No. 1 nonabsorbable suture to repair the autologous posterior capsule to the capsular tissues provided by the allograft. Finally, the medial and lateral collateral ligaments are repaired as the posterior capsule (Fig. 18.11). The patella is reduced if it was not originally deattached suturing parapatellar ligaments. Two suction drains are inserted, and after lavage of the wound with saline solution, a meticulous suture repair of the quadriceps is required. A layered closure of the subcutaneous tissues and skin is then performed.

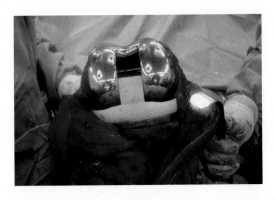

FIGURE 18.11

Intraoperative photograph made with the knee flexed showing how the both collateral ligaments where reconstructed suturing soft tissues from the receptor with the soft tissues provided by the donor.

POSTOPERATIVE MANAGEMENT

After reconstruction, the knee is placed in full extension and secured with a knee immobilizer or locked hinged postoperative brace. After 2 days, the drains are removed and the wound is inspected. Ice or a cryotherapy device is used to help minimize postoperative swelling and discomfort. Postoperatively, a physical therapist instructs patients on brace use, crutched walking, and quadriceps contractions. The goals during the first postoperative week are to minimize swelling and obtain passive complete extension. Passive flexion exercises are started 2 weeks postoperatively with the goal of obtaining at least 60 degrees of flexion. At 4 weeks postoperatively, active assisted knee motion is initiated until full active extension and 90 degrees of flexion are obtained. The patient is allowed partial weight bearing at 8 to 12 weeks, according to the stability obtained during the reconstructive procedure.

PEARLS AND PITFALLS

- The procedure is best performed by an orthopedic oncologic surgeon with experience in knee reconstructive surgery.
- All previous biopsy sites and all potentially contaminated tissues, including any needle biopsy tracks, should be removed en bloc.
- Reconstruction of the ligaments and joint capsule must be meticulous and precise since the longevity of these grafts is related, in part, to the stability of the joint.
- Uniform cortical contact, compression of the osteotomy gap, and rotational stability were noted to be better when internal fixation with plates and screws was used.
- To avoid collapse of the femoral component in the metaphyseal allografts area, a noncemented stem is added to the prosthesis.
- Locking compression plate is now used for the majority of our patients since we believe that it imparts greater mechanical stability to the reconstruction.

COMPLICATIONS

A major advantage of this technique is the ability to customize the operation at the time of surgery. The implant combined with allograft provides additional stability not present in an osteoarticular allograft. In addition, by resurfacing the proximal tibia with an implant, a degenerative articular cartilage is not a contraindication. The technique does restore bone stock, and patient recovery is similar as obtained after a revision arthroplasty. In addition, this surgery could be revised repeating the procedure or eventually with an arthrodesis. To perform this type of surgery, a surgeon has to be fully trained in all aspects of reconstructive surgery and, in addition, have access to a bone bank where large fragment, fresh-frozen allografts are available. Nonunion is a potential complication, usually solved with autologous bone grafting. Other complications could be related to prosthesis implant such as loosening. Fracture of the allograft usually will require a second operation, sometimes regrafting with a second allograft prosthetic composite (APC) or an endoprosthesis.

RESULTS

Reconstructions using the combination of an allograft and a prosthesis (composite biological implant) have become increasingly popular (2–9). This technique has developed due to reported complications with more conventional procedures such as custom metallic implant arthroplasties or osteoarticular allografts. The advantage of allograft-prosthesis composites is that the bone stock is replaced and secure attachments for tendon insertions are provided without the need to rely on allograft articular cartilage and the allograft does not need to be perfectly size-matched to the host bone. Allografts provide tendinous attachments for reconstructions and function better than when they are attached to an endoprosthetic device.

Although this is a technique that may be used in almost every joint in which there is a prosthesis available, such as proximal femur (3,4), proximal tibia (5,6), and proximal humerus (7), there are no series of patients reported including exclusively of APC of distal femur. The results of this technique are usually reported in larger series that include other various types of reconstructions (8–10).

Finally, in patients with severe bone loss due to a failed endoprostheses that require a revision, an allograft-prosthetic composite may serve as an appropriate long-term replacement without significant loss of function (11).

REFERENCES

1. Muscolo DL, Ayerza M, Aponte-Tinao LA. Massive allograft used in orthopaedics oncology. *Orthop Clin North Am.* 2006;37:65–74.
2. Gitelis S, Piasecki P. Allograft prosthetic composite arthroplasty for osteosarcoma and other aggressive bone tumors. *Clin Orthop.* 1991;270:197–201.
3. Zehr RJ, Enneking WF, Scarborough MT. Allograft-prosthesis composite versus megaprosthesis in proximal femoral reconstruction. *Clin Orthop.* 1996;322:207–223.
4. Langlais F, Lambotte JC, Collin P, et al. Long-term results of allograft composite total hip prostheses for tumors. *Clin Orthop.* 2003;414:197–211.
5. Donati D, Colangeli M, Colangeli S, et al. Allograft-prosthetic composite in the proximal tibia after bone tumor resection. *Clin Orthop Relat Res.* 2008;466:459–465.
6. Biau DJ, Dumaine V, Babinet A, et al. Allograft-prosthesis composites after bone tumor resection at the proximal tibia. *Clin Orthop Relat Res.* 2007;456:211–217.
7. Black AW, Szabo RM, Titelman RM. Treatment of malignant tumors of the proximal humerus with allograft-prosthesis composite reconstruction. *J Shoulder Elbow Surg.* 2007;16:525–533.
8. Mnaymneh W, Emerson RH, Borja F, et al. Massive allografts in salvage revisions of failed total knee arthroplasties. *Clin Orthop Relat Res.* 1990;260:144–153.
9. Mankin HJ, Gebhardt MC, Jennings LC, et al. Long-term results of allograft replacement in the management of bone tumors. *Clin Orthop.* 1996;324:86–97.
10. Biau D, Faure F, Katsahian S, et al. Survival of total knee replacement with a megaprosthesis after bone tumor resection. *J Bone Joint Surg Am.* 2006;88:1285–1293
11. Wilkins RM, Kelly CM. Revision of the failed distal femoral replacement to allograft prosthetic composite. *Clin Orthop.* 2002;397:114–118.

19 Arthrodesis of the Knee

Christopher P. Beauchamp

With the availability of modern reconstructive techniques that can achieve a mobile knee reconstruction, knee arthrodesis is now seldom chosen as a primary reconstructive solution. In fact, intra-articular extension of a tumor, necessitating an extra-articular resection, was once considered to be reconstructable only with an arthrodesis. Today, extra-articular resections can sometimes be reconstructed with a mobile knee provided extensor continuity can be maintained. When a fusion is desirable, there are many different ways to successfully achieve it. The techniques described in this chapter all have advantages and disadvantages. There is no single method that is superior to all others. Surgical experience with similar procedures, such as intramedullary nail fixation, may influence the choice of fixation. Plate fixation because of severe obesity may be a preferable choice in certain patients. The following will describe a variety of techniques to achieve a successful arthrodesis.

INDICATIONS

- The most common indication today is for salvage of a failed arthroplasty.
- Patients who are young, overweight, and have high physical demands can be considered for primary arthrodesis.
- An arthrodesis is sometimes chosen for young patients with benign or low-grade malignant neoplasm.
- Patients with a quadriceps paralysis and arthritis or a neuropathic joint are also considered candidates for knee fusion

CONTRAINDICATIONS

- Acute untreated infections are a contraindication to arthrodesis using plates or rods.
- Fusion of the ipsilateral hip or contralateral knee also makes knee arthrodesis an unattractive treatment choice.

PREOPERATIVE PREPARATION

Preoperative planning includes the following:

1. Radiographic measurement of limb lengths. The ideal final limb length should aim for a discrepancy of 1 to 2 cm. This prevents the foot from brushing against the floor during swing phase.
2. Plain radiographs with markers or a CT scan are used to determine the canal/IM rod diameter if nail diameter is a potential issue.
3. CT and MRI are used to calculate the plane of resection for tumors.
4. Surgical approach is determined by previous incisions or biopsy site. It is generally longitudinal, anterior, medial, or lateral.
5. Soft tissue coverage is often an issue especially with salvage of an infected prosthesis. Local flaps usually cover most defects about the knee; free tissue transfer is seldom needed.
6. Infected reconstructions are best treated in two stages. The first stage debriding the joint and removing the prosthesis and inserting an antibiotic spacer. The second stage being the definitive arthrodesis. The assumption being the infection is eradicated after the first stage, and the history of infection does not influence the reconstruction method.

TECHNIQUE

There are a number of reconstructive techniques to achieve a knee fusion. Each method has advantages and disadvantages. There is no single best method and it is helpful to be familiar with all methods of reconstruction. Fortunately, the principles are similar to other orthopedics procedures and this form of reconstructions should be within the capabilities of most orthopedic surgeons.

There are three main techniques including intramedullary fixation with a rod device, external fixation, and internal fixation with plates.

The factors that go into the decision making regarding the particular method include

- Age, weight, activity level, infection presence/risk, bone quality, and patient compliance.
- The remaining bone stock also is a factor. Arthrodesis for arthritis or failed total knee arthroplasty usually has enough bone in the femur and tibia to permit bone contact at the fusion site. Defects created following tumor resection are most commonly reconstructed with a segmental allograft. In the past autografts, ipsilateral fibula and hemicortical grafts were used to span the defect.

Intramedullary Fixation

There are a number of different devices available for this technique. Resection arthrodesis of the knee for defects secondary to tumor resection has been well described by Enneking and others over the years. Initially, a Kunschner nail or a Sampson nail was used; these were custom made and could be modified in the operating room. Today, most IM nail providers have a long version (Fig. 19.1). These are usually inserted in an antegrade manner. The Sampson rod was extensively used for resection arthrodesis of the knee. It was inserted in a retrograde manner using a perforator adapter that is attached to the proximal end of the rod, and the greater trochanter was penetrated by this beveled tip. The rod was driven proximally through a small incision to allow for the reduction of the knee, and the rod was then driven down the shaft of the tibia. The proximal portion of the rod was curved and the tibial portion was straight. The rod was fluted providing some rotational stability.

There are a number of modular rods. The Neff nail is designed to permit the insertion of a long intramedullary nail through a single knee incision (Fig. 19.2). The rod consists of a femoral and a tibial component so that size differences between the two bones could be accommodated. The two devices are attached to each other via a Morse taper. The device itself could not provide any compression and removal of the implant if necessary is difficult without taking down the fusion. The Wichita nail is also a two piece design with differing diameters in the femur and tibia. The two connect together and a compression nut allows for compression across the arthrodesis site. The femoral and tibial stems are locked allowing compression to be applied (Fig. 19.3).

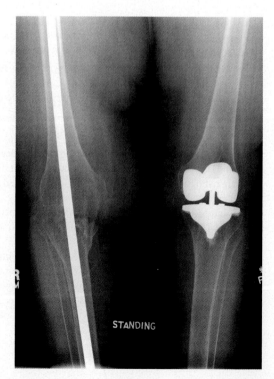

FIGURE 19.1

A 67-year-old female with an absent extensor mechanism and posttraumatic arthritis had been treated with cast immobilization for 4 months. Her very stiff arthritic knee with a contracted quadriceps mechanism was treated with a long, distally unlocked reconstruction nail, successfully fusing the knee at 16 weeks.

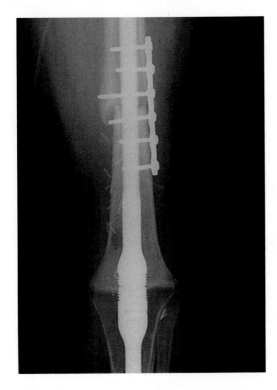

FIGURE 19.2

The patient was 26-year-old when first treated for a giant cell tumor of the distal femur. Initially treated with curettage and cementation, it recurred 9 months later. A repeat biopsy and review of the original outside pathology revealed the diagnosis of giant cell rich osteosarcoma. The patient had extensive intra-articular involvement, and the extensor mechanism and distal quadriceps had to be sacrificed. The treatment options were knee arthrodesis versus above knee amputation. A Neff nail is inserted first into the femur and then the tibia, and the two rods are joined at the arthrodesis site. This is a difficult to remove device if there was a need to do so.

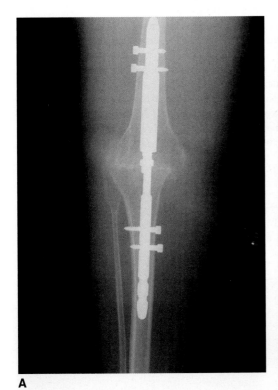

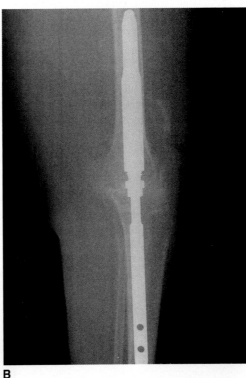

A   **B**

FIGURE 19.3

A,B: A 56-year-old patient had lower extremity partial paralysis secondary to an old cauda equina injury. The patient is ambulatory but with a sever deformity and instability of her knee with secondary arthritic pain. It was felt that she was not a candidate for a knee arthroplasty and her knee was fused with a Wichita nail, a modular two piece interlocked nail. The implant has the capability of applying compression to the fusion site with a wrench turning a bolt at the site of the femoral and tibial junction. It too is a challenge to remove without considerable disruption to the fusion site.

SURGICAL TECHNIQUE (NEFF NAIL OR WICHITA NAIL)

- The patient is positioned supine with a bump under the ipsilateral buttock.
- The limb is draped free to allow access to the greater trochanter and buttocks.
- A sterile tourniquet is used.
- The incision is chosen and the extensor mechanism is exposed. The patella is excised and retained for bone grafting.
- The patellar ligament and anterior capsule are reflected off the proximal tibia; the medial and lateral collateral ligaments and capsule are reflected as necessary.
- In the case of a failed joint replacement, the prosthesis and cement are removed. If infected, the space is filled with antibiotic cement.
- The canal of the femur is prepared and retrograde reaming is performed up to the desired diameter.
- A femoral stem is inserted to the correct depth. The stem is then locked in the case of a Wichita nail. The tibia is then prepared and the tibial stem is next inserted and locked. The femoral and tibial components can be of differing diameters.
- The knee is reduced and held in the correct rotation while the two stems are assembled. The junction is fixed with a set screw in the case of a Neff nail or compressed with a nut for a Wichita nail.
- Bone graft is packed into the junction and any defects present.
- Adjuvant fixation in the form of a supplemental plate is possible in most cases as there is room in the distal femur and proximal tibia metaphysis.
- Small intercalary arthrodesis grafts are possible with a Neff or Wichita nail.

LONG ARTHRODESIS NAIL (CUSTOM NAIL OR STRYKER T2 NAIL)

- The femur and tibia are prepared with antegrade and retrograde reaming.
- A reamer and guide rod can be passed retrograde through the greater trochanter and an incision is made in the buttock to deliver the guide rod.
- The proximal femur is further reamed to the level of the lesser trochanter.
- A rod is inserted through the greater trochanter and advanced down the femur.
- If needed, an intercalary allograft is then placed over the rod, the knee is reduced, and the rod is advanced into the tibia.
- Careful attention is paid to both graft host junctions so there are no gaps and the bone contact is complete. This can usually be fine-tuned using a fine saw blade.
- Once the alignment is adjusted, compression is applied to the limb by locking the distal nail and then slapping the nail in a retrograde fashion. This brings the arthrodesis ends together, and the nail is then locked.
- If the rod has the capability of applying further compression (Stryker T2), it is applied at this time.
- Additional rotational stability and compression can be applied using supplemental DC plates. Bone graft is then applied to the graft host junctions.

PLATE FIXATION

Plate fixation can provide good rigid fixation and is helpful in some circumstances. It is not recommended as initial treatment for an infected failed total knee but can be used for the definitive treatment (Fig. 19.4). In patients with a short segment, intercalary allograft plate fixation provides better

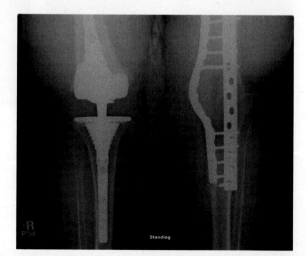

FIGURE 19.4

A 48-year-old female, BMI 55, with an infected failed knee treated with a first-stage articulated spacer, converted to an arthrodesis with dual plates.

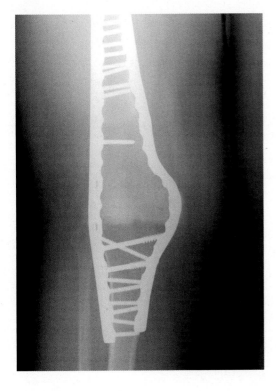

FIGURE 19.5

A 20-year-old male with a stage 3 giant cell tumor had complete destruction of the distal femur. He had a BMI of 45. He was treated with an intercalary allograft arthrodesis with dual plate fixation.

compression than a rod (Fig. 19.5). Combined rod and plate fixation has been described as well (Figs. 19.2 and 19.6B,C).

Plate Fixation Technique

- The knee is exposed anteriorly; the patella and patellar ligament are reflected laterally.
- The knee is flexed and a distal femoral and proximal tibial cut are made. The bones can then be coapted and additional saw cuts can be made to fine-tune the final bone contact point.
- Apply a broad dynamic compression anterolaterally with or without a compression outrigger.
- Contour and apply a dynamic compression plate medially using an outrigger for additional compression.
- Bone graft, locally obtained, is then applied to the fusion site.

Pearls and Pitfalls

- Ensure that the soft tissue envelope is adequate. Arthrodesis for failed joint replacement is usually due to infection and most of these patients have soft tissue problems that must be addressed first. If the ultimate reconstruction of an infected prosthesis is an arthrodesis, then I do it in two stages. The first stage with an antibiotic spacer, usually not articulated, is done with a flap, either local or free.
- If you are using an intramedulary device, select the largest implant you can fit. A delayed union with a broken rod is difficult to repair.
- Getting rotation in the correct position can be difficult. It is helpful to prepare and drape both extremities for comparison. Mark limb alignment prior to performing any osteotomies, especially with a tumor resection.
- Pay careful attention to the graft host junctions. If you can leave a gap or empty moat around the rod at the distal femur and proximal tibia, the opposing bone surfaces can be trimmed repeatedly with a saw to ensure a perfect fit. This is very similar to trimming wallpaper by cutting both overlapping panels at one with a single cut. As the bones are compressed together, a saw blade passed through the fusion site will cut both sides ensuring a perfect fit with 100% contact. Be careful to not nick the rod.
- An intercalary arthrodesis fixed with a rod increases the risk of a delayed or nonunion as the fixation is not rigid. Do not hesitate to supplement fixation with a compression plate.
- Always anticipate the need to remove the device(s) you are implanting. Choose a device that will not be difficult or nearly impossible to remove.

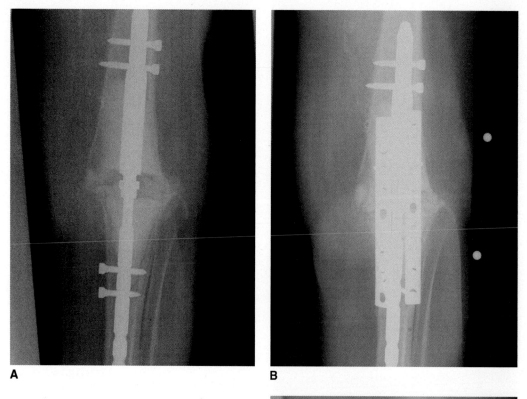

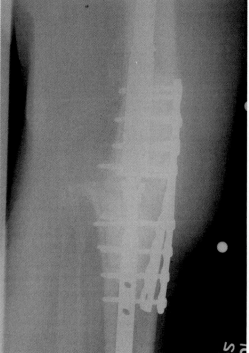

FIGURE 19.6

A–C: A Wichita nail with secondary plates to treat a delayed union. A 71-year-old male underwent unsuccessful two-stage exchange for an infected total knee. He refused amputation and a two-stage arthrodesis was performed. The definitive arthrodesis was done with a Wichita nail, supplemented with antibiotic cement. He did not unite and was rescued with two plates and bone graft. The supplemental cement provided excellent fixation.

RECOMMENDED READING

Arroyo JS, Garvin KL, Neff JR. Arthrodesis of the knee with a modular titanium intramedullary nail. *J Bone Joint Surg Am.* 1997;79:26–34.

Charnley J, Lowe HG. A study of the end-results of compression arthrodesis of the knee. *J Bone Joint Surg Br.* 1958;40: 633–635.

De Vil J, Almqvist KF, Vanheeren P, et al. Knee arthrodesis with an intramedullary nail: a retrospective study. *Knee Surg Sports Traumatol Arthrosc.* 2008;16:645–650.

Donley BG, Matthews LS, Kaufer H. Arthrodesis of the knee with an intramedullary nail. *J Bone Joint Surg Am.* 1991;73: 907–913.

Enneking WF, Shirley PD. Resection arthrodesis for malignant and potentially malignant lesions about the knee using an intramedullary rod and local bone grafts. *J Bone Joint Surg Am.* 1977;59:223–236.

Falahee MH, Matthews LS, Kaufer H. Resection arthroplasty as a salvage procedure for a knee with infection after total arthroplasty. *J Bone Joint Surg Am.* 1987;69:1013–1021.

MacDonald JH, Agarwal S, Lorei MP, et al. Knee arthrodesis *J Am Acad Orthop Surg.* 2006;14:154–163.

McQueen DA, Cooke FW, Hahn DL. Knee arthrodesis with the wichita fusion nail: an outcome comparision. *Clin Orthop Relat Res.* 2006;446:132–139.

Nichols SJ, Landon GC, Tullos HS. Arthrodesis with dual plates after failed total knee arthroplasty. *J BoneJoint Surg Am.* 1991;73:1020–1024.

Pritchett JW, Mallin BA, Matthews AC. Knee arthrodesis with a tensionband plate. *J Bone Joint Surg Am.* 1988;70: 285–288.

Puranen J, Kortelainen P, Jalovaara P. Arthrodesis of the knee with intramedullary fixation. *J Bone Joint Surg Am.* 1990;72:433–442.

Stiehl JB, Hanel DP. Knee arthrodesis using combined intramedullary rod and plate fixation. *Clin Orthop.* 1993;294: 238–241.

Waldman BJ, Mont MA, Payman KR, et al. Infected total knee arthroplasty treated with arthrodesis using a modular nail. *Clin Orthop.* 1999;367:230–237.

Wolf RE, Scarborough MT, Enneking WF. Long term followup of patients with autogenous resection arthrodesis of the knee. *Clin Orthop.* 1999;358:36–40.

Vince KG. Revision knee arthroplasty technique. *Instr Course Lect.* 1993; 42:325–339.

Weiner SD, Scarborough M, VanderGreind RA. Resection arthrodesis of the knee with an intercalary allograft. *J Bone Joint Surg Am.* 1996;78:185–192.

20 Surgical Technique of Proximal Tibia Megaprosthesis

Mario Mercuri and Costantino Errani

The proximal tibia is the second most common site involved with primary tumors of the skeleton. En bloc resection is a limb-sparing option for low-grade and most high-grade bone sarcomas, for selected cases of stage 3 benign tumors (e.g., giant cell tumor), and occasionally for metastatic lesions. Surgical options for reconstruction include megaprosthesis, osteoarticular allograft, allograft-prosthesis composite, and rotationplasty.

Modular prosthetic replacement is a relatively simple technique and has become the method of choice for reconstruction after bone tumor resection at the proximal tibia. However, the long-term survival of megaprostheses is poor; mechanical failure and infection remain the major problems. A gastrocnemius transposition flap is necessary to obtain soft tissue coverage and reconstruction of the extensor mechanism to reduce risk of infection and rupture of the patella tendon (1).

Resection for lesions of the proximal tibia can be classified into intra-articular and extra-articular. If the tumor does not involve the joint, an intra-articular resection is indicated; otherwise, an extra-articular resection can be performed (2).

INDICATIONS

- All patients with tibial sarcomas should be considered potential candidates for limb-sparing procedures.
- Indications for endoprostheses depend on age, site, type of resection, life expectancy, and the patient's functional demands.
- This reconstruction technique is indicated in adult patients and adolescents at the end of growth.
- Expandable prostheses can be used in pediatric age (7 to 12 years) and may be lengthened over time, thus correcting limb-length discrepancy (3).

CONTRAINDICATIONS

- Contraindications to resection include pathologic fractures, neurovascular involvement, contamination from a poorly performed biopsy, and local sepsis.
- When a limb-sparing procedure is possible, endoprostheses are not indicated in patients under 7 years old (4).

PREOPERATIVE PLANNING

Resection of proximal tibia requires the careful analysis of the preoperative staging studies. An accurate preoperative staging of the tumor by plain film radiographs, computed tomography (CT), magnetic resonance, and bone scintigraphy is mandatory before surgery to determine resectability by evaluating the exact extent of the lesion and its relationship to neurovascular bundles (Figs. 20.1 to 20.3).

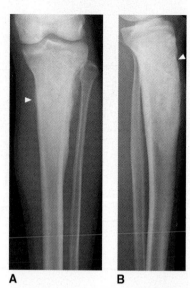

FIGURE 20.1

A,B: Typical radiograph picture of osteosarcoma of the left proximal tibia in a boy aged 15 years (*arrowheads*).

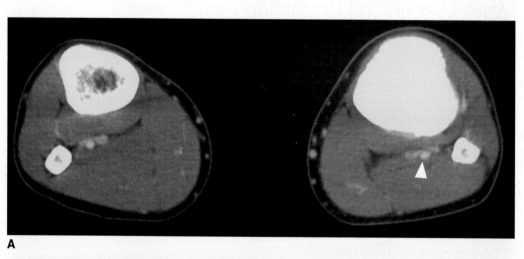

A

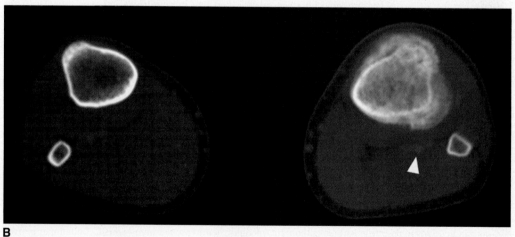

B

FIGURE 20.2

A,B: Axial CT scan for bone and soft tissue of the left proximal tibia show a relationship between tumor and neurovascular bundles (*arrowheads*).

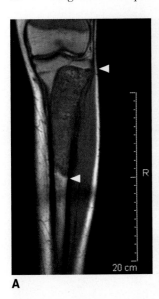

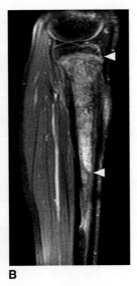

A

B

FIGURE 20.3

A,B: MRI with T1-weighted anteroposterior view and T2-weighted lateral view of the left proximal tibia evaluate the intramedullary extent of the tumor and the relation to the soft tissues (*arrowheads*).

THE TECHNIQUE

Surgeons must meticulously follow the principles of oncologic surgery: the tumor must be removed en bloc with noncontaminated surgical margins (wide-margin resection).

Position and Draping

The patient is placed supine on the operating table and the entire extremity is prepared and draped. A blood-less field should be obtained with a tourniquet after exsanguination by gravity; however, it is important not to squeeze or manipulate the lesion using elastic wrappings when preparing the patient. The tourniquet must be removed after excision of the lesion but before closing the tissue planes.

Incision and Dissection

An anteromedial longitudinal incision is used just proximal to the superior pole of the patella to the distal third of the tibia, including the previous biopsy incision with a 1 cm border between the biopsy scar and the resection incision (Fig. 20.4). The procedure begins by making an arthrotomy to inspect the joint. If the joint fluid is normal and no tumor can be seen within the joint, an intra-articular resection can be continued. If intra-articular tumor involvement is suspected, the capsule should be closed and an extra-articular resection must be performed. Popliteal vessels are identified by detaching the medial gastrocnemius muscle and splitting the soleus muscle (Fig. 20.5). The soleus must be released from its origin on the proximal tibia just distal to the lower border of the popliteus. It is necessary to leave some soleus on the tibia as a soft tissue margin and to pay

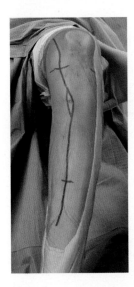

FIGURE 20.4

An anteromedial approach, including a biopsy excision, is performed from the medial peripatella to the distal third of the tibia.

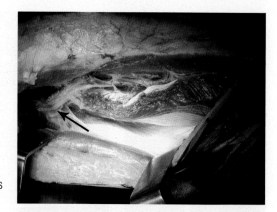

FIGURE 20.5

The medial gastrocnemius is mobilized and the soleus split to expose neurovascular structures (*arrow*).

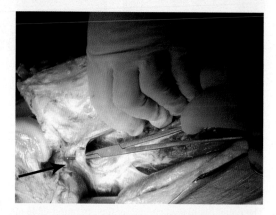

FIGURE 20.6

Ligation of the anterior tibial artery and vein (*arrow*).

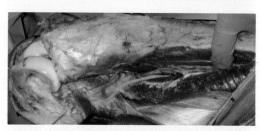

FIGURE 20.7

A neurovascular bundle visualized from the knee joint to the tibial osteotomy.

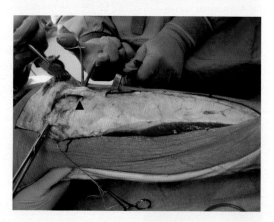

FIGURE 20.8

After the capsular incision, the patellar tendon is sectioned 2 cm proximal to the tibial tubercle (*arrowheads*).

attention to the posterior tibial nerve and vessels that are just deep to the soleus. The anterior tibial vessels are branches from the posterior vessels and enter the anterior compartment at the inferior border of the popliteus muscle. If the anterior tibial artery is adjacent to the tumor, it should be ligated at its origin in the posterior compartment (Fig. 20.6). Therefore, the posterior neurovascular bundle should be visualized from the knee joint to as far distally as needed to perform the tibial osteotomy (Fig. 20.7). The popliteal muscle is always sacrificed; patella tendon must be transected from the tibial insertion as far as possible avoiding contamination (Fig. 20.8). The capsule of the knee joint can be sectioned close to the femoral insertion and leaving the menisci

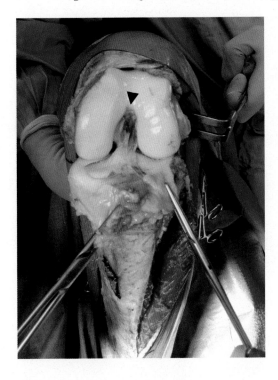

FIGURE 20.9

Cruciate ligaments are sectioned close to the femoral insertions (*arrowhead*).

with the proximal tibia tendon. The medial and lateral collateral ligaments and the cruciate ligaments, which pull the tibia anteriorly on the femur, are divided close to the femoral insertion (Fig. 20.9). On the medial side, the insertions of the sartorius, gracilis, and semitendinosus are transacted leaving their insertions on the tibia. On the lateral side, the origins of the anterior compartment muscles should be left on the tibia. After exposure of the peroneal nerve, depending on where the tumor has its extraosseous component, the proximal fibula will or will not be preserved.

If the tumor does not involve the pericapsular tissues of the tibiofibular joint, an intra-articular resection is indicated and the lateral collateral ligament should be saved. This increases the stability of the joint after reconstruction; otherwise an extra-articular resection of the tibiofibular joint must be performed to avoid the risk of contamination. Lastly, the posterior capsule of the knee is transected. At this stage, the osteotomy of the tibia can be performed at least 2 cm distal to the tumor, using the preoperative measurements determined by magnetic resonance imaging (MRI) (Fig. 20.10). Moreover, if it does not influence the reconstruction, a wider margin can be achieved.

The proximal tibia is still attached to the leg by interosseous membrane and soft tissues. The dissection plane is based on the preoperative exams (MRI and CT), confirmed during the surgery by palpation. It is necessary to leave the tumor covered with normal tissue; and so, the soft tissue resection depends on the extent of the extraosseous tumor.

After tibial osteotomy, the surgeon should examine the specimen to ensure adequate surgical margin; moreover, the length of the resected specimen should be carefully measured for later reconstruction (Fig. 20.11). The distal medullary canal is curetted and sent to the pathologist for frozen section analysis to exclude the possibility of an inadequate margin (Fig. 20.12).

Now the tourniquet can be deflated and hemostasis obtained.

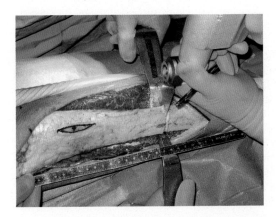

FIGURE 20.10

Tibial osteotomy 3 cm distal to the tumor completes the resection.

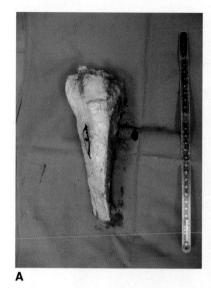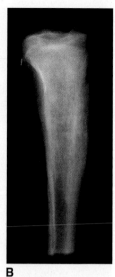

FIGURE 20.11

A,B: A resected specimen of an osteosarcoma.

A   **B**

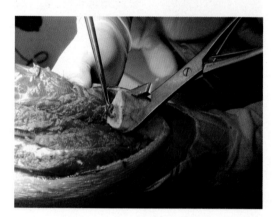

FIGURE 20.12

A curettage of the distal medullary canal frozen section analysis.

When the arthrotomy reveals a contamination of a joint, it is necessary to perform an extra-articular resection. The surgical technique is similar to the intra-articular resection, except that the knee joint is included with a proximal tibia. The neurovascular popliteal structures are dissected off the distal femur, and the medial and lateral gastrocnemius must be transected from their origins on the femur. The quadriceps muscle can be transected just proximal to the knee joint and the femur osteotomized with a power saw; or at the discretion of the treating surgeon, the patella can be preserved by an extra-articular coronal osteotomy of the patella, thereby keeping the extensor apparatus intact.

Reconstruction

The reconstruction of the bone defect is similar to the intra-articular tibial resection.

The latest generation of prostheses has a porous coating on the stem, to induce the growth of the host bone and therefore increase prosthesis fixation (bone ingrowth). The porous surface of the prosthesis body increases the formation of fibrous tissue, thereby improving soft tissue anchorage to the implant and reducing the periprosthetic dead space.

The choice of "fixation" of the megaprosthesis to the host bone depends on the experience of the surgeon. The use of uncemented press-fit prostheses is more widespread, because of the general youth of the patients treated.

Before performing tibial osteotomy, reference landmarks are determined to maintain correct leg rotation during reconstruction. Particular attention should be paid to the alignment of the residual extensor mechanism to avoid patellar subluxation-dislocation.

The patella tendon is sutured to the prosthesis with Dacron tape (Fig. 20.13). When possible, medial gastrocnemius transfer is necessary to provide suitable coverage of the prosthesis and restore continuity of the extensor mechanism. It is mobilized distally and rotated anteriorly to cover the prosthesis; it is then sutured to the remaining leg muscles. The patellar tendon and anterior capsule are sutured to the transferred medial gastrocnemius muscle with nonabsorbable sutures (Fig. 20.14). Proper tension on the quadriceps mechanism

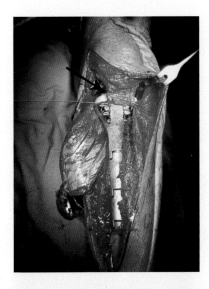

FIGURE 20.13

The patellar tendon is sutured to the loop on the proximal tibia prosthesis.

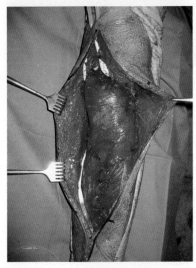

FIGURE 20.14

The medial gastrocnemius muscle is transposed to cover the prosthesis and to provide a soft tissue reconstruction of the extensor mechanism.

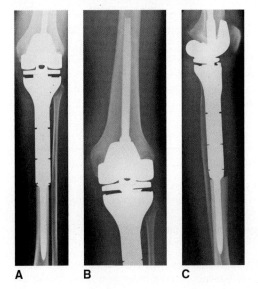

A   B   C

FIGURE 20.15

A–C: An anteroposterior and lateral plain radiograph of a proximal tibia megaprosthesis.

is determined by bending the knee through a 30- to 40-degree range motion. It is important to achieve accurate hemostasis and close all the tissue planes to avoid "dead space." The use of drains and compressive bandage is preferable to prevent hematomas (2,4). Routine orthogonal radiographs may be obtained immediately after surgery to confirm prosthesis orientation (Fig. 20.15).

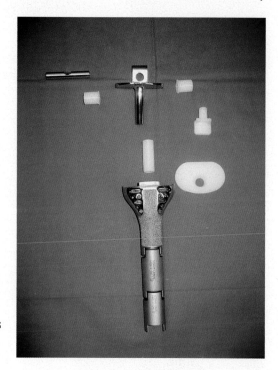

FIGURE 20.16

A proximal tibial component of Modular Prosthesis (Stryker) with a porous coating body to allow soft tissue attachments.

PEARLS AND PITFALLS

- Modular prostheses are used to reconstruct joint segments, or rare occassions an entire bone segment. These prostheses are available in various sizes and assembled in the operating theatre according to specific needs (Fig. 20.16).
- There are several advantages to this reconstruction: a relatively easy reconstruction technique, fast mobilization, and good function. The disadvantages are related to the difficulty in suturing the soft tissues to the metal prosthesis, as is for the patella tendon in proximal tibia replacement.
- Biologic reconstruction of the extensor mechanism is recommended. Therefore, the continuity of the patella tendon should be preserved, when possible, avoiding inadequate margins to reduce the risk of rupture.

POSTOPERATIVE MANAGEMENT

- Prophylactic antibiotics treatment with first generation cephalosporin is recommended during and continued for at least 6 days after surgery.
- Rehabilitation following proximal tibia megaprosthesis must be avoided for 4 weeks because reconstruction of the extensor mechanism requires a period of immobilization in a long-leg cast.
- An intensive rehabilitation of the quadriceps is necessary after the cast has been removed and knee flexion is increased only after full active extension has been obtained (2,4).

COMPLICATIONS

Complications of prosthetic reconstructions may appear early or late.

- Early complications include skin necrosis, wound dehiscence, infection, thromboembolism, neuropraxia, and articular instability. Surgical techniques with careful manipulation and reconstruction of the soft tissues may reduce these complications.
- Late complications include aseptic loosening, hematogenous infection, fatigue fracture, polyethylene component wear, and local recurrence.

Mechanical failure is multifactorial and the leading reason for implant revision. Experience with the use of custom-made prostheses has shown substantial risks of stem fracture, because older stem designs were too short and narrow. Stems over 9 mm are now used and rarely fracture. Aseptic loosening is the main cause of failure of proximal tibia megaprostheses. Several studies have shown that the worst prognosis for prostheses survival is related to the extent of bone and soft tissue resection (5,6) and that most loosened prostheses may undergo limb-sparing revision (7).

Late infection is the second most common complication and can worsen patient prognosis, postponing the beginning of adjuvant therapy (chemoradiotherapy), and is the most common cause of secondary amputations.

Adequate soft tissue coverage can be difficult after a proximal tibia reconstruction leading to a higher risk of infection. The use of a gastrocnemius muscle transfer helps prevent skin necrosis and secondary infection. Grimer et al. (8) reported an initial 36% infection rate that dropped to 12% with the use of a medial gastrocnemius flap.

Regarding pediatric age, more operations are needed if we use expandable prostheses, not only for lengthening but also for managing the complications of expandable components: fractures, infection, wear, and loosening. The use of closed expandable prostheses is a noninvasive system to lengthen a limb of a child without having to perform an operation, and so the incidence of complications associated with lengthening can be reduced (3).

The rate of local recurrence is slightly higher in conservative surgery than in amputation. Nevertheless, in terms of survival there are no differences between patients treated with reconstructive surgery and those treated by amputation. Adequacy of the resection margins and a good response to chemotherapy are important favorable prognostic factors for local control of the disease.

RESULTS

Long-term results of this kind of reconstruction have shown that endoprosthetic survival is 86%, 80%, and 69% at 3-, 5- and 10-year follow-up. Functional results in children are similar to those reported for adults, according to the average Musculoskeletal Tumor Society rating (3). Renard et al. (9) showed how functional results were significantly better after limb-sparing surgery in comparison with amputation. Biau et al. (10) recommend a weight control program and patient education to reduce risk of implant revision. Development of imaging systems and improvement in surgical techniques are the key to reducing the rate of complications. Current prosthetic implants are light, resistant, and inert systems for skeletal reconstruction. We believe that all patients with proximal tibial sarcomas should be considered potential candidates for limb-salvage surgery by endoprosthetic reconstruction.

REFERENCES

1. Campanacci M. *Bone and Soft Tissue Tumors*. Wien-New York, NY: Springer; 1999.
2. Michael AS, Springfield D. *Surgery for Bone and Soft-Tissue Tumors*. Philadelphia, PA: JB Lippincott; 1998.
3. Longhi A, Errani C, De Paolis M, et al. Primary bone osteosarcoma in the pediatric age: state of the art. *Cancer Treat Rew*. 2006;32:423–436.
4. Malawer MM, Sugarbaker HS. *Musculoskeletal Cancer Surgery*. Dordrecht, The Netherlands: Kluwer Academic Publishers; 2001.
5. Mittermayer F. Long-term followup of uncemented tumor endoprostheses for the lower extremity. *Clin Orthop*. 2001;388:167–177.
6. Kabo JM, Yang RS, Dorey FJ, et al. In vivo rotational stability of the kinematic rotating hinge knee prosthesis. *Clin Orthop*. 1997;336:166–176.
7. Mittrmayer F, Windhager R, Dominkus M, et al. Revision of the Kotz type of tumour endoprosthesis for the lower limb. *Soc Bone Joint Surg Br*. 2002;84-B:401–406.
8. Grimer RJ, Carter SR, Tillman RM, et al. Endoprosthetic replacement of the proximal tibia. *J Bone Joint Surg Br*. 1999;81:488–494.
9. Renard AJ, Veth RP, Schreuder HW, et al.: Function and complications after ablative and limb-salvage therapy in lower extremity sarcoma of bone. *J Surg Oncol*. 2000;73:198–205.
10. Biau D, Faure F, Katsahian S, et al. Survival of total knee replacement with a magaprosthesis after bone tumor resection. *J Bone Joint Surg Am*. 2006;88(6):1285–1293.

21 Transepiphyseal Resection and Intercalary Reconstruction

D. Luis Muscolo, Miguel A. Ayerza, and Luis A. Aponte-Tinao

Patients are selected for this procedure according to the following criteria: (a) intrachemotherapy tumor progression, (b) tumor growth toward the epiphysis, and (c) amount of epiphysis to be preserved in order to allow fixation of the osteotomy junction. Prechemotherapy and postchemotherapy MRI studies are compared to evaluate tumor response. Tumors with no clinical or MRI evidence of progression during chemotherapy are considered potential candidates for transepiphyseal resections (Figs. 21.1 and 21.2).

INDICATIONS

- Tumors growing in the metaphyseal area with no or partial compromise of the epiphysis
- A residual epiphysis of ≥1 cm should be obtained in order to allow fixation of the osteotomy junction and safe oncologic margins.
- Tumors with no evidence of progression clinically or on magnetic resonance imaging (MRI) studies during chemotherapy
- This technique is designed in order to resect the tumor, preserving the patient's own articular cartilage, cruciate, and collateral ligaments and without altering the normal joint anatomy.

CONTRAINDICATIONS

- Patients in whom preoperative imaging studies demonstrate evidence of epiphyseal compromise of the tumor
- Intrachemotherapy tumor progression

PREOPERATIVE PREPARATION

Patients are usually treated with chemotherapy and, after the induction period, definitive surgery of the primary lesion is performed. Magnetic resonance images are done with a 1.5-T Magnetom Vision unit (Siemens, Erlangen, Germany) at the time of the diagnosis and after chemotherapy in order to evaluate tumor response. The whole limb is evaluated using a body coil. In order to determine epiphyseal tumor spread and its relation to the articular cartilage, images are obtained using an additional knee coil. These images are reviewed on paired longitudinal T1-weighted and short tau inversion recovery images. The extent of the epiphyseal involvement is calculated with coronal, sagittal, and axial images defining the end of the tumor as the point in which marrow signal intensity changed from normal to abnormal (1–7). All scans are performed by the same radiologist.

233

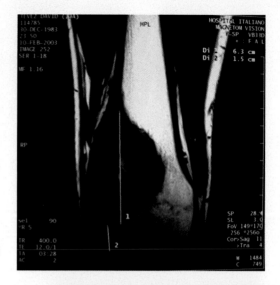

FIGURE 21.1

Coronal MRI that illustrates the preoperative assessment of tumor extension.

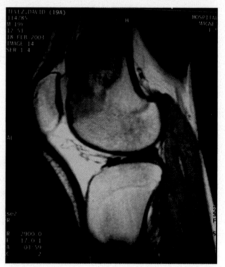

FIGURE 21.2

Sagittal MRI that shows that tumor extension is more anterior, leaving the posterior part of the condyles free of tumor.

TECHNIQUE

All operations are performed in a clean-air enclosure with vertical airflow and usually with spinal anesthesia. The patient is placed on the operating table in the supine position. A sandbag is placed under the ipsilateral buttock. A long midline incision is made beginning in the midthigh and a medial parapatellar arthrotomy is performed that enables a wide exposure of the distal femur and the knee joint. The biopsy tract is left in continuity with the specimen (Fig. 21.3). The distal femur is approached via the interval between the rectus femoris and vastus medialis. If there is an extraosseous component, a cuff of normal muscle must be excised. Proximal femoral osteotomy is performed at the appropriate location as determined by the preoperative imaging studies. All remaining soft tissues at the level of transaction are cleared. The osteotomy is performed after the posterior and medial structures have been protected and retracted and perpendicular to the long axis of the femur. Following the osteotomy, the distal femur is pulled forward to expose the soft tissue attachments of the popliteal space. The popliteal artery is mobilized, and the geniculate vessels are ligated and transected. The gastrocnemius is released and the posterior capsule is opened. The cruciates and collateral ligaments are identified and remain intact attached to the epiphysis that is saved. The next step is to mark the intraepiphyseal cut (Fig. 21.4). The osteotomy is planned 1 to 2 cm from the lower edge of the tumor growth, defined as the point at which marrow signal intensity changed from abnormal to normal. At the time of surgery, measurements obtained with preoperative MRI are correlated with anatomical landmarks: the epicondyles, the intercondylar notch roof, and the articular cartilage limits in the femur. Following the osteotomy the distal femur is passed off the operative field (Fig. 21.5). After resection of the tumor, insertion of an allograft segment tailored to fit the bone defect is performed. After the donor bone is thawed in a warm solution, it is cut to the proper length (Fig. 21.6). The intraepiphyseal osteotomy is temporarily secured with threaded Kirschner wires that are inserted through the distal part of both condyles and into the allograft. Then the osteotomy is stabilized by internal fixation with cancellous screws compressing the metaphyseal bone (Figs. 21.7 and 21.8). Before the proximal osteotomy is stabilized, the posterior capsule is repaired suturing autologous capsular tissues with capsular tissues provided by the allograft. The diaphyseal osteotomy

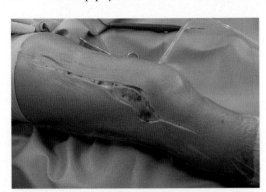

FIGURE 21.3
Intraoperative photograph showing the long midline incision that in this case is extended laterally to include the biopsy tract.

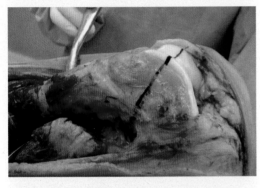

FIGURE 21.4
Intraoperative photograph with the intraepiphyseal osteotomy marked. The cruciates and collateral ligaments are identified and remained intact in the epiphysis that is saved.

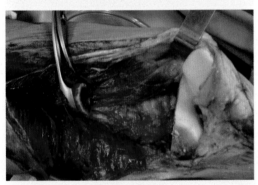

FIGURE 21.5
Intraoperative photograph showing the bone defect after both osteotomies are performed.

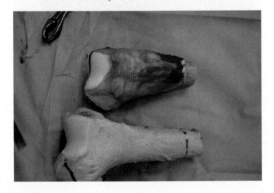

FIGURE 21.6
Intraoperative photograph after the donor graft was thawed in a warm solution and is marked according to the bone that was resected in order to cut the proper length to fit the bone defect.

is stabilized by internal fixation with an anterior short plate, and to minimize the risk of fracture an additional lateral condylar buttress plate is placed to cover the entire length of the allograft (Figs. 21.9 and 21.10). Two suction drains are inserted, and after lavage of the wound with saline solution, a meticulous suture repair of the quadriceps is required. A layered closure of the subcutaneous tissues and skin is the performed.

POSTOPERATIVE MANAGEMENT

External splinting with a brace with the knee in full extension is used until the wound heals. After 2 days, the drains are removed and the wound is inspected. Passive range-of-motion exercises are begun at 2 weeks after the operation. The patient is allowed partial weight bearing at 8 to 12 weeks.

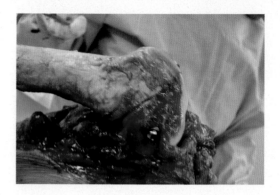

FIGURE 21.7

Intraoperative photograph showing how the osteotomy is stabilized by internal fixation with cancellous screws compressing the metaphyseal osteotomy.

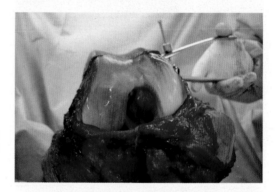

FIGURE 21.8

Intraoperative photograph after metaphyseal osteotomy is performed showing the congruence of the donor and the recipient and how both cruciate ligaments femoral insertion are preserved.

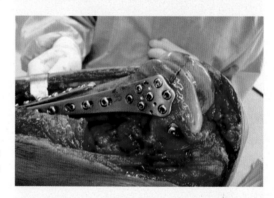

FIGURE 21.9

Intraoperative photograph after the diaphyseal osteotomy is fixed with an anterior short plate, and a buttress condylar plate is placed to minimize the risk of fracture covering the entire length of the allograft.

PEARLS AND PITFALLS

- It is important to have stringent preoperative criteria for selecting patients who are suitable for this technique.
- The procedure is best performed by an orthopedic oncologic surgeon with experience in knee reconstructive and sport medicine surgery.
- All previous biopsy sites and all potentially contaminated tissues should be removed en bloc, including needle biopsy tracts.
- The major neurovascular bundle must be free of tumor.
- Intraoperative guidelines or parameters for epiphyseal osteotomies are based on measurements obtained with preoperative MRI.
- All areas not clearly defined by MRI to be edema should be considered tumoral and included in the specimen resected.
- In order to avoid allograft fracture the internal fixation should cover as much as possible of the graft.
- Uniform cortical contact, compression of the osteotomy gap, and rotational stability were noted to be better when internal fixation with plates and screws was used.
- Locking compression plate is now used for the majority of our patients because we believe that it imparts greater mechanical stability to the reconstruction.
- As stability obtained by the reconstruction is high, no cast is used to immobilize the limb, and the postoperative rehabilitation begins at 2 weeks after operation.

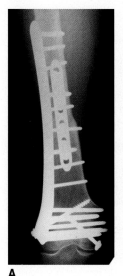 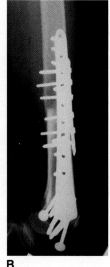

A   **B**

FIGURE 21.10

Anteroposterior (**A**) and lateral (**B**) radiographs 12 months after tumor resection and intercalary allograft of the distal femur showing healing of both osteotomies without altering the preoperative joint anatomy and preserving distal femoral articular cartilage and ligaments from the patient.

COMPLICATIONS

As the imaging techniques improve, many tumors contained within the metadiaphyseal region of long bones may be treated by wide resection but with epiphyseal preservation (8–13). Intercalary segmental allografts can be fixed to small epiphyseal host fragments, obtaining immediate limb stability and allowing active adjacent joints motion. This avoids complications associated with osteoarticular allograft, such as cartilage degeneration, joint collapse, or instability. After healing of host-donor junctions, the graft may be incorporated progressively by the host. This reconstruction can also be combined with a vascularized fibular graft to accelerate osseous union at the osteotomies sites (12).

Surgeons willing to attempt this procedure should be aware of two main and dangerous difficulties, first, to clearly define tumor margins with MRIs. Presurgical identification of epiphyseal tumor extension should include even areas of intermediate signal intensity that may turn out to be hemorrhage or edema at pathological specimen evaluation (1–7). Questionable bone marrow areas, after extensive imaging studies, should be considered as tumor invasion and included in the resection. Second, there are difficulties in correlating presurgical MRI information with real tumor limits at the time of surgery. Future application of computer-aided techniques may prove valuable to help define with precision tumor margins at time of resection.

RESULTS

Only a few small series of patients with metaphyseal osteosarcomas around the knee treated with salvage of the epiphysis and reconstruction have been reported (8–13). Reconstructive procedures included physeal distraction before removing the tumor (9), distraction osteogenesis after tumor resection (13), autoclaved autogenous bone with a vascularized fibula (8), and frozen allograft with (11) or without vascularized fibula autograft (12). All these studies reported different complications; however, no recurrences at the retained epiphysis were diagnosed.

Allograft results after transepiphyseal resection can be compared with results obtained with intercalary allografts in larger series. Ortiz-Cruz et al. (14) reported 87 (84%) of 104 patients who were followed for at least 2 years who had a successful result, with 92% rate of limb salvage. They did not find any differences in nonunion in diaphyseal or metaphyseal bone, or with different internal fixation. Cara et al. (15) reported a lower rate of satisfactory functional outcomes, with an excellent or good result in only 14 (61%) of 23 patients. They reported nonunion only in the diaphyseal osteotomies. In a recent report (16) that reviewed 59 patients followed for a mean of 5 years, the 5-year survival rate was 79%, with no differences in allograft survival in patients receiving or not receiving adjuvant chemotherapy. The nonunion rate for diaphyseal junctions was higher (15%) than the rate for metaphyseal ones (2%). Although some patients required reoperations because of allograft complications, it seems that the use of intercalary allograft clearly has a place in the reconstruction of a segmental defect created by the resection of a tumor in the diaphyseal and/or metaphyseal portion of the femur or tibia.

REFERENCES

1. O'Flanagan SJ, Stack JP, McCee HM, et al. Imaging of intramedullary tumor spread in osteosarcoma: a comparison of techniques. *J Bone Joint Surg Br*. 1991;73:998–1001.
2. Hoffer FA, Nikanorov AY, Reddick WE, et al. Accuracy of MR imaging for detecting epiphyseal extension of osteosarcoma. *Pediatr Radiol*. 2000;30:289–298.
3. Norton KI, Hermann G, Abdelwahab IF, et al. Epiphyseal involvement in osteosarcoma. *Radiology*. 1991;180: 813–816.
4. Onikul E, Fletcher BD, Parham DM, et al. Accuracy of MR imaging for estimating intraosseous extent of osteosarcoma. *Am J Roentgenol*. 1996;167:1211–1215.
5. Saifuddin A. The accuracy of imaging in the local staging of appendicular osteosarcoma. *Skeletal Radiol*. 2002;31: 191–201.
6. San Julian M, Aquerreta JD, Benito A, et al. Indications for epiphyseal preservation in metaphyseal malignant bone tumors of children: relationship between image methods and histological findings. *J Pediatr Orthop*. 1999;19:543–548.
7. Zimmer WD, Berquist TH, McLeod RA, et al. Magnetic resonance imaging of osteosarcomas. Comparison with computed tomography. *Clin Orthop*. 1986;208:289–299.
8. Amitani A, Yamazaki T, Sonoda J, et al. Preservation of the knee joint in limb salvage of osteosarcoma in the proximal tibia. *Int Orthop*. 1998;22:330–334.
9. Canadell J, Forriol F, Cara JA. Removal of metaphyseal bone tumors with preservation of the epiphysis. Physeal distraction before excision. *J Bone Joint Surg Br*. 1994;76:127–132.
10. Kumta SM, Chow TC, Griffith J, et al. Classifying the location of osteosarcoma with reference to the epiphyseal plate helps determine the optimal skeletal resection in limb salvage procedure. *Arch Orthop Trauma Surg*. 1999;119: 327–331.
11. Manfrini M, Gasbarrini A, Malaguti C, et al. Intraepiphyseal resection of the proximal tibia and its impact on lower limb growth. *Clin Orthop*. 1999;358:111–119.
12. Muscolo DL, Ayerza MA, Aponte-Tinao LA, et al. Partial epiphyseal preservation and intercalary allograft reconstruction in high-grade metaphyseal osteosarcoma of the knee. *J Bone Joint Surg Am*. 2004;86:2686–2693.
13. Tsuchiya H, Abdel-Wanis ME, Sakurakichi K, et al. Osteosarcoma around the knee. Intraepiphyseal excision and biological reconstruction with distraction osteogenesis. *J Bone Joint Surg Br*. 2002;84:1162–1166.
14. Ortiz-Cruz EJ, Gebhardt MC, Jennings LC, et al. The results of transplantation of intercalary allografts after resection of tumors: a long- term follow- up study. *J Bone Joint Surg*. 1997;79A:97–106.
15. Cara JA, Laclériga A, Cañadell J. Intercalary bone allografts: 23 tumor cases followed for 3 years. *Acta Orthop Scand*. 1994;65:42–46.
16. Muscolo DL, Ayerza MA, Aponte-Tinao LA, et al. Intercalary fémur and tibia segmental allografts provide an acceptable alternative in reconstructing tumor resections. *Clin Orthop*. 2004;426:97–102.

22 Internal Fixation of Metastatic Lesions of the Distal Femur

Adam J. Schwartz and David J. Jacofsky

Metastatic bone lesions involving the distal femur are less frequently encountered than those affecting the pertrochanteric region or diaphysis. While only 4% of all metastatic bone lesions ultimately result in pathologic fracture, those affecting the femur may portend a seven- to eightfold increased risk, particularly those resulting from primary breast carcinoma.

The goal of treatment is to provide immediate fracture stability, allowing for rapid patient mobilization and full weight-bearing with return to function. Patients with distal femoral metastasis may seek medical attention prior to pathologic fracture, and in such cases, nonoperative management may be a reasonable alternative to surgical intervention if symptoms and osseous stability permit.

Patients presenting after fracture through a metastatic lesion, however, are rarely treated nonoperatively. The results of nonoperative treatment in this patient population are less than optimal, leading to decreased mobility, prolonged hospital stays, and increased risk of pulmonary and cardiovascular complications. Depending on the histology of the lesion, the presence of metastatic lesions involving other organ systems, and the patient's overall health, median life-expectancy may range anywhere from 6 months to >48 months, and the surgeon should assume that the patient may not survive long enough for the fracture to heal. As a consequence, the initial surgical stabilization of the fracture should be adequate to provide immediate weight bearing. If adequate stability cannot be achieved by internal fixation alone or supplementation with polymethylmethacrylate (PMMA) cement, an alternative treatment option should be employed, such as prosthetic distal femoral replacement.

Patients at risk of pathologic fracture are generally treated according to fracture risk. The most common method of determining the likelihood of fracture is the use of a popular classification system described by Mirels (1). Nonoperative management typically consists of external beam radiotherapy, hormone therapy, and/or the administration of bisphosphonates. This regimen, while effective, is generally more successful in non–weight-bearing portions of the appendicular skeleton, such as the distal upper extremity.

Nonoperative treatment of patients with a symptomatic lesion of the distal femur, or those who have already sustained a pathologic fracture, however, is less likely to result in effective pain control or adequate function. For this subset of patients, internal fixation with or without PMMA augmentation provides reliable pain relief and rapid mobilization (2). Various authors have advocated en bloc resection of solitary lesions resulting from primary thyroid and renal cell carcinoma (3–9). Althausen et al. (3) cited presentation with a long disease-free interval between nephrectomy and first metastases and appendicular skeletal location as favorable prognostic factors (3). The authors advocate aggressive surgical resection rather than internal fixation in such cases.

INDICATIONS

Indications for surgical stabilization of metastasis to the distal femur include

- Failure of nonoperative management
- Fracture pattern amenable to rigid initial fixation and early mobilization.

CONTRAINDICATIONS

Treatment of metastatic lesions resulting in pathologic fracture of the distal femur must be individualized. Relative contraindications to open reduction and internal fixation include

- Life expectancy <3 months
- Active infection
- Acute deep venous thrombosis or pulmonary embolism (placement of a vena caval filter may be considered preoperatively in certain cases)
- Severely compromised bone quality proximal or distal to the level of fracture.

Additionally, in cases of severe fracture comminution, extremely poor bone quality, or extensive neurovascular envelopment, outcomes may be compromised (10).

PREOPERATIVE PREPARATION

A comprehensive review of the preoperative evaluation and preparation of patients with metastatic lesions to the distal femur is provided elsewhere (11) In general, patients should undergo a thorough preoperative medical evaluation, including history and physical examination as well as laboratory evaluation. Physical examination should focus on ruling out concomitant lesions that may affect treatment options, carefully inspecting the skin and surrounding soft tissues, and performing a complete neurovascular evaluation. In addition, the examination of the patient without a history of metastatic disease should include palpation of the thyroid, breast, and prostate as potential sites of primary carcinoma (12).

Investigations

For those patients presenting with a pathologic fracture as the initial symptom of metastatic disease, the workup should include laboratory analysis (including complete blood count, liver enzymes, alkaline phosphatase, erythrocyte sedimentation rate, and serum protein electrophoresis), chest radiograph, whole body technetium-99m-phosphate scintigraphy, and computed tomography of the chest abdomen and pelvis. This protocol has been shown to identify 85% of primary lesions (12). Attention should also be paid to the patient's overall nutritional status and healing potential.

Adjuvant Therapy

Perioperative treatment with bisphosphonates decreases the incidence of pathologic fracture secondary to metastasis (13). Radiation therapy is also employed postoperatively to reduce pain and obtain local control of microscopic disease (14). Radiation therapy is generally delayed until the wound has adequately healed, typically 2 to 4 weeks postoperatively.

If surgery is to be delayed more than 24 to 72 hours, placement of a simple bridging external fixator will prevent fracture shortening, and may also be used as an aid to reduction at the time of definitive fixation. The surgeon should make every effort to avoid placement of the fixator in a location that would compromise future skin incisions. A simple frame can be constructed with two 4.5-mm half pins in the anterior femur, and two 4.5-mm half pins into the medial tibial shaft.

Classification

In general, fractures of the distal femur are classified from high-quality anteroposterior and lateral radiographs alone. Occasionally, however, it is necessary to obtain specialized views or further imaging. Traction views are particularly helpful if there is a high degree of comminution, or if there exists ligamentous involvement resulting in a significant sagittal deformity. Computed tomography scans are also used liberally for fractures that extend to the articular surface. Magnetic resonance imaging can also be helpful to determine the extent of disease, although hematoma makes interpretation difficult once a fracture has occurred. Advanced imaging often helps delineate those patients with disease too extensive for open reduction alone and may help determine the need for prosthetic replacement.

Various classification systems are available that describe fractures of the distal end of the femur. The most common classification currently used is that of Reudi et al. (Fig. 22.1; Table 22.1) Type A fractures involve the extra-articular aspect of the distal femur only and are subclassified according to the amount of comminution present. Type B fractures consist of simple articular fragments, medial, lateral, and coronal (also referred to as the Hoffa fragment). Type C fractures are characterized by involvement of both the metaphyseal and intra-articular aspect of the distal femur.

TABLE 22.1   Advantages and Disadvantages of the Various Methods of Surgical Fixation Based Upon Preoperative Fracture Classification

Device	Indicated For OTA Type(s)	Advantages	Disadvantages
95-degree blade plate	A1–3, C1–2	Resists varus collapse Fixed-angle device	May displace large posterior fragments Technically demanding Load-bearing device
Dynamic condylar screw	A1–3, C1–2	Resists varus collapse Fixed-angle device	May displace large posterior fragments Technically demanding Load-bearing device
Standard buttress plate	B1–3	Ease of insertion Improved fixation of intra-articular fragments Easily supplemented with PMMA	Load-bearing device Does not resist varus collapse Resulting stress-riser at tip of plate
Distal femoral locking plate	B1–3	Resists varus collapse Fixed-angle device Improved fixation of intra-articular fragments Easily supplemented with PMMA	Load-bearing device Resulting stress-riser at tip of plate
Retrograde femoral nail	A1–3, C1–2	Load-sharing device Ease of insertion Easily supplemented with PMMA Can stabilize very distal fragments	May displace large posterior fragments Poor fixation of intra-articular fragments Resulting stress-riser at nail tip
Antegrade femoral nail	A1–3, C1–2	Load-sharing device Ease of insertion Easily supplemented with PMMA Potential to stabilize entire femur, including femoral neck	Cannot stabilize distal fragments (<9 cm from joint line) Poor fixation of intra-articular fragments

Utilizing a preoperative templating system as described by the AO Group is extremely useful for planning the intraoperative sequence of fixation, particularly when dealing with pathologic fractures due to metastatic lesions. The mental exercise of formulating an operative plan allows the surgeon to anticipate intraoperative problems before they occur. Templating each individual screw will alert the surgeon to areas that are likely to gain poor purchase into the pathologic bone and potentially require supplemental fixation with PMMA cement.

Multiple fixation devices, including 95-degree fixed-angle plates, retrograde or antegrade femoral nails, and locked plates, should be available at the time of surgery. The advantages and disadvantages of each are explained in Table 22.1. In general, pathologic fractures are more effectively treated with load-sharing devices such as intramedullary nails, to allow for immediate weight-bearing with less concern for hardware failure. In some cases, however, such as very distal fractures, or those with a high degree of intra-articular involvement, a plate and screw construct is preferable. Plates are also indicated when the intramedullary canal is already occupied by another device, which is quite common in patients with established metastatic disease.

Biopsy

The need for histologic confirmation of solitary lesions prior to surgical stabilization cannot be overemphasized (12,14,15). It is estimated that primary sarcomas may account for up to 10% to 20% of solitary lesions in patients with a history of previously treated malignancy (16). If the surgeon is unsure of the correct diagnosis, needle or open biopsy prior to internal fixation is an effective means of histologic confirmation. As noted above, treatment of solitary metastasis from renal or thyroid carcinoma with en bloc resection may result in improved patient life expectancy, even in the face of existing pulmonary metastasis. Consultation with an orthopedic oncologist is recommended if wide resection is potentially indicated or a solitary lesion exists (Fig. 22.2).

Informed Consent

Prior to any surgical procedure, the surgeon should have an open discussion about the various treatment options with the patient. The surgeon should set realistic expectations, and it should be explained that prosthetic replacement is a possibility if adequate stabilization cannot be obtained intraoperatively. Prior to any attempt at internal fixation of a pathologic distal femur fracture, the surgeon should be prepared to abort the

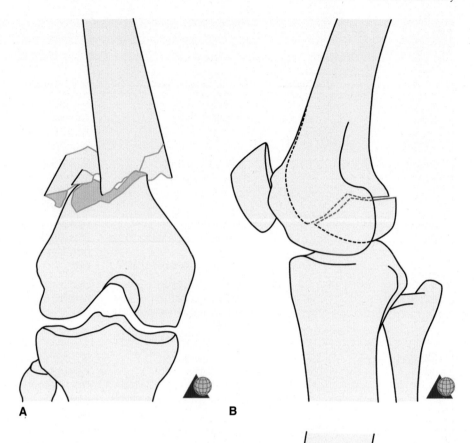

FIGURE 22.1

Classification system of distal femur fractures according to
Muller. Type A fractures involve the extra-articular aspect of the
distal femur only and are subclassified according to the amount
of comminution present (**A**). Type B fractures consist of simple
articular fragments, medial, lateral, and coronal (also referred to
as the Hoffa fragment) (**B**). Type C fractures are characterized by
involvement of both the metaphyseal and intra-articular aspect of
the distal femur (**C**).

procedure and proceed with prosthetic replacement if he or she does not feel comfortable allowing the patient
to immediately weight-bear on the construct. The goal of internal fixation in these cases is to return the patient
to preinjury function as soon as possible and to provide excellent pain relief for the remainder of the patient's
life. As a general rule, the surgeon should leave the operating room under the assumption that the fracture will
never heal (15).

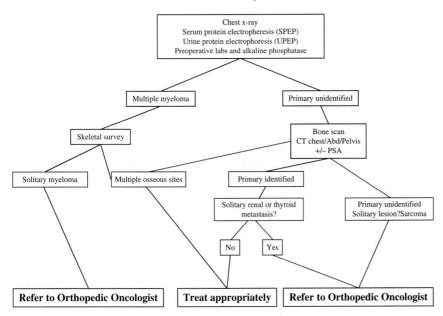

FIGURE 22.2

Evaluation of patient with destructive bone lesion.

TECHNIQUES

Positioning and Draping

The patient is positioned on a radiolucent table with the entire lower extremity accessible from the anterior-superior iliac spine to the foot. Fluoroscopic anteroposterior and lateral images of the fracture site are obtained prior to skin preparation, and the position of the c-arm is checked to ensure the ability to image the entire extremity. The extremity is then prepped and draped in the usual fashion, taking care to include the hip in the event that more proximal fixation is required. In general, a tourniquet is not used for internal fixation of pathologic fractures of the distal femur.

For fractures involving the articular surface, exposure should be large enough for the surgeon to confidently visualize the articular surface and accurately assess the reduction. If the fracture is extra-articular, it is not necessary for the exposure to include an arthrotomy; however, the surgeon should always be prepared to extend the incision if intraoperative findings change the operative plan.

Plate Fixation

Plate fixation, with supplemental PMMA cement augmentation, may be used for fixation of most types of metastatic distal femur fractures. Plate fixation provides rigid internal fixation and allows for immediate patient mobilization. Two exceptions are (a) highly comminuted fractures involving the metaphyseal portion of the distal femur (Type A3), where it is preferable to utilize an intramedullary, load-sharing device; and (b) articular fractures with a high degree of comminution (Types C2, or C3) that will not permit immediate weight-bearing postoperatively. In the latter situation, it is preferable to proceed directly to prosthetic joint replacement with an oncologic prosthesis.

Incision and Exposure

The lateral approach is the workhorse for plate and screw fixation of pathologic distal femur fractures. This approach begins just anterior to the insertion of the lateral collateral ligament and may be extended proximally along the entire shaft of the femur. If visualization of the articular surface is required, the incision may extend distally to the tibial tubercle, and a lateral parapatellar arthrotomy is performed. A blunt retractor is placed over the medial condyle to retract the extensor mechanism, allowing for excellent visualization of the medial and lateral condyles. Generally, the vastus lateralis is split longitudinally during the exposure, although one can lift it off the intermuscular septum if they so desire. Perforating vessels will require cautery and ligation if a vastus-lifting approach is utilized.

The use of minimally invasive percutaneous plate osteosynthesis, and transarticular retrograde plate osteosynthesis approaches have been shown to improve fracture healing and reduce the need for supplemental bone graft (17), but have less of a role in the treatment of pathologic fractures. The minimally invasive techniques are more difficult to utilize in the setting of pathologic distal femoral fractures, especially those requiring curettage, or supplementation with PMMA cement. In this patient population, the primary goal is rigid internal fixation allowing immediate patient mobilization. The incision should be large enough to permit the surgeon to achieve these goals in every case.

Plate Fixation Devices

Various plates are currently available that provide excellent initial fixation of pathologic distal femoral fractures. Historically, the 95-degree blade plate was the workhorse of periarticular distal femoral fractures, due to its broad, fixed-angle distal surface. Standard buttress plates with nonlocking screws have a higher rate of failure, particularly in this patient population with poor bone stock. The dynamic condylar screw is similar to the 95-degree blade and provides a fixed-angle construct (Fig. 22.3). The advantage when compared to the 95-degree blade plate is the greater ease of insertion and lesser risk of condylar disruption.

More recently, the introduction of locking plates has provided an attractive alternative to previous implant designs (Fig. 22.4). Locking plates are not as technically demanding as the 95-degree blade plate or dynamic condylar screw because the distal fixation screws are introduced individually, allowing more room for error and equal or superior distal fragment fixation. Additionally, screw threads form a frictional bond with the plate, providing a fixed-angle construct, which is particularly advantageous when poor bone quality results in inadequate screw purchase. Newer plate designs also provide a highly conforming profile, allowing for greater ease of insertion, and acting as an aid to fracture reduction.

As a general rule, at least one femoral cortex must be intact to provide adequate stability for immediate postoperative weight bearing (16). As a result, plate fixation is more effective in cases of impending pathologic fracture, when cement augmentation of the deficient cortex provides immediate stability and a fixed-angle construct. If such stability cannot be achieved, then fixation with a load-sharing intramedullary device is more reliable.

The following general steps are followed to help ensure stable fixation of pathologic distal femoral fractures using plates and screws:

Restoration of Length

Regardless of the implant selected, it is helpful to apply traction and utilize the principle of ligamentotaxis as an aid to reduction. Manual traction is generally sufficient to restore length for fractures that are treated within 24 hours of injury. For surgeons working without multiple assistants, however, this technique may be overly demanding or impossible. In this situation, a temporary bridging external fixator and femoral distractor device are excellent alternatives that provide prolonged traction and stability (see discussion above). After gross mechanical alignment is achieved, the fracture may be reduced using various clamps, ball-spiked pushers, or a dental pick.

Reduction and Stabilization of the Articular Surface

For Type B or C fractures, with intra-articular involvement, it is important to adequately visualize the joint surface. A lateral parapatellar arthrotomy and mobilization of the extensor mechanism as described above allow for excellent inspection of the joint surface. Large fragments may be reduced with a large pelvic clamp and fixed with 6.5 mm partially threaded cannulated screws. Smaller articular fragments may be held provisionally with 2.0-mm K-wires, or bioabsorbable pins. Fixation may be improved with the use of countersunk 3.5 mm fully-threaded cortical screws, or variable-pitch headless compression screws. Severely comminuted intra-articular fractures in this setting may not be amenable to fixation and immediate weight bearing, even with augmentation from PMMA. In this case, prosthetic replacement is preferred.

Once articular reduction and stability is achieved, the plate device is then secured to the distal fragment. This part of the procedure is different for each individual type of plate fixation device. The 95-degree blade plate and the condylar compression screw both rely on accurate placement of the distal portion of the plate. Three K-wires are typically placed: one parallel to the distal aspect of the medial and lateral femoral condyles, one along the patellofemoral articulation, and a final "summation" wire that represents a tract parallel to both of the previously placed wires. The condylar compression screw can rotate into varying amounts of flexion or extension, whereas the 95-degree blade plate cannot. As a result, the technique required for insertion of the 95-degree blade is much more demanding and requires accurate placement in the axial, coronal, and sagittal planes. Once the path for the 95-degree blade is determined, the chisel is inserted with or without predrilling the lateral cortex. The blade plate is then inserted and secured to the remaining distal block with screws just proximal to the blade.

Distal femoral buttress plates, or distal femoral locking plates, are similarly secured to the distal fragment. It is important to remember that locking screws will not compress the plate to the bone; the position of the plate cannot be changed once the screws engage the threads in the plate. For this reason, it is important for the surgeon to confirm proper plate placement prior to the insertion of locking screws into the distal fragment.

Reduction of the Articular Segment to the Shaft Segment

The next step in plate fixation of distal femoral fractures is to reduce the articular fragment to the proximal shaft segment. It is important to maintain proper length and rotation prior to fixation of the plate to the

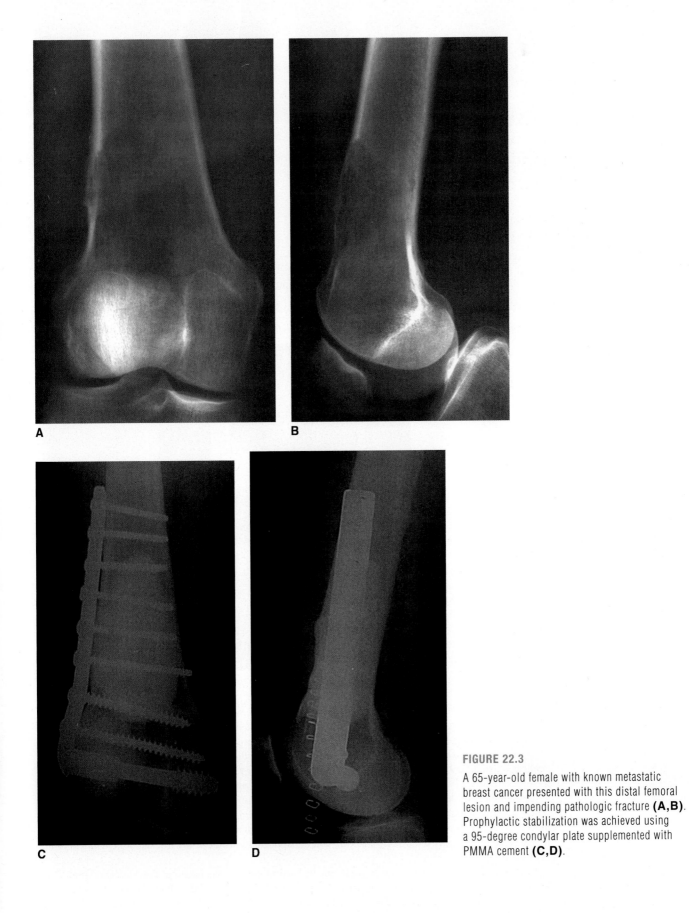

FIGURE 22.3

A 65-year-old female with known metastatic breast cancer presented with this distal femoral lesion and impending pathologic fracture **(A,B)**. Prophylactic stabilization was achieved using a 95-degree condylar plate supplemented with PMMA cement **(C,D)**.

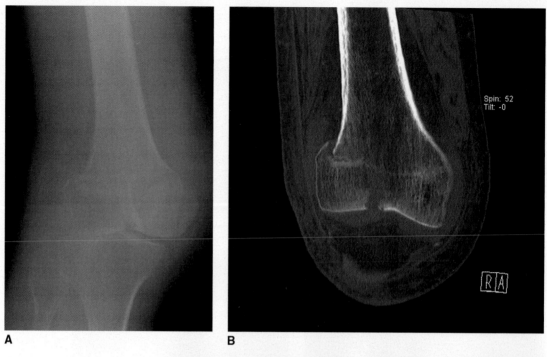

A

B

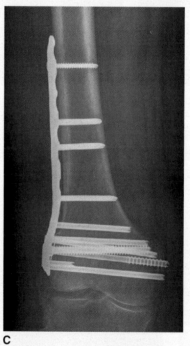

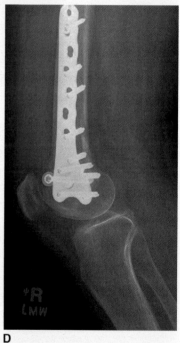

C

D

FIGURE 22.4

A 79-year-old male with a 40 pack-year history of smoking and lung cancer presented with an intra-articular distal femur fracture (**A**). Prior to fracture, the patient had undergone a bone scan that identified this site as one of many areas of metastatic bone disease. Although there was tumor present, the preoperative CT scan (**B**) demonstrated relatively good preservation of the periarticular bone. Excellent fixation was achieved with a periarticular locking plate (**C,D**), although a modular endoprosthesis was available at the time of surgery.

proximal segment. Due to destruction of landmarks and bone remodeling from neoplastic activity, this may be difficult to achieve by direct visualization alone. The Bovie cautery cable, held proximally over the center of the femoral head, and distally over the center of the ankle joint, may be used to demonstrate restoration of the mechanical axis. The cable should lie over the center of the knee joint, or just medial, which can be confirmed using fluoroscopy. One method of confirming proper rotation is to obtain a fluoroscopic view of the opposite lesser trochanter while holding the patella facing superiorly (2). This image may be obtained at the beginning of the case, and the image is saved for future reference. During plate fixation of the distal articular segment to the shaft, the surgeon may then use a 4.5-mm Schanz pin placed into the proximal fragment to rotate the proximal fragment. With the patella facing superiorly on the operative limb, the surgeon may then confirm proper rotation by ensuring that the appearance of the lesser trochanter is identical to the opposite limb.

Prior to draping, a radiopaque meter stick may be used to measure the length of the unaffected limb. This length is documented and used as a reference, especially for fractures with a high degree of metaphyseal comminution. The AO tensioning device may be used in reverse orientation to gain additional length prior to definitive fixation of the proximal fragment to the plate. A 4.5-mm fully threaded cortical screw is placed just proximal to the plate device, and the tensioner is applied in reverse orientation to distract the fracture to the desired length.

Augmentation of Fixation Using PMMA Cement (If Necessary)

Please refer to the discussion below, "Cement Augmentation."

Intramedullary Nailing   Various criteria have been employed to determine whether an intramedullary nail is the ideal implant for distal femoral fractures (17–19). While many authors recommend the use of load-sharing intramedullary implants for the fixation of all types of pathologic distal femoral fractures, exceptions should include those fractures with significant articular comminution and fractures within 9 to 10 cm of the articular surface (19).

The approach for intramedullary nailing is the same for pathologic distal femoral fractures as for nonpathologic fractures. The approach may either split the patellar tendon or proceed just medial or lateral to it. We recommend insertion of the guide pin directly through the skin into the anticipated starting location of the opening reamer. The position of the guide pin is confirmed on AP and lateral fluoroscopic images. This location generally corresponds to a point just anterior to Blumensaat's line on the lateral image and in line with the anatomic axis of the femur on the AP view. Once the position of the guide pin is confirmed, a small incision is centered around the pin. The exposure may be modified to include a small medial or lateral incision over the pathologic lesion to allow for curettage and PMMA insertion. Some authors advocate venting the femoral shaft with multiple holes to prevent the formation of fat or tumor emboli during intramedullary reaming.

The technique of intramedullary nailing of pathologic distal femur fractures proceeds in a similar fashion to that employed in the traditional trauma setting. Due to the likelihood of progressive bone destruction, the maximum number of locking screws are typically placed. In addition, most orthopedic oncologists recommend against the use of short nails and advocate placement of cephalomedullary devices whenever possible. This strategy may preemptively address future lesions of the femoral neck. Special attention should be paid to the diameter of the femoral canal preoperatively, however, as the risk of causing a fracture is increased with an intact diaphysis. In addition, it is often necessary to supplement nail fixation with screws for intra-articular fractures.

Though intramedullary nailing may provide reliable fixation of pathologic distal femoral fractures, many authors have expressed concern over the high rate of fat embolism, intra-articular fragment displacement during retrograde nailing, and seeding of the knee joint with metastatic tumor cells (2). The potential for these potentially devastating complications to occur should be discussed with the patient prior to surgery. Likewise, postoperative irradiation of the entire surgical field, including the knee joint, should be performed in this setting.

Cement Augmentation   A variety of techniques have been described for supplementing internal fixation with PMMA cement. The particular technique selected depends largely on the type of implant used for fracture fixation and the fracture pattern.

For intramedullary nails, the technique described by Varriale et al. (20) is effective, safe, and has been shown to reduce the incidence of intraoperative complications. This technique involves passage of the femoral nail in the typical fashion, followed by the creation of a drill hole in the metaphyseal bone. A 30-mL syringe filled with PMMA in the liquid phase (cooled to allow for prolonged working time) is then used to pressurize the cement into the pathologic bone, surrounding the intramedullary nail. This technique was compared to intramedullary cementation prior to passage of the nail in the calf model, and demonstrated superior mechanical performance, as well as a decreased incidence of complications associated with nail passage through previously placed cement (20).

Plate devices are also amenable to supplemental fixation with PMMA cement. The two techniques most commonly used involve placement of the PMMA cement either before or after the fixation device is placed (17). The liquid cementation technique calls for the removal of screws with poor bony purchase. The screws are aligned and marked on a towel, so that the surgeon can quickly replace them prior to cement curing. The cement is mixed and pressurized into the screw holes, which can be widened using a drill bit, if necessary. The screws are then replaced into their respective holes.

Another technique involves the impaction of cement through the fracture site, if an actual fracture has occurred. The fracture is cleaned of any callus or hematoma. After plate fixation to the distal fragment, the proximal and distal canals are debrided of medullary contents. The cement is then impacted into the canal, both proximally and distally, taking care to avoid contact with the fracture site. The plate is then secured to the proximal fragment in the usual fashion, drilling and tapping the screws into the previously placed cement.

POSTOPERATIVE MANAGEMENT

Patients with metastatic disease have limited life expectancy. Patients should be mobilized immediately, with the goal of returning to preoperative functional status as soon as possible. With adequate preoperative planning, the procedure should have provided the patient with the ability to ambulate early.

PEARLS AND PITFALLS

We would direct the reader to the article by Beauchamp et al. (15) for an excellent review of the common complications involved with treating metastatic bone lesions. The most common pitfalls involved in treating pathologic fractures of the distal femur are

- Inaccurate Diagnosis
- Inadequate Fixation
- Underestimating the Potential for Intraoperative Complications
- Failure to Anticipate Future Adjacent Lesions

Careful preoperative planning and good intraoperative decision making may help avoid these complications. Certain histologic types of metastatic disease, including renal and thyroid carcinoma and multiple myelomatous lesions, may result in highly vascularized lesions, leading to potentially disastrous intraoperative blood loss. It is vital to recognize the potential for this complication to occur, as preoperative embolization has been shown to dramatically reduce bleeding in this situation. Given the often copious intraosseous blood supply, bleeding during surgery for a distal femoral lesion may not always respond to the inflation of a tourniquet, and often the surgical location precludes tourniquet use altogether.

Patients with metastatic lesions to the femur are at an increased risk of developing a second lesion more proximal to the level of fixation. Some authors would advocate the use of an antegrade cephalomedullary device for distal femoral fractures whenever possible to protect the femoral neck from future lesions (16). While this strategy would certainly work well for most fracture patterns, we recommend that implant selection remain individualized, based on the fracture pattern and patient circumstances.

COMPLICATIONS

Infection

Infection rates as high as 7% after fixation of nonpathologic distal femoral fractures are reported. Factors predisposing patients to increased infection risk are open fracture, poor nutritional status, prolonged operative times, inadequate stability, and lack of surgeon experience (2). Due to the often compromised health of patients with malignancy, the infection rates after treatment of pathologic fractures are at least this high. Prior irradiation to the surgical bed may also further compromise host tissue and increase complication rates. Use of preoperative prophylactic antibiotics, typically third-generation cephalosporins or vancomycin, reduce the incidence of surgical site infection.

Failure of Fixation

Failure of fixation is typically the result of poor preoperative planning and failure to recognize the extent of bone loss surrounding the pathologic lesion. Highly comminuted A3 or C3 fractures are at an increased risk for overload and fatigue failure of the implants. The surgeon should leave the operating room with the expectation that the fracture will not heal and with the confidence that the procedure performed will provide the patient with adequate stability to permit immediate weight bearing.

Fat or Tumor Embolism

Fat and tumor embolism is a potentially devastating complication, leading to pulmonary collapse and death. Many authors have expressed concern regarding the high incidence of fat embolism in patients treated with intramedullary nailing for pathologic femur fractures. The rate of fat or tumor embolism is estimated to be as high as 10% in this patient population. Strategies to reduce the rate of fat embolism have included the placement of unreamed nails, venting the femur with multiple cortical holes prior to reaming, and overreaming the femoral canal by 2 mm or more (21).

RESULTS

While many authors have demonstrated excellent long-term results after internal fixation of distal femoral fractures of all types (1,19,22–25), there is a relative paucity of literature with particular focus on pathologic distal femoral fractures resulting from metastatic bone disease. Benum et al. (26) reviewed the results of 14 patients with osteoporotic distal femoral fractures treated with plate and screw fixation supplemented with PMMA cement. Only two patients in their series developed a nonunion (26). Healey et al. (23) treated 14 pathologic distal femoral fractures due to metastasis with retrograde nailing. All but three patients achieved immediate weight bearing and adequate pain control. The authors concluded that the failures were related to technical errors rather than implant selection (23).

Scholl et al. (27) reviewed 11 patients with 12 pathologic distal femoral fractures stabilized with retrograde femoral nailing. With an average follow up of 17 months, all patients were sufficiently satisfied with the outcome. One patient underwent shortening of the limb by 2 cm due to hardware failure (27).

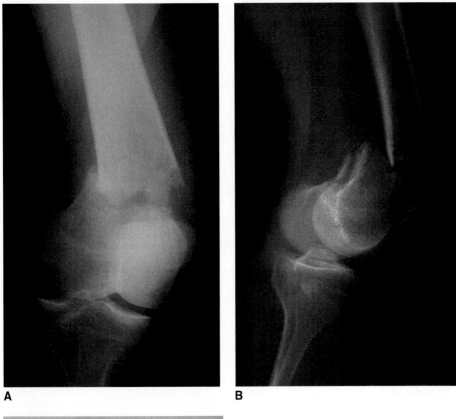

A   B

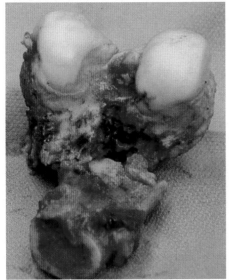

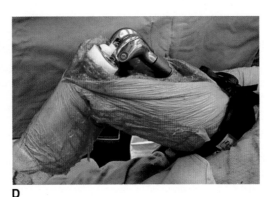

C   D

FIGURE 22.5

A–D: A low-demand 60-year-old male with advanced metastatic colon cancer presented with a transverse distal femoral fracture through a metastatic lesion. Reconstruction with a modular endoprosthesis allowed for immediate mobilization and weight bearing postoperatively.

Struhl et al. (28) reported the results of 17 distal femoral fractures in 15 patients suffering from severe osteoporosis treated with a 95-degree dynamic compression screw and plate device supplemented with PMMA cement. All patients had sufficient initial stability to allow early mobilization and weight bearing. At an average follow-up of 2 years, all patients demonstrated complete bony union with average range of motion of 100 degrees. There were no malunions or hardware failures (28).

CONCLUSIONS

Decision making in patients with metastatic disease of the distal femur can be challenging. Confirmation of diagnosis of lesions, when indicated as described above, is critical to avoiding medical errors. Overall care of the patient with metastatic disease is of paramount importance to optimize outcomes. The initial surgical stabilization of the fracture should be adequate to provide immediate weight bearing. If adequate stability cannot be achieved by internal fixation alone or supplementation with PMMA cement, an alternative treatment option should be employed, such as prosthetic distal femoral replacement (Fig. 22.5).

REFERENCES

1. Mirels H. Metastatic disease in long bones: a proposed scoring system for diagnosing impending pathologic fractures. *Clin Orthop*. 1989;249:256–264.
2. Levine AM, Aboulafia AJ. Pathologic fractures. In: Browner, ed. *Skeletal Trauma: Basic Science, Management, and Reconstruction*, 3rd ed. Philadelphia, PA: WB Saunders Co.; 2003:1957, Chapter 16.
3. Althausen P, Althausen A, Jennings LC, et al. Prognostic factors and surgical treatment of osseous metastases secondary to renal cell carcinoma. *Cancer*. 1997;80(6):1103–1109.
4. Do MY, Rhee Y, Kim DJ, et al. Clinical features of bone metastases resulting from thyroid cancer: a review of 28 patients over a 20-year period. *Endocr J*. 2005;52(6):701–707.
5. Fuchs B, Trousdale RT, Rock NG, et al. Solitary bony metastasis from renal cell carcinoma: significance of surgical treatment. *Clin Orthop Relat Res*. 2005;(431):187–192.
6. Jung ST, Ghert MA, Harrelson JM, et al. Treatment of osseous metastases in patients with renal cell carcinoma. *Clin Orthop Relat Res*. 2003;(409):223–231.
7. Kollender Y, Bickels J, Price WM, et al. Metastatic renal cell carcinoma of bone: indications and technique of surgical intervention. *J Urol*. 2000;164(5):1505–1508.
8. Linn P, Mirza AN, Lewis VO, et al. Patient survival after surgery for osseous metastasis from renal cell carcinoma. *J Bone Joint Surg Am*. 2007;89(8):1794–1801.
9. Tickoo SK, Pittas AG, Adler M, et al. Bone metastases from thyroid carcinoma: a histopathologic study with clinical correlates. *Arch Pathol Lab Med*. 2000;124(10):1440–1447.
10. Ward WG, Holsenbeck S, Dorey FJ, et al. Metastatic disease of the femur: surgical treatment. *Clin Orthop Relat Res*. 2003;415(Suppl):S230–S244.
11. Bibbo C, Patel DV, Benevenia J. Perioperative considerations in patients with metastatic bone disease. *Orthop Clin North Am*. 2000;31(4):577–595.
12. Rougraff BT, Kneisl JS, Simon MA. Skeletal metastasis of unknown origin: a prospective study of a diagnostic strategy. *J Bone Joint Surg Am*. 1993;75:1276–1281.
13. Boissier S, Ferreras M, Peyruchaud O, et al. Bisphosphonates inhibit breast and prostate carcinoma cell invasion, an early event in the formation of bone metastases. *Cancer Res*. 2000;60:2949–2954.
14. Frassica DA, Thurman S, Welsh J. Radiation therapy: orthopedic management of metastatic disease. *Orthop Clin North Am*. 2000;31(4):557–566.
15. Beauchamp CP. Errors and pitfalls in the diagnosis and treatment of metastatic bone disease. *Orthop Clin North Am*. 2000;31(4):675–685.
16. Jacofsky DJ, Haidukewych GJ. Management of pathologic fractures of the proximal femur: state of the art. *J Orthop Trauma*. 2004;18(7):459–469.
17. Krettek C, Helfet DL. Fractures of the distal femur. In: Browner, ed. *Skeletal Trauma: Basic Science, Management, and Reconstruction*, 3rd ed. Philadelphia, PA: WB Saunders Co.; 2003:1957, Chapter 53.
18. Butler MS, Brumback RJ, Ellison TS, et al. Interlocking intramedullary nailing for ipsilateral fractures of the femoral shaft and distal part of the femur. *J Bone Joint Surg Am*. 1991;73:1492–1502.
19. Leung KS, Shen WY, So WS, et al. Interlocking intramedullary nailing for supracondylar and intercondylar fractures for the distal part of the femur. *J Bone Joint Surg Am*. 1991;73:332–340.
20. Varriale PL, Evans PE, Salis JG. A modified technique for the fixation of pathologic fractures in the lower femur. *Clin Orthop Relat Res*. 1985;199:256–260.
21. Roth SE, Robello, Kreder, Whyne. Pressurization of the metastatic femur during intramedullary nail fixation. *J Trauma*. 2004;57(2):333–339.
22. Chiron HS, Casey P. Fractures of the distal third of the femur treated by internal fixation. *Clin Orthop*. 1974;100:160–170.
23. Healy JH, Lane JM. Treatment of pathologic fractures of the distal femur with the Zickel supracondylar nail. *Clin Orthop*. 1990;250:216–220.
24. Olerud S. Operative treatment of supracondylar-condylar fractures of the femur: technique and results in fifteen cases. *J Bone and Joint Surg Am*. 1972;54:1015–1032.
25. Schatzker J, Horne G, Waddell J. The Toronto experience with the supracondylar fracture of the femur, 1966–72. *Injury*. 1974;6:113–128.
26. Benum P. The use of bone cement as an adjunct to internal fixation of supracondylar fractures of osteoporotic femurs. *Acta Orthop Scand*. 1977;48:52–56.
27. Scholl BM, Jaffe KA. Oncologic uses of the retrograde femoral nail. *Clin Orthop Relat Res*. 2002;Jan (394): 219–226.
28. Reudi T, Buckley R, Moran C. AO Principles of Fracture Management, 2nd. Ed. AO Publishing, Switzerland. 2007; Chapter 6, Femur pages 787–788.

RECOMMENED READING

Giles JB, DeLee JC, Heckman JD, et al. Supracondylar-intercondylar fractures of the femur treated with a supracondylar plate and lag screw. *J Bone Joint Surg Am*. 1982;64:864–870.
Hage WD, Aboulafia AJ, Aboulafia DM. Incidence, location, and diagnostic evaluation of metastatic bone disease. *Orthop Clin North Am*. 2000;31(4):515–528.

Healy WL, Brooker AF Jr. Distal femoral fractures: comparison of open and closed methods of treatment. *Clin Orthop Relat Res.* 1983;174:166–171.

Healy JH, Shannon F, Boland P, et al. PMMA to stabilize bone and deliver antineoplastic and antiresporptive agents. *Clin Orthop Relat Res.* 2003;October (415;suppl):S263–S275.

Kregor PJ, Morgan SJ. Fractures of the distal femur. In: Baumgaertner MR, Tornetta P III, eds. *Orthopedic Knowledge Update: Trauma 3.* Rosemont, IL: American Academy of Orthopedic Surgeons; 2005:397–408.

Mize RD, Bucholz RW, Grogan DP. Surgical treatment of displaced, comminuted fractures of the distal end of the femur. *J Bone Joint Surg Am.* 1982;64:871–878.

Peter RE, Schopfer A, Le Coultre B, et al. Fat embolism and death during prophylactic osteosynthesis of a metastatic femur using an unreamed nail. *J Orthop Trauma.* 1997;11(3):233–234.

Schatzker J, Lambert DC. Supracondylar fractures of the femur. *Clin Orthop.* 1979;138:77–83.

Shelbourne KD, Brueckmann FR. Rush pin fixation of supracondylar and intercondylar fractures of the femur. *J Bone Joint Surg Am.* 1982;64:161–169.

Struhl S, Szporn MN, Cobelli NJ, et al. Cemented internal fixation for supracondylar femur fractures in osteoporotic patients. *J Orthop Trauma.* 1990;4:151–157.

23 General Considerations

Peter F. M. Choong

Tumor resections about the ankle are uncommon because primary and secondary malignancies infrequently develop in this region. Should they occur, then the two sites that have the greatest impact on ankle function are the distal tibia and the talus. In the nononcologic setting, the greater use of ankle prostheses has witnessed the potential for greater numbers of revision surgery. Advances in technique, biologic reconstructions, prosthetic design, and experience with ankle joint replacement coupled with a better understanding of the indications and contraindications have increased the popularity of limb-sparing surgery for distal tibial and ankle tumors. Whether surgery is for tumor or complex arthroplasty, procedures about the ankle require special care because of the confluence of neurovascular structures anteriorly and medially around the ankle, the relative thinness of the investing skin of the ankle, and the need for the ankle to sustain the entire body weight when standing or moving.

INDICATIONS

Primary malignancies of the distal tibia are few. Of these, osteosarcoma and Ewing sarcoma are by far the commonest. Both these tumors distinguish themselves by the soft tissue component, which frequently accompanies the tumor's development (Fig. 23.1A,B). In the confined area of the ankle, extraosseous extension of the tumor may compromise the ability to undertake limb-sparing surgery. The main reasons are the lack of a robust layer of soft tissue around the ankle to provide the necessary structures to include in a wide margin and the vulnerability of the neurovascular structures that hug the ankle joint. Successful surgical management has a great reliance on chemotherapy or radiotherapy to assist in the containment and reduction of the soft tissue component of both these tumors.

If limb-sparing surgery is possible, then careful dissection would be required to prevent injury to the vital structures and the overlying skin or transgression of the tumor boundaries. In planning a wide resection of

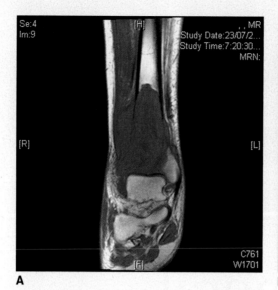
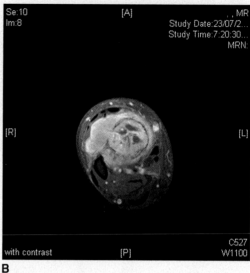

FIGURE 23.1

A: T1-weighted coronal MRI of a distal right tibial Ewing sarcoma in a 36-year-old male. Note the prominent lateral soft tissue component, which is a feature of this tumor and which may complicate a tumor of the lower leg because of the confined anatomy in this region. **B:** T2-weighted contrast-enhanced fat-suppressed axial magnetic resonance image of a distal right tibial Ewing sarcoma in a 36-year-old male. Extension of the soft tissue component anteriorly and along the interosseous membrane will compromise the anterior tibial neurovascular structures.

the distal tibia, care must be taken to accurately calculate the amount of residual tibia remaining after tumor resection. This will determine the type of reconstruction possible. For example, short resections lend themselves to almost all varieties of reconstructions including biologic reconstructions (Fig. 23.2A–H), prosthetic reconstructions, and combinations of these (1–6). Long resections, however, make prosthetic reconstructions with megaprostheses difficult because of the lack of tibial length to contain the stem of a megaprosthesis. Unlike the femur where long resections of either the proximal or distal femur may be converted to total femoral resections, no device or reconstruction is readily available for extended tibial resections. In this regard, appropriate

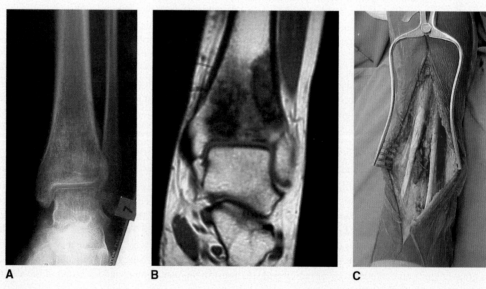

FIGURE 23.2

A: Anteroposterior radiograph of a distal tibial osteosarcoma characterized by a mixed sclerotic and lytic appearance. **B:** T1-weighted coronal magnetic resonance image demonstrates excellent soft tissue contrast and marrow definition. The tumor extends down to the articular margin and in this case has complicated the joint by invading it. **C:** Anterior incision to expose the tumor identified in **(B)**. Note that the biopsy tract between tibialis anterior and extensor digitorum tendons has been isolated and left in continuity with the tumor.

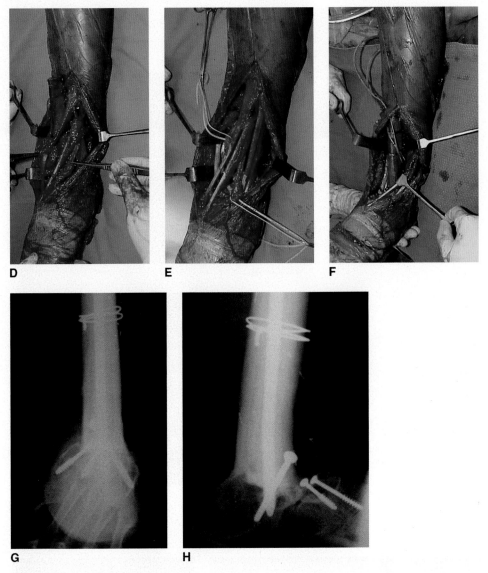

FIGURE 23.2 (*Continued*)

D: The distal tibia and fibula have been osteotomized and the tumor specimen is being mobilized to be delivered to the medial side of tibialis anterior tendon. The extensor hallucis tendon and anterior tibial neurovascular structures, which are lateral to the anterior tibialis tendon, are indicated by the forceps.
E: The tumor has been extracted and the major structures around the ankle are clearly visible. From left to right, tibialis posterior tendon (retracted), posterior tibial vessels and nerves (*yellow sling*), tibialis anterior tendon, extensor hallucis longus tendon, anterior tibial neurovascular structures, extensor digitorum longus tendons, and peroneus tertius tendon. **F:** Defect between calcaneus and tibia spanned by allograft arthrodesis. Anteroposterior **(G)** and lateral **(H)** radiographs at 8 years after allograft arthrodesis reconstruction. Reconstruction was supported by intramedullary rod fixation with supplementary interfragmentary screw fixation between the distal allograft and calcaneus. The navicular was fused to the cuneiform bones with interfragmentary screws.

care must be taken to exclude the presence of intramedullary skip lesions. If limb-sparing surgery cannot be undertaken with oncologically sound margins or the potential for postoperative complications outweigh the benefits of this surgery, then below knee amputation should be seriously considered (Fig. 23.3A–C). The function possible with appropriately fitted amputation prostheses, after below knee amputation, is generally excellent.

Metastatic carcinoma infrequently involves the distal tibia or tarsal bones. These lesions are either sclerotic, lytic, or a combination of these. Extraosseous extension of tumor may occur but typically is not as prominent as for primary malignancies, thus allowing local surgical treatment such as excisional curettage with maximal preservation of host bone (Fig. 23.4A–G). As with all metastatic diseases, if the diaphysis of the tibia is affected and there is a risk of development of other lesions, then protection of the entire bone with a durable construct should be planned.

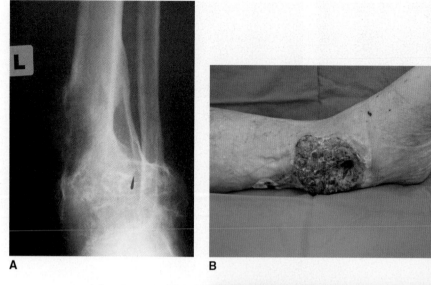

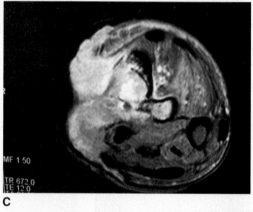

FIGURE 23.3

A: A 73-year-old male with chronic osteomyelitis following a distal tibial fracture sustained over 30 years previously. The sequestrum and involucrum are clearly visible on the oblique radiograph. **B:** The discharging sinus related to the chronic osteomyelitis is now complicated by extensive skin ulceration secondary to the development of a squamous cell carcinoma. **C:** T1-weighted fat-suppressed image with marked intramedullary tibial enhancement demonstrating significant marrow replacement after destruction of the overlying cortical bone. There is involvement of all three compartments of the leg and permeation of the carcinomatous change along the dermis and skin has occurred for a quite a distance from the epicenter of the ulcer.

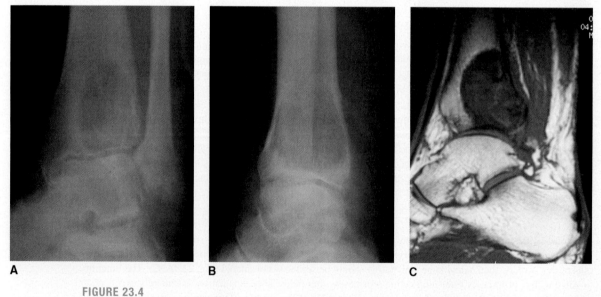

FIGURE 23.4

Anteroposterior **(A)** and lateral **(B)** plain radiographs of a melanoma deposit in a distal tibia. T1-weighted sagittal **(C)** and coronal.

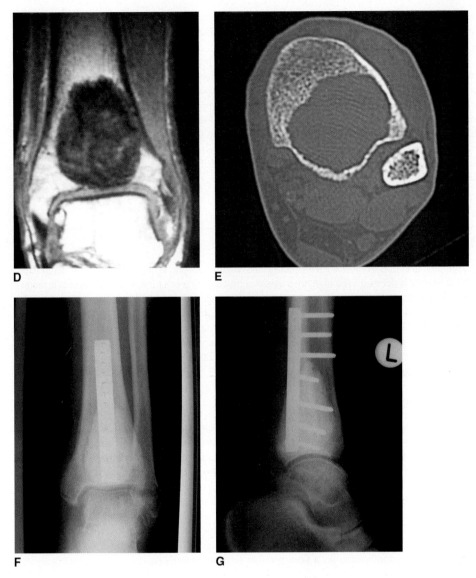

FIGURE 23.4 (Continued)

(D) images showing an intramedullary lesion with minimal breach of the tibial cortex. The perimeter of the tumor is clearly visible with this sequence, which highlights the contrast between tumor and fatty marrow. **E:** Axial computed tomographic scan highlighting the excellent delineation of trabecular destruction with this imaging modality. **F,G:** Surgical treatment of an osseous melanoma deposit with curettage, cementation, and internal fixation.

CONTRAINDICATIONS

- Deep infection in the setting of primary malignancy is a contraindication to reconstruction. This is particularly relevant for tumors of the distal tibia where limb-sparing surgery is often associated with soft tissue resection that includes skin, and reconstructions that require major bone allograft transplants or autograft transfers. Soft tissue closures that occur under tension or that require complex soft tissue transfers are vulnerable to wound complications, which can be amplified in the presence of preexisting infection. Implantation of allograft or prosthetic devices is absolutely contraindicated in the setting of infection.
- Extensive involvement of the tibia may preclude reconstruction on the basis of having no reliable bone on which to perform a reconstruction. Most reconstructions are stabilized with internal fixation such as plate or intramedullary fixation against host bone. Such fixation is usually relied upon to provide initial strength and stability and therefore requires sound and dependable fixation to host bone. If fixation to host bone is tenuous, then supplementary external splintage such as via ischial weight-bearing casting is recommended.
- Involvement of the vascular structures at the level of the distal tibia is a contraindication to limb-sparing surgery if the artery that is compromised is a dominant vessel. Vascular bypass operations while possible are associated with a higher failure rate with more distal reconstructions. Because the major nerves and vessels of the lower leg run together, it is unusual for involvement of one member of the neurovascular bundle, not

to include the others. Therefore, involvement of any member of the neurovascular structures usually means involvement of the others and the risks of an insensate foot and ischemic foot after resection or reconstruction may be unacceptably high.

- Patients who present with metastatic sarcoma have a very poor prognosis. It is debatable whether patients with systemic disease and a complex distal tibial primary tumor should undertake resection and reconstruction. In this setting, there are few reconstructions that will permit immediate and full weight bearing to allow patients the same level of mobility and independence as others who have undergone knee or hip resections and reconstructions. Moreover, the risks of complications and the prolonged recuperation of any distal tibial reconstruction may not be considered worthwhile in the context of a limited life expectancy. In contrast, a below knee amputation may permit earlier mobilization and the fitting of an amputation prosthesis, which the patient may capitalize on to achieve reliable, independent and complication free weight-bearing mobility.

INVESTIGATIONS

Plain Radiographs

Biplane radiographs are important for determining the nature of the malignancy in the distal tibia (Fig. 23.5A,B). If the risk is deemed to be high, then non–weight-bearing precaution between crutches is recommended. Standard (1:1) magnification radiographs also permit comparison with radiographs of allograft bone that is stored in bone banks. This is important if osteoarticular allografts are required, where size matching is important. Radiographs also provide a modality for assessing response to neoadjuvant chemotherapy with ossification of the soft tissue component during chemotherapy being one sign of response. The degree of response, however, can be more accurately measured using metabolic imaging such as positron emission tomography (PET) or thallium scanning.

Nuclear Bone Scans

Technetium methyl diphosphonate (MDP) bone scans are excellent for determining the multifocality of disease (Fig. 23.5C). It may be used to screen for the presence of additional bone lesions in the same or other bones. This is important not only for defining systemic spread, but also because skip lesions within the same bone have the same prognostic significance as metastatic disease. Widespread skip lesions within the tibia may preclude limb-sparing surgery.

In contrast to technetium MDP bone scans, which reflect the response of the bone to the tumor, thallium and PET scans reflect the metabolic activity of the tumor itself. In this regard, thallium and PET scans are useful for identifying that part of the tumor with the most active tumor, which should be targeted for biopsy. Further, the ability to identify metabolically active tumor makes thallium and PET scans useful for determining the response to neoadjuvant chemotherapy. As a postoperative screening modality, thallium and PET scans are useful for differentiating between tumor and postoperative granulation tissue.

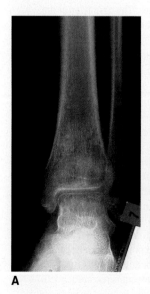 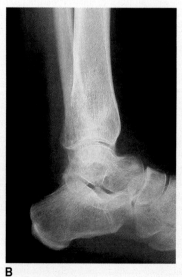 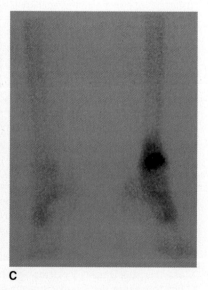

A   B   C

FIGURE 23.5

Plain anteroposterior **(A)** and lateral **(B)** radiographs of a distal tibial osteosarcoma. **C:** Technitium bone scan demonstrating increased bone formation/turnover at the site of distal tibial osteosarcoma.

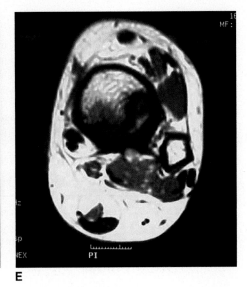

D   E

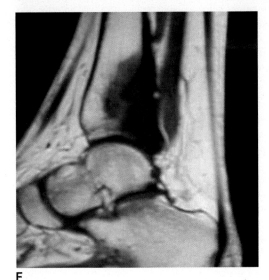

FIGURE 23.5 (*Continued*)

D: Computed tomographic scans are an excellent modality for highlighting calcium
containing structures. This technique provides excellent definition of trabecular
and cortical bone and can be used for gross and subtle bone changes. **E,F:**
T1-weighted axial and sagittal magnetic resonance images of a distal tibial tumor.
This technique provides unsurpassed soft tissue contrast, which is essential for
planning bone and soft tissue surgical margins. Although magnetic resonance images
can show cortical bone well, computed tomography provides clearer definition of the
structure.

F

Computed Tomography

Computer tomography is excellent for defining cortical bone destruction (Fig. 23.5D). This is particularly
useful when considering the reconstructive options for metastatic disease of the distal tibia. Further, the ability
to accurately measure the dimensions of the tibia in three dimensions allows closer anatomic matching when
considering osteoarticular allograft use or when planning for custom-made implants.

Magnetic Resonance Imaging

Magnetic resonance imaging (MRI) is critical for assessing the extraosseous extension of tumor
(Fig. 23.5E,F) because of the close proximity of the tibial neurovascular structures at the level just proximal
and distal to the ankle joint. Defining the planes that divide these vital structures from the tumor is important
for planning surgical margins if limb-sparing surgery is to be attempted. Alternately, recognizing involvement
of the neurovascular structures may lead to an early decision for amputation rather than risking tumor contamination from oncologically inadequate surgery. The proximal extent of tumor and the amount of involved tibia
are also important information that MRI can provide, which will lead to a decision between amputation and
limb-sparing surgery.

Involvement of foot bones by sarcoma increases the risk of amputation. MRI is an excellent modality for
determining this information because of its excellent multiplanar capability that allows clear visualization of all
the tarsal and metatarsal bones. The easily defined cortical outlines and fatty marrow signal in the foot bones
means that any cortical breach or bone involvement will be readily appreciated.

Angiography

Standard angiography, computerized tomographic angiography, and magnetic resonance angiography are techniques that may be exploited to determine the involvement of the anterior and posterior tibial vessels by distal tibial or ankle tumors. The vessels anterior to the ankle lie directly on bone and therefore may be more vulnerable than those posterior to the medial malleolus, which are often separated from bone by the tibialis posterior tendon and flexor hallucis longus.

Angiography is also useful for determining the vascularity of the uncommon metastatic lesion that arises below the knee. This is particularly important when planning treatment of renal, thyroid, and myelomatous deposits.

ANATOMIC CONSIDERATIONS

The distal part of the lower leg and ankle are the narrowest parts of the lower limb with the relationship of the vital neurovascular tendons and bones occurring in a very confined space. Where a tumor is located in relation to these structures will determine whether limb-sparing surgery or amputation should be chosen.

Distal Fibula

The distal fibula is a subcutaneous bone with its closest relations being the skin on its lateral and anterior side, peroneal tendons posteriorly, and the tibia and distal syndesmosis on its medial aspect. Tumors arising from the distal fibula are usually resectable with preservation of the limb because all its neighboring structures are expendable. Even the syndesmosis may be sacrificed with part of the attached tibia without loss of ankle stability because of the availability of a variety of bone and ligamentous reconstructions.

Distal Tibia

The distal tibia has from medial to lateral the anterior tibial tendon, extensor hallucis longus tendon, anterior tibial vessels and nerve, and peroneus tertius tendon as its anterior relations. Medially, the tibia is a subcutaneous structure; posteriorly, the tendons of tibialis posterior and flexor hallucis longus hold the posterior tibial vessels and nerve away from the bone. Laterally it has the syndesmosis and the fibular. All these structures are held tightly to the lower end of the tibia by a very resilient retinaculum, which gives rise to compression when a distal tibial tumor is associated with a prominent soft tissue component. Under this circumstance, careful scrutiny of MRI scans is recommended to determine if a plane of dissection is available between the neurovascular structures and the tumor. While the neurovascular structures mandate preservation in limb-sparing surgery, all the tendinous structures about the ankle may be sacrificed with adequate functional support being provided postoperatively by the use of ankle-foot orthoses.

Talus

The talus is an integral part of the ankle joint. Sacrifice of this structure alone (talectomy/astragalectomy), however, still permits limb-sparing surgery with the distal tibia articulating with the superior surface of the calcaneus (Fig. 23.6 A–C). Should this be required, appropriate refashioning of the medial and lateral malleoli is required to prevent troublesome impingement symptoms and shoe wear problems.

Ankle Joint And Capsule

The ankle joint is a hinge type joint with a mortise comprised of the malleoli and the tibial plafond, and the talus acting as the tenon. The stability of the joint is due not only to its shape but also the presence of very strong medial and lateral collateral ligaments, the tibiofibular joint with anterior, interosseous, and posterior tibiofibular ligaments. The joint capsule is thinned anteriorly and posteriorly allowing movement in plantar and dorsiflexion. An effusion may be discernable when it bulges the capsule at these areas giving rise to fullness on either side of the Achilles tendon or medial and lateral to the tendons that run anteriorly across the joint. Although the fibrous capsule attaches superiorly to the articular margins of the tibia and malleoli and inferiorly to the articular margin of the talus, the synovial cavity may extend superiorly as far as the interosseous tibiofibular ligament. The extent of the synovial cavity and the firm attachment created by the inferior syndesmosis are important considerations when planning tumor resections.

NEUROVASCULAR STRUCTURES

The arterial supply to the foot comes by way of the anterior and posterior tibial arteries. The former enters the foot as the dorsalis pedis artery while the latter forms the lateral plantar artery. Both form arches distally in the

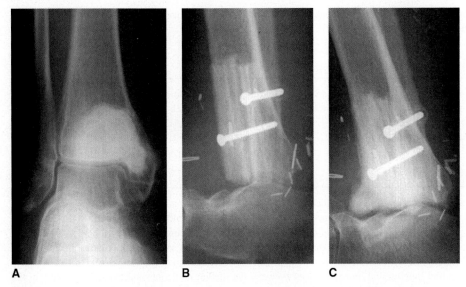

A   B   C

FIGURE 23.6

A: A recurrent giant cell tumor of the distal tibia with involvement of the ankle joint in a 46-year-old female. **B:** The tumor was excised with wide en bloc margins including the distal tibia and talus. This defect was reconstructed with a double-barrelled vascularized fibular graft. **C:** Twelve months after surgery, the fibular grafts have united with the distal tibia and there has been remodeling of the distal fibulas to match the upper surface of the calcaneus.

foot and communicate with each other via a metatarsal anastamosis. A medial tarsal artery joins the two main arteries at the midfoot. The rich network of communications normally ensures adequate blood supply to the foot and toes; however, one or either artery may be dominant and this information is vital to the planning of surgery. The caliber of vessels is very small by the time the foot is reached and bypass operations to reconstruct transacted or excised portions of artery at the distal tibia are at risk of occlusion from spasm, thrombosis, or embolism. The veins form a mirror image of the arterial supply.

The nerves to the foot enter superficially as the saphenous, superficial fibular and sural nerves and more deeply as the deep fibular nerve anteriorly and behind the medial malleolus as the medial and lateral plantar divisions of the posterior tibial nerve. Dissections around the ankle that are at risk of injuring these nerves will result in sensory deficits. This is more important with dissection around the medial malleolus where the sensory deficit may be on the plantar weight-bearing surface of the foot.

SURGICAL CONSIDERATIONS

Major reconstruction about the distal tibia and ankle is challenging because the construct has to sustain the entire body weight over a very small area. For this to succeed, stability at the proximal and distal end of the reconstruction has to be ensured to allow safe and dependable transfer of weight or stress across the construct. Proximal stability is usually dependent on the union of host diaphyseal bone to allograft or autograft bone. There are a number of factors that may negatively influence union namely, chemotherapy, which is known to inhibit bone healing; movement at the osteotomy site; the tibial diaphysis, which is primarily cortical; and the junction of the middle and distal thirds of the tibia, which is at the watershed of its blood supply and therefore is prone to nonunion. Surgery should aim for rigid internal fixation and supplementary grafting to maximize union.

The distal end of the reconstruction may be part of an intercalary reconstruction where allograft or autograft bone must unite with the distal tibial epiphysis, or part of an allograft arthrodesis where the union is between graft and talus, or graft and calcaneus, or an osteoarticular reconstruction where a tibial allograft will articulate with the native talus, or an allograft prosthetic composite where a standard prosthesis is combined with an allograft distal tibia to create an articulating ankle joint. Whether it is a fixed or mobile reconstruction, stability of the distal reconstruction is key to its success. Union of bone surfaces needs to be solid and dependable, while a mobile reconstruction has to be stable throughout its range. Because of the anatomic complexity of the ankle joint, stiffness should be accepted, as this may provide greater stability.

Supplementary fixation in terms of casting or bracing should be considered to enhance the development of union across osteotomy surfaces, as well as to support the repair or development of scar tissue around mobile joints. Osteoarticular allografts or allograft prosthetic composites are similar to neuropathic joints. Special attention should be paid to educating the patient on avoiding unnecessary trauma to the joint if the longevity of the reconstruction is to be preserved.

POSITIONING

The patient should be positioned supine and the limb draped free on the operating table for surgery on the distal tibia and ankle. This will permit a direct anterior and medial approach to the ankle, which is important to access the two main neurovascular bundles of the foot. A tourniquet should be applied and inflated or deflated according to surgeon preference.

INCISION

A universal anterior incision will allow adequate access to the distal tibia and ankle joint (Fig. 23.7A,B). If there is no soft tissue component to be concerned about and an intra-articular ankle resection is possible, then opening the ankle joint from the front and continuing the dissection around the sides to the back will allow delivery of the distal tibia or talus through the incision without the need to create a further incision. If however, there is a posteriorly directed soft tissue component that may be threatening the medial neurovascular structures, then a second longitudinal incision placed between the medial malleolus and the Achilles tendon will allow adequate exposure (Fig. 23.7C,D).

The skin and soft tissue is usually firmly applied about the lower leg and ankle. The disused leg is also often associated with peripheral edema. These together with the trauma of surgery are likely to result in further soft

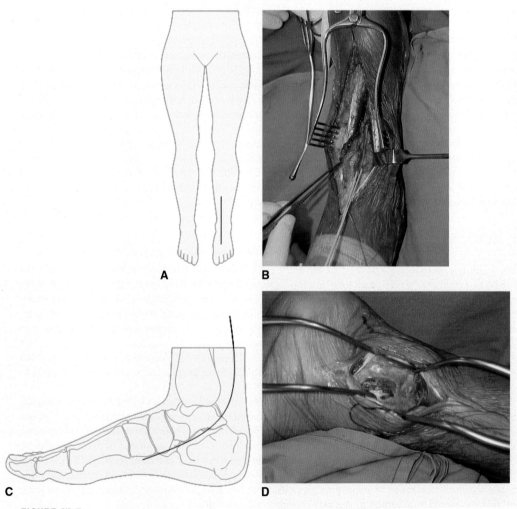

FIGURE 23.7

A universal anterior incision **(A)** permits exposure of the major structures of the ankle **(B)**. **C,D:** If there is a large medial component of the tumor that requires special attention during dissection to protect the medial tibial neurovascular bundle, this can be accessed by a separate curved medial incision centered on the medial malleolus and passing to the tubercle of the navicular and proximally along the tibial diaphysis.

tissue swelling, which may cause retraction of the skin edges following incision. Careful resuture of the wound is required to ensure that the tension under which the wound is closed is kept to a minimum. If two incisions are used, it is important that the skin bridge is as wide as possible to minimize skin flap necrosis, which is a constant risk because the soft tissue layer around the ankle is normally thin. Further, the closure of one wound may widen the second wound on the opposite side of the leg, so careful closure of both wounds must be observed.

COMPLICATIONS

- The poor tissue vascularity combined with significant dissection increases the risk of deep and superficial infection. The immunosuppressive effect of chemotherapy and the subcutaneous nature of bone and its reconstruction make the patient highly susceptible to infection. Prophylactic antibiotics, careful wound handling, and copious amounts of wound lavage should be utilized to minimize the risk of infection. Deep infection in the setting of chemotherapy should be managed with amputation because ongoing sepsis will not permit safe delivery of chemotherapy. Superficial infection will require treatment on its own merits.
- The vascular supply of the foot is at considerable risk with major resection and reconstruction about the ankle. Care must be taken to ensure ongoing perfusion during surgery and tissue should be handled with care. It is easy to deform the lower leg and ankle once a tumor has been resected and this may lead to arterial spasm or thrombosis. Digital or forefoot gangrene is a complication of arterial obstruction at the ankle that may lead to amputation. Tourniquet control should be kept to a minimum.
- Poor drainage from venous obstruction may lead to problematic edema. Sometimes this can be bad enough to threaten the viability of the foot or lead to chronic venous hypertension and ulceration. Acute venous obstruction may lead to tissue ischemia and necrosis.
- Skin necrosis is a real risk with complex surgery about the lower leg and ankle. The subcutaneous tissue, which transmits skin vascularity, is insubstantial and the trauma of dissection may be sufficient to raise tissue ischemia. This and the postoperative swelling may exacerbate any subcritical skin perfusion leading to significant wound edge or skin flap necrosis. In anticipation of potential wound edge ischemia, patients need to be warned of the possibility for split skin grafting of open wounds if closure is likely to lead to wound compromise.
- Injury of the deep or superficial fibular nerves as they pass from lower leg to foot will cause variable numbness on the dorsum of the foot. This is less important than the numbness in the sole of the foot, should the medial or plantar nerves be injured. This is more important because of the exposure of the plantar skin to weight bearing and the risk of trophic ulceration. If sacrifice of these nerves is anticipated, consideration should be given to nerve grafting or repair to preserve at least deep sensation.

REFERENCES

1. Abudu A, Grimer RJ, Tillman RM, et al. Endoprosthetic replacement of the distal tibia and ankle joint for aggressive bone tumors *Int Orthop*. 1999;23:291–294.
2. Ebeid W, Amin S, Abdelmegid A, et al. Reconstruction of distal tibial defects following resection of malignant tumors by pedicled vascularised fibular grafts *Acta Orthop Belg*. 2007;73:354–359.
3. Lee SH, Kim HS, Park YB, et al. Prosthetic reconstruction for tumors of the distal tibia and fibula *J Bone Joint Surg Br Vol*. 1999;81B:803–807.
4. Natarajan MV, Annamalai K, Williams S, et al. Limb salvage in distal tibial osteosarcoma using a custom mega prosthesis *Int Orthop*. 2000;24:282–284.
5. Niimi R, Matsumine A, Kusuzaki K, et al. Usefulness of limb salvage surgery for bone and soft tissue sarcomas of the distal lower leg. *J Cancer Res Clin Oncol*. 2008;134:1087–1095.
6. Shalaby S, Shalaby H, Bassiony A. Limb salvage for osteosarcoma of the distal tibia with resection. arthrodesis, autogenous fibular graft and Ilizarov external fixator *J Bone Joint Surg Br Vol*. 2006;88B:1642–1646.

24 Ankle Arthrodesis

Norman S. Turner

Ankle arthrodesis is commonly performed on patients with end-stage ankle arthritis. A solid ankle arthrodesis can provide a patient with a durable, pain-free, functional extremity, which enables them to be productive with work and active in low-impact sports such as biking, swimming, or golfing. However, as the arthrodesis is extended to the adjacent joints, the functional limitations increase.

Patients with end-stage arthritis are often treated nonsurgically with activity modification, anti-inflammatory medicines if tolerated, and bracing prior to considering surgery. When these treatments do not provide adequate pain relief, then surgical treatment is indicated. Ankle replacements can also be performed on appropriate patients with end-stage ankle arthritis.

INDICATIONS

- Posttraumatic arthritis and rheumatoid arthritis are the most common cause of arthritis in the ankle.
- It can also be seen in patients who have had long-standing pigmented, villonodular synovitis, or synovial chondromatosis.
- Patients who have cartilage loss as a sequela of radiation, infection, or failed reconstruction of their ankle will be candidates for an arthrodesis.
- An arthrodesis can be used in attempted limb salvage for patients who require significant resection of the ankle joint and is not reconstructable with other options.
- In patients undergoing extensive tumor resection and reconstruction with allograft, an arthrodesis may be used as a salvage procedure.

CONTRAINDICATIONS

- Ankle arthrodesis is contraindications in patients with poor vascular supply to their lower extremity. These patients should undergo a vascular workup and reconstruction if appropriate prior to the arthrodesis.
- Patients with poor soft tissue around the ankle are a relative contraindication for an ankle arthrodesis and may require soft tissue coverage.
- Acute infection is a contraindication to arthrodesis. However, this may be treated with a debridement and antibiotics; then, a staged arthrodesis if there is extensive arthritis is warranted.
- In patients with minimal arthritis, an arthrodesis is not indicated and nonsurgical treatment should be utilized.

Prior to surgery, a medical examination in the elderly patient is recommended to optimize healing potential. Also, an evaluation by physical therapy prior to surgery can be beneficial in determining the patient's ability to be non–weight-bearing after surgery and may aid in determining if placement in a nursing facility will be needed.

PREOPERATIVE PREPARATION

The evaluation of the patient begins with a complete history and physical exam. Occasionally, the patient will have minimal pain with extensive radiographic changes so identification of the painful joint must be made. The soft tissues around the ankle are evaluated for previous incisions or soft tissue reconstructions. This may affect the exposure and may affect the type of fixation that is planned.

Imaging

The alignment of the ankle is closely evaluated with both physical and radiographic exams. Radiographic analysis begins with weight-bearing anteroposterior and lateral views, as well as a mortise view. This enables the surgeon to determine the bone quality, deformity, and bony defects. These views are essential for preparation for surgery. This will assist in determining the amount of bone that needs to be resected. It will also help in preparation if bony reconstruction requires bone graft from either the iliac crest or the allograft. If there is a mild deformity, frequently, this can be corrected through the arthrodesis site. However, if there is a severe deformity, it may require other procedures to balance the foot.

Exposure Options

The exposure for the arthrodesis can be determined by the deformity. If there is a mild deformity, you may be able to precede with either an arthroscopic or minimally invasive procedure where small incisions are used to débride the joint surface and then percutaneous fixation is placed. However, if there is a significant deformity of >10 degrees of varus or valgus, then a transfibular approach is frequently used.

Fusion Options

Preoperative planning is critical in determining what type of fixation will be needed. The goal of the surgery is to have broad congruent surfaces that are compressed and rigidly fixed in an optimal position in order to provide the best chance of solid fusion. The fixation options include internal compression screws, plate and screw fixation, or external fixator. Occasionally, an intramedullary rod can be used. However, this requires the fusion of the subtalar joint as well as the ankle joint. External fixators can be used especially in patients with history of infection or when there is poor bone quality or soft tissues. The advantage of internal fixation in patients receiving chemotherapy is that you do not have the risks of pin site infection in an immunocompromised individual.

Informed Consent

Preoperative counseling is important to prepare the patient for realistic expectations of what an ankle arthrodesis will provide. It provides significant pain improvement but does not give them a normal extremity. It is important that a patient understands the risk of infection, nonunion, adjacent joint arthritis, and neurovascular complications. Also, preoperative counseling should include a detailed description of the postoperative course so that the patient understands the length of immobilization as well as use of walking aids and prepares appropriately.

TECHNIQUE

Position and Draping

After general or spinal anesthetic, the patient is positioned on a radiolucent table in a supine position with a bump under the hip so that the foot is internally rotated and the toes are pointing toward the ceiling. A sterile tourniquet is placed on a thigh. The foot and ankle is prepped and draped in a standard fashion. The knee should be palpable. The patella and the tibial tubercle should be palpable in order to assist with positioning of the arthrodesis site (Fig. 24.1).

Incision and Exposure

If a minimal deformity is present, then a *minimal exposure technique* can be performed. In this technique, the foot is exsanguinated and the thigh tourniquet is inflated. A 2-cm incision is made just medial to the anterior tibial tendon with dissection through the skin and the subcutaneous tissue down the capsule (Figs. 24.2 and 24.3). The capsule is split longitudinally exposing the joint. A curved clamp can then be placed within the joint and palpated anterolaterally. An incision is made over the anterior lateral aspect of the ankle with dissection through the skin and the subcutaneous tissue. Careful dissection through the subcutaneous tissue is performed in order to identify and protect the superficial peroneal nerve branches. Dissection is then carried deep to the capsule (Fig. 24.4). The capsule incised longitudinally.

   Through these two incisions, you have access to the ankle joint which is then prepared using osteotomes and curettes removing the remaining cartilage as well as the subchondral bone until cancellous-type bone is visualized. The joint surfaces are feathered with an osteotome to increase surface area. The contours of the surfaces are maintained to improve bony apposition. A laminar spreader placed within the joint from one incision enables you to have excellent visualization of the joint through the other incision and can assist with your preparation of the joint surfaces (Fig. 24.5).

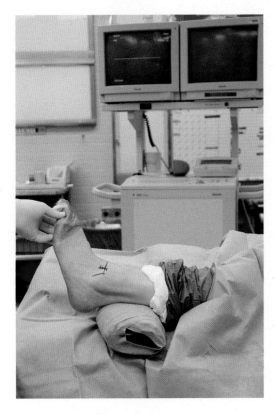

FIGURE 24.1

This illustrates the proper patient positioning for an arthrodesis. In order to minimize malpositioning of the arthrodesis, you should be able to palpate the tibial spine from the tubercle to the ankle.

After adequate preparation has been obtained, the foot is then positioned into neutral dorsiflexion, plantar flexion, slight external rotation, and 5 degrees of valgus. This can be held temporarily with a smooth Steinmann pin or can be held manually. Percutaneous large fragment cannulated screws are then placed. The alignment helps determine which screw is placed first. If the patient has a tendency toward varus, a lateral screw will be placed (Fig. 24.6). If the tendency is toward valgus, the medial screw will be placed first in order to optimize the alignment. Intraoperative imaging will verify the position, making sure the subtalar joint is not perforated, and then a partially threaded cannulated screw can be placed to obtain compression across the arthrodesis site (Fig. 24.7). A second pin is then placed percutaneously from the medial malleolus or the lateral tibial plafond into the talus.

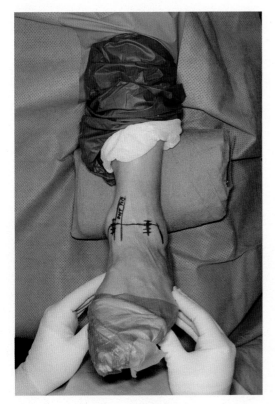

FIGURE 24.2

The location of the incisions for a minimal exposure ankle arthrodesis is seen. The medial incision is just medial to the anterior tibial tendon. The lateral incision is located over the anterolateral aspect of the ankle.

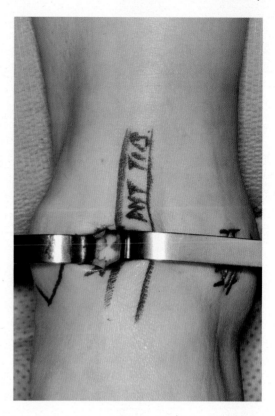

FIGURE 24.3

A 2-cm incision is made just medial to anterior tibial
tendon. This gives exposure to the medial ankle.

Again, intraoperative imaging in multiple planes is used to verify the position and then a partially threaded cannulated screw is placed (Fig. 24.8). A third screw is frequently placed percutaneously from the posterior malleolus into the talus (Fig. 24.9). Intraoperative imaging verifies it and a partially threaded cancellous screw is placed.
Three screws usually give excellent stability to the joint and other screws are not needed (Fig. 24.10A,B).

The tourniquet is then released. Hemostasis is obtained. The wounds are then closed with 3-0 absorbable
suture and 4.0 nylon sutures. A sterile dressing is applied and then a compressive bulky Robert Jones dressing.

A transfibular approach is recommended for patients with rigid deformity of >10 degrees, avascular necrosis
of the talus or in cases that require a wide exposure. The foot is exsanguinated and the thigh tourniquet is inflated.

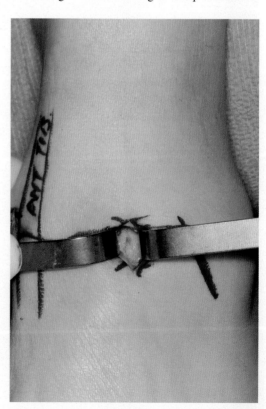

FIGURE 24.4

The lateral incision is made at the anterolateral aspect
of the ankle. Care to protect the superficial peroneal
nerve is needed.

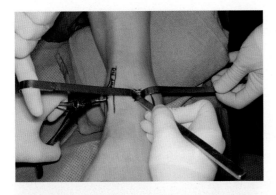

FIGURE 24.5

The laminar spreader is placed in the medial incision so the ankle can be prepared through the lateral incision. The laminar spreader is then placed laterally so the medial aspect of the joint can be prepared.

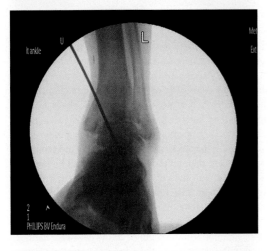

FIGURE 24.6

The medial pin is placed first since the patient had the tendency to drift into the valgus.

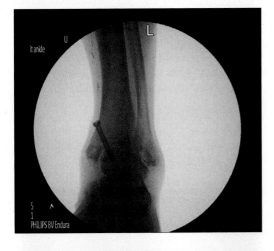

FIGURE 24.7

The screw is placed over the pin and checked to verify that the subtalar joint is not violated.

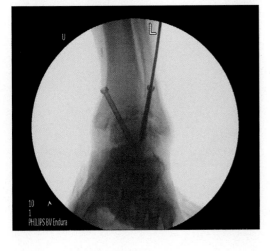

FIGURE 24.8

The lateral screw is placed in similar fashion.

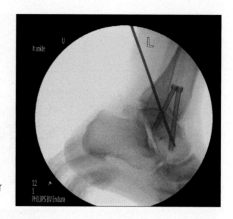

FIGURE 24.9

The posterior screw is placed percutaneously from the posterior malleolus to the talus.

A curvilinear incision is made along the course of the fibula and extending toward the base of the fourth metatarsal (Fig. 24.11). Dissection carries through the skin and the subcutaneous tissue down to the fibula. The soft tissues remain intact on the posterior aspect of the fibula. The soft tissue is reflected off of the fibula anteriorly. The fibula is osteotomized approximately 8 cm from the tip and 1 cm of bone is then removed (Fig. 24.12). The anterior syndesmotic ligaments are resected and the fibula is then externally rotated. The medial half of the fibula is then removed and is used as bone graft. The remaining lateral aspect of the fibula is vascularized, because of the posterior attachments of the soft tissue (Fig. 24.13). This approach gives excellent exposure to the ankle joint. An incision is made over the anteromedial aspect of the ankle with care to protect the saphenous vein and nerve. Through these two incisions, the joint surfaces are then prepared. The joints can be prepared either by keeping the contours of the tibia and the talus intact or with flat cuts that are made so that the foot will be in neutral dorsiflexion/plantar flexion, slight valgus, and slight external rotation. Bone can be resected as needed to correct the deformity. After preparation of the surfaces, temporary smooth Steinmann pin can be used to assist with holding the alignment while images are obtained with a C arm. Cannulated screws, noncannulated screws, or plate and screws can be placed based upon surgeon's preference. After the hardware has been placed, the fibula is placed as an onlay graft and is secured with two partially threaded 4/0 cancellous screws (Fig. 24.14). Bone graft can be used as needed and at the discretion of the surgeon (Fig. 24.15A,B). The tourniquet is then released. Hemostasis is obtained. The wound is closed with 3-0 absorbable suture and 4-0 nylon sutures. Sterile dressings and a compressive Robert Jones dressing is applied.

In patients who require an extensive tumor resection, your careful preoperative planning will assist in preparing the joint surfaces and determining the bone defect. The main goal is to have congruent surfaces with excellent bony apposition and rigid fixation in an optimal position to provide the best possible functional results to the patient.

In patients treated with external fixation, the joint surfaces are prepared as above. Then an external fixator with either half pins or fine wires is placed in a standardized fashion. Compression is applied through the arthrodesis site.

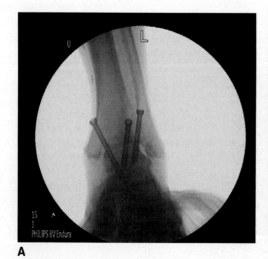
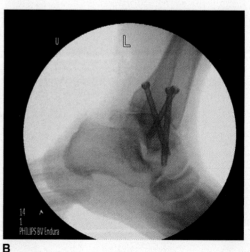

A   **B**

FIGURE 24.10

A,B: AP and lateral view of the three screws placed across the arthrodesis site. Careful inspection of the subtalar joint verifies that it was not penetrated.

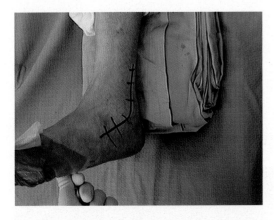

FIGURE 24.11

Curvilinear incision that is made along the course of the fibula and extends to the base of the fourth metatarsal is shown.

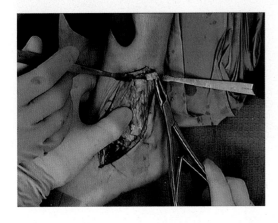

FIGURE 24.12

The fibula is osteotomized 8 cm from the tip of the fibula and 1 cm of bone is removed.

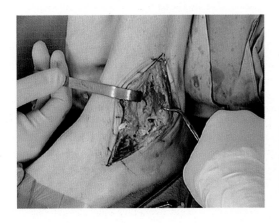

FIGURE 24.13

After the anterior syndesmotic ligaments are transected, the fibula is externally rotated and the medial half of the fibula is removed and used as bone graft. The posterior soft tissues are intact so the fibula is vascularized.

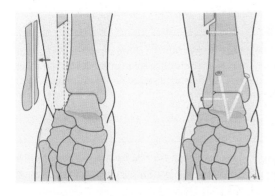

FIGURE 24.14

This illustrates how the fibula will be used as an onlay graft.

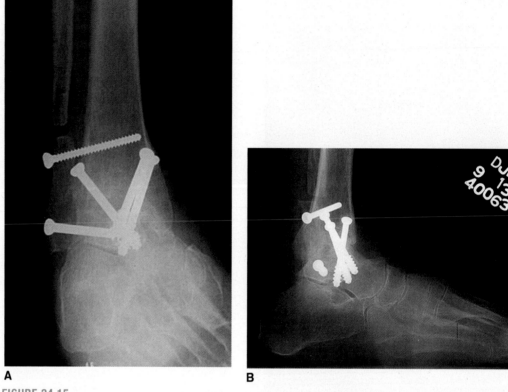

FIGURE 24.15

A,B: This shows AP and lateral radiograph of the ankle arthrodesis performed with a transfibular approach.

POSTOPERATIVE MANAGEMENT

Postoperative management consists of a period of immobilization. Usually, the patient is placed in a compressive Robert Jones dressing with a posterior plaster splint until the swelling has subsided. The patient is admitted to the hospital and the lower extremity is kept elevated. They are strictly non–weight-bearing. A non–weight-bearing cast is then applied. The patient usually returns 2 to 3 weeks after surgery for cast change and suture removal. Another non–weight-bearing cast is applied.

Six weeks after surgery, the cast is then removed. Imaging is obtained to determine if weight-bearing can be started. The leg is then placed in a cast for another 4 to 6 weeks. At approximately 3 months after surgery, the patients are allowed to increase their weight-bearing as tolerated in a removable boot if clinical and radiographic healing is present. In patients treated with an external fixator, clinical and radiographic follow-up is performed every 3 to 4 weeks. Once radiographic healing has been obtained usually around 3 months after surgery, the fixator is removed.

Physical therapy can be helpful in patients preoperatively to education them on non–weight-bearing. During the hospitalization, the therapist will work with the patient on strict non–weight-bearing. Once the cast is removed, the patient is allowed to increase his or her activities in a removable walking boot. At approximately 4 months after surgery, the patient can return to his or her shoe. Occasionally, a rocker bottom sole with a sach heel is needed to improve the gait and function. Patients are allowed to begin swimming and water aerobics at 3 months after surgery, start riding a stationary bike at 3 to 4 months after surgery, and return to playing golf with a cart at 4 to 6 months after surgery.

RESULTS

Using contemporary techniques for ankle arthrodesis, a union rate of over 90% has been reported. This procedure enables patients to improve their activities and function. Gait analysis after ankle arthrodesis shows that patients do take a shorter stride and have a shorter time interval during single stance on the arthrodesis side. Patients are able to return to low impact activities as tolerated.

COMPLICATIONS

The most common complication after ankle arthrodesis is a nonunion, and the rate has been reported to be approximately 10% ranging from 0% to 30%. Publications within the last 15 years using contemporary fixation has shown that the nonunion rate is <10%.

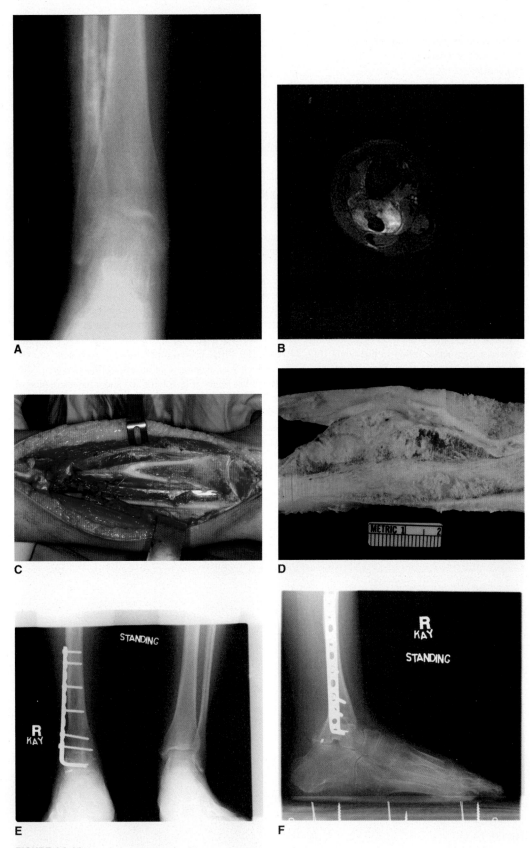

FIGURE 24.16

A: The AP radiograph of the ankle shows an aggressive destructive lesion of the distal fibula. **B:** The MRI of the fibula shows a heterogenic mass with soft tissue extension. **C:** The remaining tibia after the fibula and one third of the lateral tibia plafond was removed. **D:** The gross specimen of the osteogenic sarcoma of the distal fibula is seen. **E,F:** The AP and lateral radiographs at 4 years from tumor resection and reconstruction with ankle arthrodesis show a well-healed ankle arthrodesis in satisfactory condition.

Factors that do increase the risk of a nonunion include

- High-energy posttraumatic arthritis
- Presence of a neuropathy
- Diabetes
- Infection
- Nicotine use

A nonunion is usually diagnosed 6 months after surgery, and a CT scan can be helpful in evaluating a patient with continued pain after his or her arthrodesis. Revision arthrodesis is the treatment for a nonunion and usually requires bone grafting. If the patient is asymptomatic or minimally symptomatic, conservative treatment with a brace can be advised.

Malunions can occur after ankle arthrodesis especially when the foot is in equinus causing hyperextension of the knee and knee pain. Special care intraoperatively to verify that the foot is in a neutral dorsiflexion/plantar flexion position will help minimize this problem. The use of an external fixator does increase the chance of a malunion. Varus positioning can cause a patient to walk on the lateral border of the foot and can be painful and may require treatment with an orthotic. Postoperative infection can occur and is seen most commonly in patients with a history of a previous surgery or diabetes. Hardware can be prominent and it may require to be removed if painful.

The long-term consequence of an ankle arthrodesis includes increasing stress on the adjacent joints that can lead to degenerative arthritic changes with time. However, these changes are not always symptomatic and may be observed. If, however, they do become symptomatic, it may require an extension of the arthrodesis.

Figure 24.16 Illustrative case 1. A 14-year-old female presented with swelling around her ankles for about 3 weeks. There was a question of some minor trauma. She was evaluated and x-rays were obtained, which showed a destructive lesion in her fibula (Fig. 24.16A). Her MRI showed a heterogenic mass with soft tissue extension (Fig. 24.16B). She underwent a biopsy, which was diagnostic of an osteogenic sarcoma. After completion of chemotherapy, she underwent a resection of her tumor (Fig. 24.16C,D) and a reconstruction of her ankle. The tumor resection required the removal of the distal fibula and a portion of the distal tibia in order to get adequate margins. After the resection, two third of the tibia plafond was intact. There were no longer any ligamentous restraints to her ankle. She, therefore, underwent an arthrodesis with a blade plate. The remaining

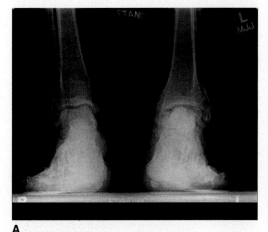

A

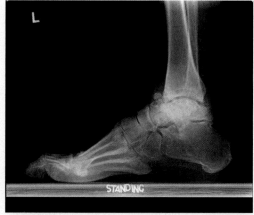

B

FIGURE 24.17

A,B: The AP and lateral radiograph of a patient with ankle arthritis after curettage and cementation of the talus for chondroblastoma is shown. **C:** The radiograph of a solid ankle arthrodesis after removal of the bone cement, bone grafting, and arthrodesis of the ankle is seen.

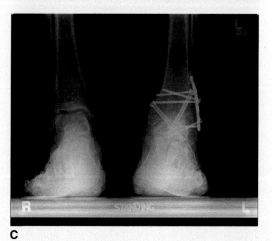

C

portion of her peroneal tendons was then tenodesed to the talus to give stability to the subtalar joint. The patient is now over 4 years from her surgery and she is without recurrence and is performing low-impact activities (Fig. 24.16 E,F).

   Figure 24.17 Illustrative case 2. A 49-year-old manual laborer who was diagnosed 15 years ago with a chondroblastoma of his talus presents with ankle pain. He underwent tumor resection with bone grafting. He had a recurrence and then underwent curettage and placement of bone cement. He did well for 12 years and now has increasing pain. His x-rays show extensive degenerative change through his ankle joint (Fig. 24.17A,B). His workup did not show any evidence of chondroblastoma recurrence. He was treated nonsurgically with bracing, activity modification, and anti-inflammatory medicines. His pain was significant enough that he ultimately underwent an ankle arthrodesis. He is 1 year from surgery with marked improvement in his pain and function (Fig. 24.17C).

RECOMMENDED READINGS

Abidi NA, Bruen GS, Conti SF. Ankle arthrodesis: Indications and techniques. *J Am Acad Orthop Surg.* 2000;8:
   200–209.
Ahmad J, Raikin, SM. Ankle arthrodesis: the simple and the complex. *Foot Ankle Clin.* 2008;13(3):381–400.
Buchner M, Sabo D. Ankle fusion attributable to posttraumatic arthrosis: a long-term followup of 48 patients. *Clin Orthop
   Relat Res.* 2003;406:155–164.
Buck P, Morrey BF, Chao EY. The optimum position of arthrodesis of the ankle. A gait study of the knee and ankle.
   J Bone Joint Surg. 1987;69A:1052–1062.
Easley ME, Montijo HE, Wilson JB, et al. Revision tibiotalar arthrodesis. *J Bone Joint Surg Am.* 2008;90A(6):
   1212–1223.
Kitaoka HB. Arthrodesis of the ankle: Technique, complications, and salvage treatment. *Instr Course Lect.* 1991;48:
   255–261.
Myerson MS, Quill G. Ankle arthrodesis. A comparison of an arthroscopic and an open method of treatment. *Clin Orthop
   Relat Res.* 1991;268:84–95.
Smith RW. Ankle arthrodesis, chapter 36. In: Kitaoka HB, ed. *Master Techniques in Orthopaedic Surgery: The Foot and
   Ankle*, 2nd ed. Philadelphia, PA: Lippincott; 2002:533–549.
Stone JW. Arthroscopic ankle arthrodesis. *Foot Ankle Clin.* 2006;11(2):361–368.

25 Prosthetic Replacement for Tumor of the Distal Tibia

Roger M. Tillman

The distal tibia is a rare site for primary malignant bone tumors. A review of 1,754 consecutive patients from our unit with osteosarcoma or Ewing sarcoma revealed that only 40 tumors were located in the distal tibia representing just over 2% of primary malignant bone tumors. When bone sarcomas do occur in the distal tibia, they present a particular challenge with regard to limb salvage surgery.

These challenges include:

The lack of soft tissue cover anteriorly. The tibia is in a subcutaneous position and, although, a fascio cutaneous flap can be turned down from the calf or, alternatively, a free flap can be applied, skin and soft tissue cover is a significant challenge particularly where there is soft tissue extension of the tumor.

The talus is a relatively small bone, and hence a difficult site to obtain secure bony fixation for the distal component of an endoprosthesis particularly as the implant usually has to provide a greater degree of ankle joint's stability than might be required from, for example, a total ankle replacement for arthritis, where the soft tissues are intact.

It is common knowledge from celebrities and media coverage of disabled athletes that function can be remarkably good following below knee amputation and therefore a limb salvage procedure that saves the limb but provides relatively poor function may not be regarded as an overall success. In most cases, there will, therefore, be a trade-off between body image and function when performing limb salvage surgery at this site in particular.

The salvage procedure from a failed distal tibial prosthetic replacement will in most cases be inferior to the result that would have been obtained had a primary below knee amputation been performed. The amputation level will be elevated to gain clearance from the previous surgical zone particularly if there has been infection or local recurrence of tumor. It may even be necessary to perform a through knee or above knee amputation under these circumstances.

INDICATIONS

Clinical situations where prosthetic surgery (or other types of limb salvage surgery) for a tumor of the distal tibia should at least be discussed with the patient are as follows:

- Primary sarcomas or highly aggressive benign bone tumors of the distal tibia with little or no extra osseous extension
- Normal neurological function and circulation in the foot
- Skeletally immature children

CONTRAINDICATIONS

- Relative contraindications include obesity, diabetes, skin conditions such as psoriasis that may predispose to infection, previous radiotherapy to the lower leg, lymphoedema, and evidence of distant metastases (although in some cases this may be regarded as an indication for limb salvage surgery as opposed to amputation).

In our practice, we advise patients that their function, in the long term, is likely to be inferior with limb salvage surgery as opposed to expected function from a modern below knee prosthesis.

PREOPERATIVE PLANNING

The basic principles are the same as for limb salvage surgery at other sites (1). Routine staging studies include

- MRI scan of the lesion (the scan must include the entire affected tibia).
- Long-leg measured radiographs to check the limb alignment and condition of proximal joints.
- Whole-body radioisotope bone scan and CT scan of the chest.
- CT pelvis and abdomen looking in particular for evidence of occult pelvic lymphadenopathy is also recommended.
- Hematological investigations are principally aimed at excluding infection or other concomitant medical conditions. Full blood count, ESR, CRP, and bone biochemistry are obligatory. The alkaline phosphatase may be elevated, but in the majority of the cases, all other investigations will be normal.

Biopsy

The biopsy site and technique are critical. We recommend a percutaneous bone biopsy via an anterior approach directly into the tibia at its subcutaneous border using a short vertical stab incision. A large transverse biopsy scar, if it has been carried out elsewhere, will often effectively preclude limb salvage surgery. If the bone is hard, then a drill hole will need to be made.

Prosthesis

Measured long-leg radiographs must be obtained for ordering an endoprosthetic replacement. All of the implants used in this unit for the distal tibia have been custom implants from Stanmore Implants Worldwide, London (Fig. 25.1). We are not aware of any modular options for the distal tibia. The tibial component is a massive replacement made of titanium alloy and cobalt chrome on the articulating surface. An intramedullary stem is used for fixation in the remaining portion of the proximal tibia. Fixation is with cement, but we recommend in all cases an HA (Hydroxyapatite) collar to aid osseointegration at the bone-prosthesis interface.

Anatomic Landmarks and Incision

The principle bony landmarks are the medial and lateral malleoli and the anterior tibial crest. A longitudinal anterior incision excising the biopsy scar and tract en bloc with the tumor is recommended and this incision can be extended onto the dorsal aspect of the foot in order to gain adequate access to the talus (Fig. 25.2).

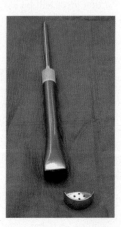

FIGURE 25.1

Photograph showing segmental replacement for proximal tibia and talar component of ankle arthroplasty.

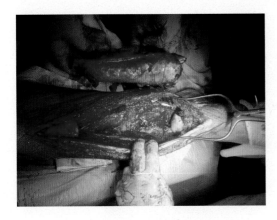

FIGURE 25.2
Surgical photograph following resection of distal tibia. Note adjacent tumor specimen.

Position

The procedure can be performed with or without the use of a tourniquet. The author recommends that a tourniquet is not in fact used but the patient should be placed in the supine position with the table in the head-down (Trendelenburg) position to drain the superficial veins in the lower leg and foot and minimize blood loss. It is essential that if the posterior tibial artery is inadvertently divided that this is immediately recognized and this will not be the case with a tourniquet in place.

Dissection and Procedure

If the surgeon is satisfied with macroscopic surgical margins (frozen section pathology may be obtained if there is doubt in this regard), then the tibia should be transected at the previously determined level, using bone retractors to carefully protect the adjacent soft tissues from the blade of the oscillating saw. The intraosseous membrane should be mobilized and the distal tibia can then be carefully removed. The talus is then prepared with a burr to receive the talar dome prosthesis, which is manufactured from cobalt chromium caladium alloy. The prosthesis currently in use is manufactured with two flanges for anchorage in the talus.

The components are cemented in place with low-viscosity polymethyl methacrylate bone cement with gentamicin (Fig. 25.3). Great care is taken to ensure that the tibial component is inserted in correct rotation. The author recommends the use of an antirotation lug (a notch is prepared for this in the tibia using a burr) as this allows the cement to harden with complete rotational stability.

Wound Closure

Wound closure is achieved where there is adequate tissue, by suturing the extensor hallucis longus across the prosthesis and attaching this to the peroneus longus to provide some anterior prosthetic cover. If there is insufficient tissue, then a combined procedure with a plastic surgical team should be performed with fabrication of a free flap or fascio cutaneous turn-down flap from the calf. The wound is closed over a single vacuum drain. I would recommend a subcuticular absorbable suture where the skin edges are healthy and suitable to accept this technique.

Interrupted fine elongated sutures are an acceptable alternative. The limb is then bandaged and rested in a plaster back slab. Postoperative elevation is essential. Prophylactic antibiotics are recommended. We do not routinely give prophylactic anticoagulants, but this should be considered in high-risk patients.

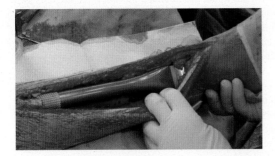

FIGURE 25.3
Surgical photograph of distal tibial replacement prosthesis with ankle arthroplasty. Note hydroxyapatite collar at the bone-prosthesis junction.

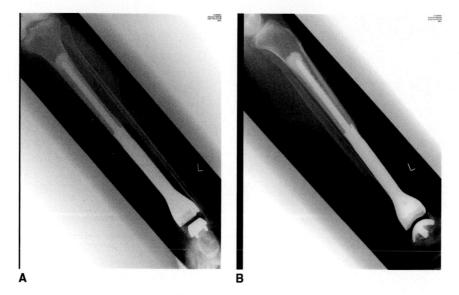

FIGURE 25.4

A,B: AP and lateral views of distal tibial segmental prosthesis with total ankle arthroplasty.

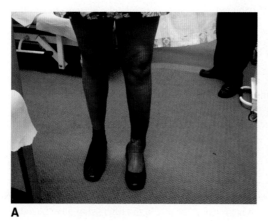
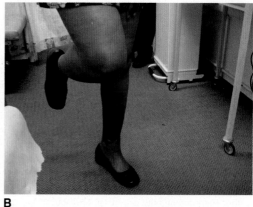

FIGURE 25.5

A: Clinical photograph taken 12 years following segmental replacement of the left distal tibia and total ankle replacement. Patient reports she is pain free and very satisfied.
B: Clinical photograph of same patient standing only on the operated leg with no pain or difficulty. Clearly not all such reconstructions will be this sucessful.

POSTOPERATIVE CARE

The patient should be mobilized, partial weight bearing, for a period of 6 weeks. If a split-thickness skin graft, fasciocutaneous flaps, or free flaps were used for wound coverage, then plaster cast immobilization may be required for up to 6 weeks to allow adequate healing. Elevation to minimize swelling at all possible times is essential. It is our practice to readmit patients for several days of intensive in-patient physiotherapy and rehabilitation for approximately 6 weeks postoperatively as we find that reliance on local physiotherapy services where therapists are inevitably less experience with the management of this type of prosthesis can be variable and sometimes unsatisfactory.

RESULTS

Papers describing prosthetic replacement of the distal tibia for tumor are rare and, indeed, there are only two published series to our knowledge, one from our own Unit in Birmingham and also a series of 5 replacements of the distal tibia by Lee et al. from Korea (1999) (2–4). This reflects the wide spread practice of advocating below knee amputations for aggressive tumors at this anatomical site due to the challenge of functionally and durable prosthetic reconstruction. Inevitably, patients will occasionally present who refuse to accept amputation and for whom the prosthetic option may be suitable.

In our own experience of only nine cases, this is a procedure that can be very durable and successful in a carefully selected and highly motivated group of patients (Fig. 25.4A,B). One female patient is now 14 years post surgery and remains very satisfied and with good MSTS score (Fig. 25.5A,B). No revisions have been required, but of course the long-term survival of the patient is dependent on oncological factors as with limb salvage surgery at any other site.

REFERENCES

1. Niimi R, Matsumine A, Kusuzaki K, et al. Usefulness of limb salvage surgery for bone and soft tissue sarcomas of the distal lower leg *J Cancer Res Clin Oncol.* 2008;134:1087–1095.
2. Natarajan MV, Annamalai K, Williams S, et al. Limb salvage in distal tibial osteosarcoma using a custom mega prosthesis *Int Orthop.* 2000;24:282–284.
3. Abudu A, Grimer RJ, Tillman RM, et al. Endoprosthetic replacement of the distal tibia and ankle joint for aggressive bone tumours *Int Orthop.* 1999;23:291–294.
4. Lee SH, Kim HS, Park YB, et al. Prosthetic reconstruction for tumours of the distal tibia and fibula. *J Bone Joint Surg Br Vol.* 1999;81B:803–807.

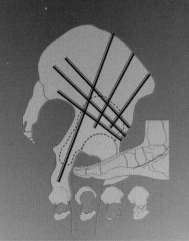

Part TWO

Upper Extremity

26 General Considerations

Kristy L. Weber

The shoulder is a relatively common location for tumor resections that involve limb-sparing operations for primary bone sarcomas as well as metastatic disease. The complex anatomy about the shoulder girdle and the need to maintain maximal function for the patient to perform activities of daily living underscore the importance of a thorough understanding of the issues related to complex surgery in this area. The options for reconstruction of the humerus and shoulder girdle after tumor resection are varied and explained in detail in the following chapters.

INDICATIONS

Resection

- Primary bone/soft tissue sarcomas or occasionally isolated bone metastasis that involve the humerus or scapula without involvement of the main neurovascular bundle are indicated for wide resection with goals to achieve lasting local control and potentially increase the patient's survival (Figs. 26.1 and 26.2).
- Widespread metastatic bone disease with a pathologic fracture of the humerus that is not amenable to internal fixation is often indicated for resection. The goal is to achieve pain relief rather than local control, thus a wide resection is often not necessary. If an intralesional or marginal resection is performed, postoperative external beam radiation is used (Fig. 26.3).

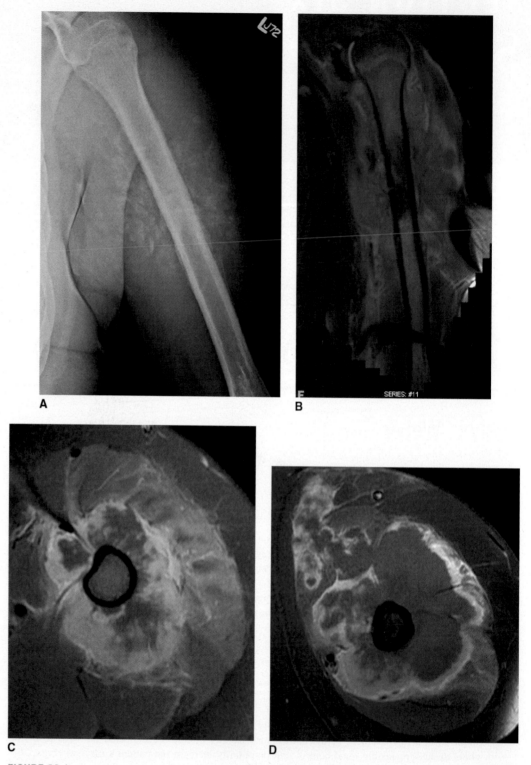

FIGURE 26.1

A: AP radiograph of the left humerus in a 17-year-old man with a humeral osteosarcoma. Note the ossification of the soft tissue tumor extension after chemotherapy. Coronal (**B**) and axial (**C,D**) postgadolinium MR images reveal the bony extent of tumor and the surrounding soft tissue mass. Careful evaluation of the medial neurovascular structures is necessary in order to determine whether the patient is a candidate for limb-sparing surgery.

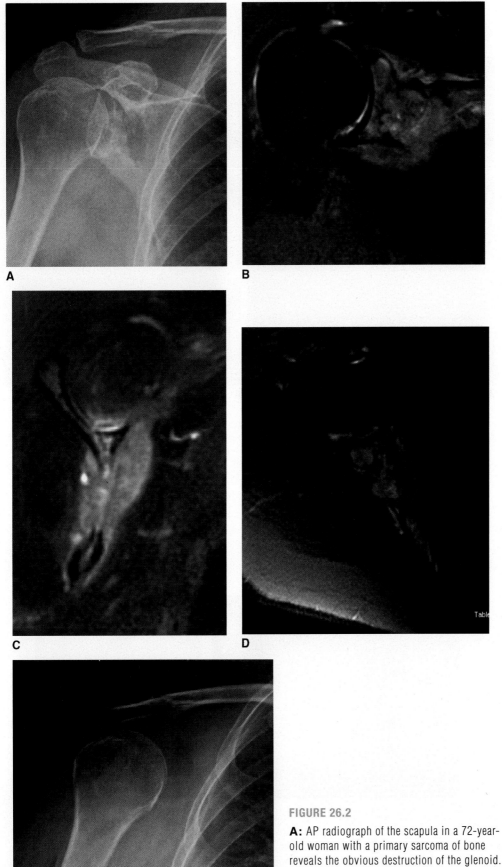

FIGURE 26.2

A: AP radiograph of the scapula in a 72-year-old woman with a primary sarcoma of bone reveals the obvious destruction of the glenoid. Coronal T2 (**B**), sagittal T2 (**C**), and axial T2 (**D**) MR images show the lateral and distal extent of the tumor. **E:** The entire scapula was removed, and the humerus was resuspended to the clavicle.

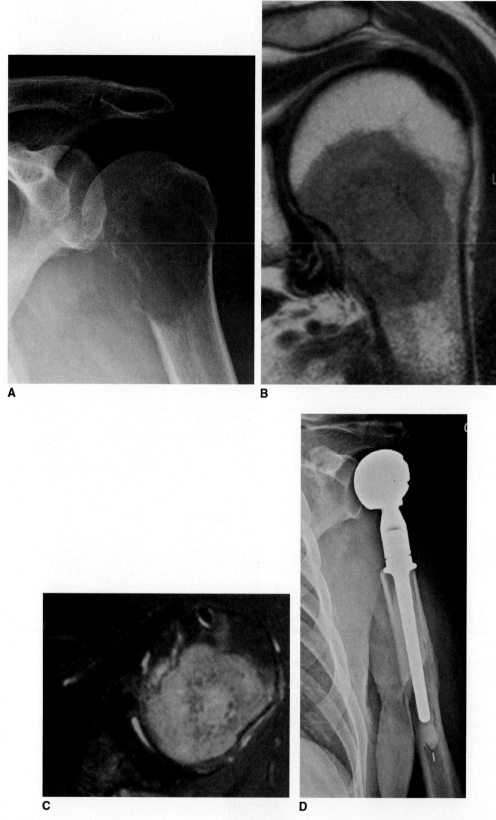

FIGURE 26.3

A: AP radiograph of a 62-year-old man with metastatic lung cancer to the left proximal humerus. The osteolytic lesion is progressive and his pain is severe despite external beam radiation. Note the cortical bone loss medially. Coronal T1 (**B**) and axial T2 (**C**) MR images reveal the localized disease in this area. **D:** Postoperative radiograph after wide resection of the metastasis with reconstruction using a megaprosthesis. There was not thought to be enough proximal bone to allow stability with intramedullary fixation.

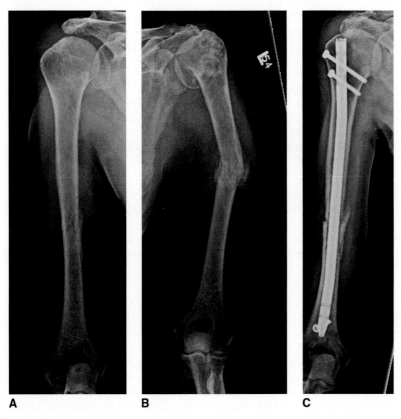

FIGURE 26.4

A: AP radiograph of the right humerus in a 62-year-old woman with widely metastatic breast cancer. Although this fracture can be treated nonoperatively, she required the use of her right upper extremity for ambulation due to painful lower extremity lesions that limited her weightbearing capacity and a prior pathologic fracture of the left humerus (**B**). **C:** Postoperative radiograph after intramedullary fixation of the right humerus. She could bear full weight on this arm after surgery.

Stabilization

- An impending or actual pathologic fracture of the humerus in a patient with multiple sites of disease where the integrity of the proximal and distal ends of the humerus are maintained is indicated for stabilization. The remaining bone should allow stable internal fixation with or without methylmethacrylate. These patients are also treated with postoperative external beam radiation (Fig. 26.4).

Reconstruction

- After an intra-articular resection of the proximal humerus for a primary sarcoma, the reconstructive options include a proximal humeral osteoarticular allograft, a megaprosthesis or an allograft-prosthesis composite (APC). The final decision is made with consideration to patient preference, surgeon experience, and functional expectations. The risks and benefits of each type of reconstruction are discussed with the patient in detail with regard to postoperative range of motion, functional restrictions, risk of infection, and risk of prosthetic loosening. These complications and outcomes are discussed in more detail in the following chapters.
- After an extra-articular resection of the shoulder for primary tumors of the humerus or scapula, reconstructive options include a total or partial scapular prosthesis with a prosthetic humeral component versus a glenohumeral arthrodesis. The arthrodesis requires use of an intercalary allograft with or without a supplemental vascularized fibular graft. The expected function of the axillary nerve and deltoid muscle after resection is an important point to consider related to decision making. Patient expectations, surgeon experience, complications of the particular procedure, and failure rates of the prosthetic reconstruction are factors in decision making.
- Prosthetic/allograft reconstructions or glenohumeral arthrodeses can be used as salvage operations for failed shoulder reconstructions performed for nononcologic conditions.
- Rarely a primary sarcoma or isolated metastasis occurs in the humeral diaphysis, sparing the shoulder and elbow joints. In this situation, a wide resection can be performed with reconstruction using a diaphyseal humeral spacer cemented into the proximal and distal humerus.

CONTRAINDICATIONS

Resection

- Patients with involvement of the neurovascular bundle about the shoulder or arm
- Patients with growth of a primary sarcoma on chemotherapy
- Patients with a primary sarcoma about the shoulder and extensive metastatic disease with a limited lifespan (<3 months)
- Patients with metastasis and a humerus lesion amenable to stabilization with internal fixation and radiation
- Patients with metastatic disease to the scapula or clavicle (usually treated with external beam radiation, cryotherapy, radiofrequency ablation or other nonoperative methods rather than resection)

Reconstruction

- Patients with active infection of the shoulder joint are contraindicated for prosthetic or allograft reconstruction of the shoulder.
- Patients with a history of treated infection of the shoulder joint or active/treated infection elsewhere in the body are relative contraindications for reconstruction using a shoulder prosthesis or allograft, but a glenohumeral arthrodesis might be appropriate.
- Patients with lack of active scapulothoracic motion are a contraindication for glenohumeral arthrodesis.

IMAGING

The preoperative imaging obtained for resection and/or reconstruction about the shoulder and humerus is the same as for other anatomic areas. Plain radiographs document the visible bone destruction and allow for templating the reconstruction or size-matching an allograft. Technetium bone scans are not necessary for preoperative planning but are helpful in identifying additional sites of metastatic bone disease around the shoulder as well as skip metastases in cases of primary bone sarcoma. Computed tomography (CT) scans are ideal to delineate the bony anatomy but have been replaced by magnetic resonance imaging (MRI) for preoperative planning in most conditions. CT scans remain useful in staging patients to determine additional sites of disease in the chest, abdomen and pelvis and for follow up surveillance. MRI scans delineate the marrow extent of disease for bone lesions and accurately outline the relationship of extraosseous tumor to the surrounding soft tissue (shoulder capsule) and neurovascular structures. MRI is often the best test to determine whether limb salvage surgery can be safely performed. An angiogram or MR angiogram is necessary in rare instances where embolization is used preoperatively for vascular metastasis (renal, thyroid) or when the detailed blood supply of the shoulder needs to be mapped for use of a vascularized fibular reconstruction of the upper extremity.

ANATOMIC CONSIDERATIONS

The shoulder girdle and proximal humerus is a complex anatomical area with close proximity between the soft tissue structures and the neurovascular structures that supply the arm. It is important to understand the anatomy and be able to assess the involvement of key structures on an MRI scan to determine the indications for limb salvage surgery versus amputation. The majority of primary bone tumors occur in the proximal humeral metaphysis with variable extension into the epiphysis and diaphysis. In skeletally immature patients, the proximal epiphyseal plate is often a barrier to tumor but not always.

The subclavian artery becomes the axillary artery at the lateral border of the first rib. The axillary artery is at risk during procedures about the shoulder as it courses inferior to the coracoid process beneath the pectoralis minor. Abduction of the arm during dissection puts the artery on stretch around the coracoid and at risk for injury. The axillary artery turns into the brachial artery that runs medial to the humerus and under the biceps with the median nerve in the upper two thirds of the arm. The profunda brachii artery runs with the radial nerve. The posterior circumflex humeral artery runs with the axillary nerve in the quadrangular space beneath the teres minor, and the anterior circumflex humeral artery crosses the anterior shoulder between the pectoralis major and the deltoid. The anterior circumflex vessels are ligated during a proximal humeral resection. The circumflex scapular vessels supply the scapula and can be damaged during dissection between the teres minor and teres major.

The axillary nerve arises from the posterior cord of the brachial plexus and courses posteriorly in the axilla on the subscapularis. It goes through the quadrangular space and abuts the surgical neck of the humerus where it is vulnerable during resection. The radial nerve also arises from the posterior cord of the plexus and courses through the triangular space and then lies in the spiral groove of the humerus between the lateral and medial triceps. The musculocutaneous nerve arises from the lateral cord of the brachial plexus and enters the coracobrachialis from the medial side 8 cm below the coracoid process and is subject to damage during retraction in this area.

The quadrangular space contains the axillary nerve and posterior circumflex humeral vessels and is bordered by the lower border of the teres minor, surgical neck of the humerus, long head of the triceps, and upper border of the teres major when viewed from posterior.

The coracoid process of the scapula is a key attachment area for structures vital to stability of the shoulder. When possible these ligaments and tendons should be maintained or reattached after reconstruction. The pectoralis minor, coracobrachialis, and short head of the biceps (latter two make the conjoined tendon) are the three muscle attachments. The coracoacromial ligament helps to form the coracoacromial arch and can help prevent superior subluxation of a proximal humeral prosthetic reconstruction. The coracoclavicular ligaments include the trapezoid and conoid (medial) ligaments and help stabilize the acromioclavicular joint.

SURGICAL CONSIDERATIONS

For resection of the proximal humerus, the patient can be supine in a beach chair position with a bump beneath the scapula and the arm extended laterally off the operative table or, alternatively, placed in the lateral position on a beanbag. If a scapular resection is to be performed alone or in combination with resection of the proximal humerus, the patient is placed in the lateral position. The entire arm is prepped and draped. For anterior approaches, the deltopectoral interval is used unless a prior biopsy or surgical incision precludes this. The anterior incision can be extended to the elbow by splitting the brachialis. The cephalic vein is maintained if possible, taking it medially or laterally with a small cuff of either deltoid or pectoralis muscle. Depending on the extent and location of tumor extension into the surrounding soft tissues, the deltoid may be released from the clavicle and acromion and later reattached. The conjoined tendon can also be released and reattached to the coracoid process. The long head of the biceps is released distal to the glenohumeral joint and reattached at resting length after the reconstruction. For a scapular resection, a longitudinal incision is made over the lateral scapula and extended over the superior surface of the arm to the anterior approach for a humeral resection if necessary. For a glenohumeral arthrodesis, careful attention is necessary to the expected postoperative position of the arm. Soft tissue coverage should be planned preoperatively if it is expected that the deltoid will be resected with the tumor. For cases involving a structural allograft, appropriate size-matching should be done preoperatively, and necessary soft tissues should be maintained on the allograft. If internal fixation is used for stabilization of metastatic disease to the humerus, intraoperative fluoroscopy is used. The appropriate rehabilitation program depends on the stability of the reconstruction and ability to bear weight on the arm.

COMPLICATIONS

Major complications during surgical resection of the humerus or shoulder girdle are usually neurovascular. Neuropraxia or actual transection of the axillary, radial or musculoskeletal nerves can cause functional deficits postoperatively. Complications related to the reconstruction include superior subluxation of a proximal humeral prosthesis or allograft if it is not secured appropriately within the glenoid with accurate tensioning of the surrounding ligaments and tendons. Postoperative function and active shoulder range of motion are improved when using an osteoarticular or APC reconstruction, as the allograft soft tissues are sutured to those remaining in the host for a more biologic repair than suturing the capsule and rotator cuff tendons to a metal prosthesis. Allograft-host nonunion can occur in patients reconstructed with an osteoarticular allograft, APC, or allograft-arthrodesis. For patients requiring a proximal humeral resection and reconstruction, the goals of sparing the limb, allowing normal elbow, wrist, and hand function, and providing a pain-free construct outweigh the common functional limitations of the reconstruction. Complications related to the various types of reconstructions are listed in the following chapters and include pain, infection, wound breakdown, aseptic loosening, hardware failure, and cartilage degeneration. Oncologic complications include local recurrence or progression of disease.

27 Total Scapulectomy and Reconstruction Using a Scapular Prosthesis

Panayiotis J. Papagelopoulos and
Andreas F. Mavrogenis

Tumors of the scapula often become quite large before being brought to a physician's attention. In the early stages, they are usually contained by a cuff of muscle (infraspinatus, subscapularis, and supraspinatus). Tumor extension to the chest wall, axillary vessels, proximal humerus, glenohumeral joint, and rotator cuff may follow during disease progression (1,3,10,13,18,19).

The first reported scapular resection was a partial scapulectomy performed by Liston in 1819 for an ossified aneurysmal tumor. Since then, most shoulder girdle resections are performed for low-grade tumors of the scapular and periscapular soft tissue sarcomas (7–10). After the initial description of the Tikhoff-Linberg resection for osteosarcoma and Ewing sarcoma of the proximal humerus or scapula in the 1980s, a variety of new techniques and modifications of shoulder girdle resections have been developed, and several classification systems have been proposed (1,2–9,11,12,14–20). The earlier systems were purely descriptive and related almost exclusively to the bones resected. In addition, they did not accommodate or reflect concepts or terminology that have developed in the past 2 decades in orthopedic oncology. The present surgical classification system was described by Malawer in 1991 (Table 27.1) (7). This classification was based on the current concept of surgical margins (intra-articular vs. extra-articular), the relationship of the tumor to anatomic compartments (intracompartmental vs. extracompartmental), the status of the glenohumeral joint, the magnitude of the individual surgical procedure, and consideration of the functionally important soft tissue components.

INDICATIONS

- Total en bloc scapulectomy and limb-salvage surgery are indicated for most low- and high-grade primary sarcomas of the scapular and soft tissue sarcomas that secondarily invade the bone when an adequate soft tissue cuff can be obtained for surgical margins, that is, Type III (intra-articular total scapulectomy), Type IV (extra-articular scapulectomy and humeral head resection), and Type VI (extra-articular humeral and total scapular resection) resections (Fig. 27.1).
- It may be performed if the potential results are equivalent to or better than amputation, with preservation of good elbow and hand function.

293

TABLE 27.1	Surgical Classification of Shoulder Girdle Resections
Type	**Classification**
I	Intra-articular proximal humeral resection
II	Partial scapular resection
III	Intra-articular total scapulectomy
IV	Extra-articular total scapulectomy and humeral head resection (the classic Tikhoff-Linberg resection)
V	Extra-articular humeral and glenoid resection
VI	Extra-articular humeral and total scapular resection

From Malawer MM. Tumors of the shoulder girdle: technique of resection and description of a surgical classification. *Orthop Clin North Am.* 1991;22:7–35.

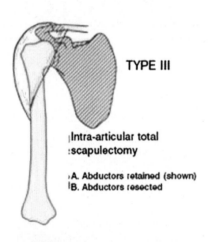

TYPE III

Intra-articular total scapulectomy

A. Abductors retained (shown)
B. Abductors resected

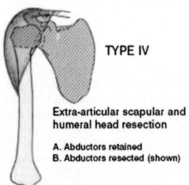

TYPE IV

Extra-articular scapular and humeral head resection

A. Abductors retained
B. Abductors resected (shown)

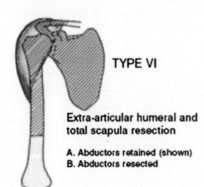

TYPE VI

Extra-articular humeral and total scapula resection

A. Abductors retained (shown)
B. Abductors resected

FIGURE 27.1

The three types of total scapulectomy according to Malawer et al (7).

CONTRAINDICATIONS

- Contraindications for the procedure include tumor extension into the axilla with involvement of the neurovascular bundle, inability to spare the required muscles, and the patient's inability or unwillingness to tolerate a limb-salvage operation.
- Although a functioning deltoid is recommended for use of a scapular prosthesis, resection of the axillary nerve should not be considered an absolute contraindication for scapular replacement (14,21).
- Relative contraindications may include chest wall extension, pathological fractures of the scapular or proximal humerus, lymph node involvement, and an inappropriately placed biopsy that has resulted in infection or extensive hematoma and tissue contamination.

PREOPERATIVE EVALUATION

Physical examination, plain radiographs, computed tomography (CT) scan, and magnetic resonance imaging (MRI) are important means for evaluation of a patient with a tumor of the shoulder girdle. The MRI can help estimate whether there will be enough soft tissue remaining for the reconstruction. For large tumors involving the proximal humerus, a venogram may also be useful if there is evidence of distal obstruction suggesting tumor thromboembolism (analogous to tumor thromboembolism seen in the iliac vessels and inferior vena cava from large pelvic sarcomas).

The goals of preoperative templating are to guide both proper sizing of the humeral and custom-made scapular components, as well as intraoperative restoration of the soft tissue balance of the shoulder joint. CT scan data are used to design the prototype model to manufacture the custom scapular prosthesis. Alternatively, nonmodular scapular prostheses are available in two sizes, adult and pediatric. Thinking of the glenohumeral articulation, either a reverse constrained shoulder replacement (i.e., the head on the scapular and a captive cup in the proximal humeral prosthesis) or a nonconstrained replacement with a shallow glenoid and a large head on the proximal humeral prosthesis (much like a Neer II prosthesis) can be performed. However, when a large amount of periscapular soft tissue is resected, a constrained shoulder joint prosthesis is indicated.

SURGERY

Limb-salvage surgery at the shoulder girdle is more difficult than a forequarter amputation. The surgical options are technically demanding and fraught with potential complications. One should be experienced with all aspects of shoulder girdle anatomy. Anatomic landmarks to be considered include the clavicle, acromion, acromioclavicular joint, scapular spine and the borders of the scapular, proximal humerus, and glenohumeral joint. We describe herein the procedure of intra-articular total scapulectomy and constrained reverse total scapular reconstructions after resection of a sarcoma of the right scapular (Fig. 27.2A,B).

Patient Positioning

The patient is placed in the lateral position on a standard operating room table secured with commonly available positioners (Fig. 27.3A,B). A Foley catheter is inserted, and preoperative antibiotic prophylaxis is administered. An axillary roll is inserted distal to the opposite axilla under the chest wall. The dependent arm is placed on a well-padded arm board in an extended position.

The arm is prepared and draped free for intraoperative manipulation. It may be placed on a bolster or a sterile Mayo stand.

Incision

A combined anterior and posterior approach is utilized (utilitarian shoulder girdle incision), as it permits wide exposure and release of all muscles attached to the scapular including the rhomboids, latissimus dorsi, and trapezius. The utilitarian shoulder girdle incision is identical to that of the Tikhoff-Linberg procedure for resection of the proximal humerus. This incision, or parts of it, permits safe exposure for resection and reconstruction of most shoulder girdle tumors and safe exposure of the axillary vessels and brachial plexus. The surgical incision should incorporate the biopsy tract and remove it with the surgical specimen.

Anteriorly, the incision begins at the junction of the inner and middle thirds of the clavicle and continues over the coracoid process, along the deltopectoral groove at the anteromedial aspect of the deltoid muscle, and down the arm over the medial border of the biceps muscle.

Posteriorly, the incision begins over the midclavicular portion of the anterior incision, crosses the suprascapular area, runs over the lateral aspect of the scapular along the neck of the glenoid, proceeds distally to

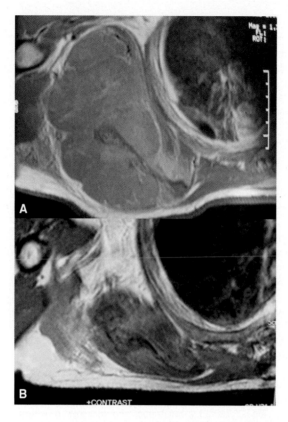

FIGURE 27.2

Ewing sarcoma of the right scapular in a 54-year-old man. **A:** MRI prior to chemotherapy shows a large tumor involving the scapular with extensive soft tissue extension. **B:** MRI after chemotherapy shows reduction of the tumor size.

the inferior tip of the scapular, and curves toward the midline. One skin flap is mobilized medially toward the vertebral border of the scapular and the other laterally to expose the entire scapular and its covering fascia and musculature. To preserve vascularity to the skin, care should be taken not to make the flaps any wider than necessary.

Approach

The operative procedure begins with the posterior incision to mobilize the scapular and explore the retroscapular area to determine if there is any involvement of the chest wall. The approach for freeing the scapular of

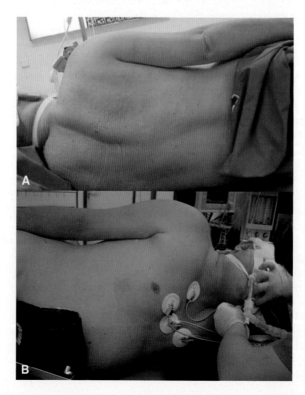

FIGURE 27.3

The patient is placed in the lateral position on a standard operating room table secured with commonly available positioners.

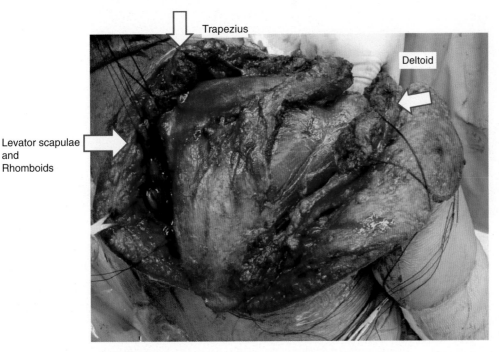

Trapezius

Deltoid

Levator scapulae
and
Rhomboids

FIGURE 27.4

The scapula is free of its superficial muscular attachments.

its superficial muscular attachments begins with release of the trapezius muscle from the scapular spine, leaving a small soft tissue cuff for a margin. The trapezius muscle is then retracted medially. The insertion of the deltoid muscle on the inferior aspect of the spine of the scapula is detached in a similar manner (Fig. 27.4). If there is no tumor involvement, the deltoid and trapezius muscles are preserved and reflected off the spine of the scapula and the acromion. The deeper musculature of the scapula is exposed. This approach is routinely used if an extra-articular resection is to be performed, that is, the classical Tikhoff-Linberg resection (Type IV). It is unusual to perform a Type III or Type IV scapular resection from the posterior approach alone unless there is minimal soft-tissue extension. The classical Tikhoff-Linberg resection does not preserve the deltoid or trapezius muscles; however, in order to provide adequate soft tissue coverage for the scapular prosthesis, these muscles must be retained (modified Type IV resection).

At the most inferior aspect of the posterior incision, the attachment of the latissimus dorsi muscle to the inferior angle of the scapula is identified and released. This maneuver allows the inferior angle to be elevated manually, so that the surgeon's hand can be placed between the chest wall and the deep musculature on the spinal border of the scapula. With gentle, upward traction on the inferior angle, the musculature on the spinal border of the scapula is released, starting most distally with the rhomboid major, then the rhomboid minor, and finally the levator scapulae (Fig. 27.5). The remaining serratus posterior, which is deep to these muscles, can then be released to give maximum mobility to the spinal border of the scapula. The margins of muscle that must remain on the scapular depend on the extent of the tumor; a 1- to 2-cm cuff of muscle is required for most tumors.

Release of the muscles adjacent to the lateral border of the scapula starts at the inferior angle of the scapula and moves superiorly through the teres major and teres minor. The circumflex scapular artery is identified

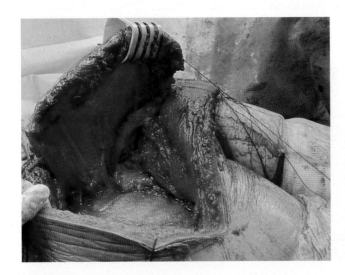

FIGURE 27.5

With gentle, upward traction on the inferior angle, the musculature on the spinal border of the scapula is incised, starting most distally with the rhomboid major, then the rhomboid minor, and finally the levator scapulae.

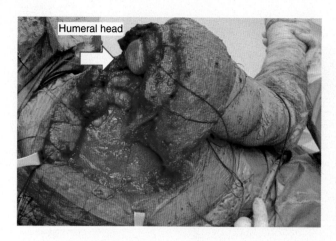

FIGURE 27.6

After complete release, en bloc removal of the scapula is performed after an intra-articular incision of the glenohumeral joint.

between these two muscles and ligated. The infraspinatus and supraspinatus muscles are then released near their insertions, permitting direct visualization of the attachment of the long head of the triceps to the scapula, and protection of the axillary nerve and the posterior circumflex humeral vessels from injury. After the capsule of the glenohumeral joint is incised, the tendon of the long head of the biceps is transected as it crosses the humeral head to its origin on the glenoid.

The anterior incision is utilized to mobilize the axillary vessels and nerve from any extraosseous component of the tumor. Begin superiorly by disarticulation of the acromioclavicular joint; the branches of the thoracoacromial trunk are ligated or coagulated for hemostasis. If there is concern about the margins, the distal clavicle may also be osteotomized and removed with the scapular. The coracoclavicular ligaments are incised to free the clavicle from the scapula. The deltoid muscle is detached at its insertion on the clavicle. The subcutaneous flap is reflected medially, and the cephalic vein is identified and ligated. The tendon of the pectoralis minor and the conjoined tendon are released from the coracoid process, and tagged for later reattachment. The pectoralis minor is reflected medially and the conjoined tendon distally to expose the clavicopectoral fascia and the underlying axillary artery and brachial plexus. For high-grade tumors of the scapula with a large soft-tissue mass, mobilization of the axillary vessels and brachial plexus through the anterior approach is necessary for safe resection. The small branches of the axillary and brachial arteries are exposed and ligated. Special attention is given to the anterior and posterior humeral circumflex vessels. Once these are ligated, along with the axillary nerve if necessary (Tikhoff–Linberg type IV resection for stage IIB sarcomas of the scapular neck, the glenoid or the humeral head), the neurovascular bundle can more easily be retracted medially, away from the site of the resection. The musculocutaneous and radial nerves are identified and can usually be preserved. The subscapularis muscle is released at its humeral insertion with care to avoid injury to the subscapular artery. Medially, the suprascapular artery is identified crossing above the transverse scapular ligament and ligated. Medial to this artery, the attachment of the serratus anterior muscle to the anteromedial border of the scapula is released. If the humeral lesion extends distal to the deltoid insertion, the entire insertion is resected with the tumor. The lateral flap is developed by reflecting the skin and subcutaneous tissue laterally.

Then, complete release and en bloc removal of the scapular are performed by an intra-articular incision of the glenohumeral joint (Type III resection) (Fig. 27.6). Alternatively, an extra-articular resection is performed by an osteotomy inferior to the glenohumeral capsule at the distal predetermined level necessary for resection of the humeral lesion (Tikhoff–Linberg, Type IV resection). The determination of either a scapulectomy (Type III resection) or an extra-articular resection of the glenohumeral joint and the scapular (Type IV resection) is made preoperatively.

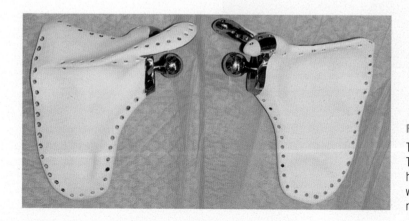

FIGURE 27.7

The scapular prosthesis. The implant shown is hydroxyapatite-coated with holes for soft tissue reattachment.

Prosthetic Reconstruction

If significant periscapular muscles remain (especially the deltoid, trapezius, rhomboids and latissimus dorsi) following a Type III or IV shoulder girdle resection, then a scapular prosthesis can be utilized. The implant is designed using the patient data; it is the same size and shape as the original scapular (Fig. 27.7). Holes are provided for soft tissue reattachment. The implant can be hydroxyapatite-coated to prevent metallosis debris. Suture holes are 3.0 mm in diameter and are positioned 10 mm apart for fixation with strong monofilament sutures (PDS 1.0 mm). The prosthesis accommodates a 22.2 mm head to link with the humeral prosthesis. The acromion area of the prosthesis is highly polished to allow some articulation between the acromion and the clavicle.

The scapular prosthesis is laid on the chest wall superficial to the remaining serratus anterior muscle. The teres major and minor muscles (if present) are then attached to the axillary border of the scapular prosthesis. Medially, the rhomboids and levator scapulae muscles are reattached. Then, the latissimus dorsi muscle is rotated over the body of the scapular prosthesis and sutured along the inner border of the scapular. The reverse constrained humeral prosthesis (Fig. 27.8) is then inserted into the proximal humerus in adequate orientation (30 degrees of retroversion). In cases of proximal humeral replacement, a polypropylene mesh or a Gore-Tex graft may be utilized to reconstruct the articular capsule to prevent migration of the head of the humerus and provide for a stable shoulder with satisfactory motion and no additional morbidity (1,7,8,19).The trapezius and the posterior deltoid muscles are then tenodesed to provide complete coverage of the prosthesis (Figs. 27.9 and 27.10). The scapular prosthesis fits between the serratus anterior and the latissimus dorsi and rhomboid muscles "as if in a sandwich." The humeral prosthesis is reduced to the scapular prosthesis and range of motion of the prosthetic shoulder joint is examined (Fig. 27.11).

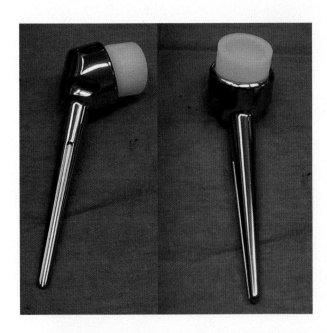

FIGURE 27.8
The reverse constrained humeral prosthesis.

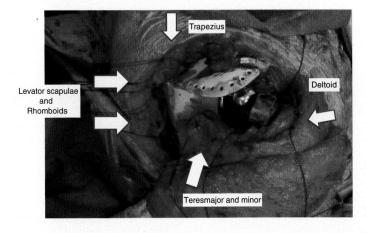

FIGURE 27.9
Reattachment of the muscles is done at the suture holes of the scapular prosthesis.

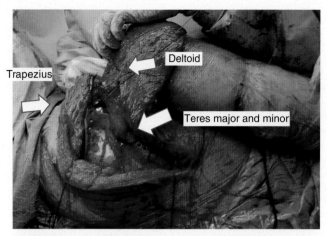

FIGURE 27.10

Strong monofilament sutures (PDS 1.0 mm) are used for the reattachment of the muscles.

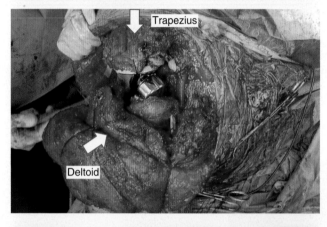

FIGURE 27.11

The humeral prosthesis is reduced to the scapular prosthesis; the range of motion and the stability of the shoulder joint are examined.

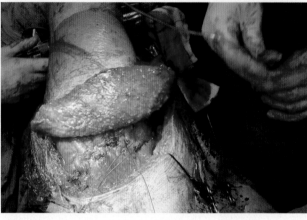

FIGURE 27.12

Tenodesis of the trapezius to deltoid and latissimus dorsi to serratus anterior muscles is done, and the fascia and subcutaneous tissue are closed in separate layers.

Final Closure

The wound is inspected for meticulous hemostasis. Large suction drains are placed at the anterior and the posterior aspects of the incision, and the fascia and subcutaneous tissue are closed in separate layers followed by the skin (Fig. 27.12). Sterile dressings are applied and the arm is secured in a sling and swathe or immobilizer.

PEARLS AND PITFALLS

- The combined anterior and posterior approach (utilitarian shoulder girdle incision) permits safe exposure for resection and reconstruction of most shoulder girdle tumors.
- The initial biopsy tract should be incorporated to the surgical incision and removed with the surgical specimen.
- The anterior component of the utilitarian incision alone can be used for resection of tumors of the proximal humerus, the proximal arm, or the axilla. The posterior component of the utilitarian incision

can be used for resections around the scapular and glenoid. It is unusual to perform a Type III or Type IV scapular resection from the posterior approach alone unless there is minimal soft-tissue extension.

- The operative procedure begins with the posterior incision to mobilize the scapular and explore the retroscapular area.

- At the superior border of the scapular, we perform disarticulation of the acromioclavicular joint; if there is concern about the margins, the distal clavicle may also be osteotomized and removed with the scapular.

- The determination of either a scapulectomy (Type III resection) or an extra-articular resection of the glenohumeral joint and the scapular (Type IV resection) is made preoperatively.

- The scapular prosthesis fits between the serratus anterior, latissimus dorsi and rhomboid muscles "as if in a sandwich."

- Malorientation of the humeral prosthesis can be avoided with adequate preoperative templating, intraoperative measurements, and skilled technique.

POSTOPERATIVE MANAGEMENT

Patients remain at bedrest on the day of surgery. Drains are removed and dressings are changed on the second to third postoperative day (Fig. 27.13A,B). A sling and swathe is applied for 4 weeks to allow healing of the reattached muscles that provide the stabilizing force to the upper extremity. A compression arm stocking may be required to prevent swelling in the immediate postoperative period. Elbow flexion and motion of the hand and wrist, are encouraged in the immediate postoperative period as tolerated. Elbow extension and shoulder range of motion exercises are initiated after the incision has healed, approximately 2 to 4 weeks after surgery (Fig. 27.14A-B). Gentle motor strengthening of the pectoralis major, latissimus dorsi, trapezius muscles, and other scapular stabilizers begins approximately 6 weeks after surgery.

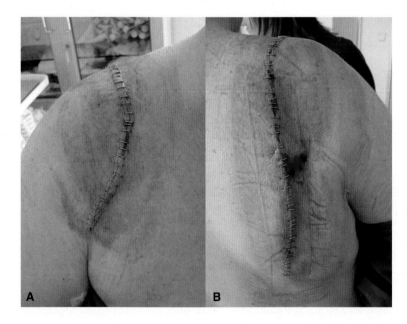

FIGURE 27.13

Postoperative clinical photographs showing (**A**) the anterior and (**B**) the posterior components of the utilitarian shoulder girdle incision.

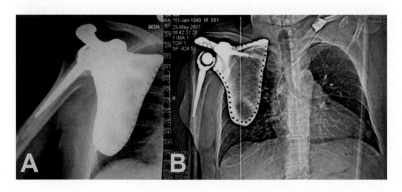

FIGURE 27.14

(**A**) Anteroposterior radiograph and (**B**) CT scout image showing the total scapular prosthesis in place.

COMPLICATIONS

Local complications including mechanical failure, infection and dislocation occur in up to 30% of patients; amputation is rare, related only to local recurrence (22).Late dislocations and neurovascular complications are not common following prosthetic reconstruction of the shoulder (2,3,7–9,13). The risk of pulmonary embolism during cementation of the proximal humerus for stabilization of the humeral prosthesis is similar to that of shoulder arthroplasty in noncancer patients. Malorientation of the humeral prosthesis can be avoided if the technique is followed precisely (4,6,9,12,14,19,20). Intraoperative measurements and guides will detect malpositioning. Psychological effects and depression are usual after major operations, especially in sarcoma patients, and should be treated by a psychiatric specialist.

RESULTS

Alternative reconstruction options and modifications of shoulder girdle resections have been reported. Initially, humeral suspension was the most popular reconstructive procedure after total scapulectomy. Until the early 1990s, there was no effort to reconstruct the shoulder girdle after resection; shoulders were left flail and the extremity was left dangling by the skin and neurovascular bundle. There was no active shoulder motion. This combined with shoulder instability led to difficulty with carrying objects and placing the hand into a functional position necessary for activities of daily living. Failure to stabilize the resulting floating humerus resulted in poor cosmesis and traction neuropraxia, which led to chronic pain and motor and sensory deficits; many patients required an external orthosis for support (2,10,12–14,19). In these cases, upper limb function was improved by using a bone-anchoring system to suture the biceps, triceps, and deltoid muscles to the clavicle. Others attempted to circumvent these problems by stabilizing the proximal humerus or remaining humeral shaft directly to the clavicle or a rib with heavy sutures or wires. An intramedullary rod or other type of functional spacer can be placed into the remaining humeral shaft with stabilization of its proximal end (4,10,12). Shoulder motion was not improved and shoulder instability remained a problem. Complications and failures were frequent and included broken sutures and wires rods eroding through overlying skin and abrading the chest wall, and superior subluxation of the implant. Patients often ended up with a flail, painful shoulder or an amputation (12). These early methods of reconstruction are referred to as nonanatomic methods because they made no attempt to reconstruct the bony structures that were resected nor restore the normal muscle force couples responsible for scapulothoracic and glenohumeral motion (19). Scapular allograft reconstruction has also been reported following total or partial scapulectomy for malignant tumors to restore cosmesis, shoulder stability, and function; however, preservation or reconstruction of rotator cuff muscles is also necessary (11). Near total scapulectomy with preservation of the glenoid to provide a fulcrum for movement of the arm for primary or secondary malignant tumors of the shoulder girdle has also been reported for reconstruction following shoulder girdle resections, however, with a considerable reduction in power and ability to lift the hand (21). A constrained shoulder joint prosthesis is indicated when a large amount of periscapular soft tissue will need to be resected; if an unconstrained prosthesis is used, severe instability usually occurs (19).

The goal of shoulder girdle reconstruction is to provide a stable and painless shoulder that allows positioning of the arm and hand in space, thereby preserving function. Patients undergoing shoulder girdle resections retain hand and elbow function, but lose shoulder motion. There is minimal functional loss following partial scapular resections (Type II); shoulder motion and strength are almost normal. However, total scapular resections (Types III and IV) result in significant loss of shoulder motion, predominantly shoulder abduction. Following prosthetic replacement of the scapular compared to those patients left without a scapular reconstruction, abduction and external rotation is partially restored (2,3,7–9,11–14,20). Elbow and hand function should be normal, again depending on the extent of the resection and remaining neurovascular status. Soft-tissue reconstruction is the key to establishing shoulder stability and obviating the need for an external orthosis.

Reconstruction with a constrained total scapular prosthesis is preferred by the current authors, because it restores most of the bony architecture necessary for reconstructing the normal muscle force couples of the scapulothoracic and glenohumeral mechanisms, both of which are important for optimal shoulder abduction and upper extremity stabilization. Wide tumor resection and scapular replacement allow for shoulder stability, a functional extremity and an optimal oncological outcome for most patients presenting with tumors around the shoulder girdle. This is accomplished through a skilled surgical technique and meticulous soft tissue reconstruction. Surgical outcomes are directly dependent on the extent of tumor involvement and surgical resection. The functional results vary considerably depending on how much periscapular muscle is retained and whether it is innervated. In general, the cosmesis is improved over simple scapulectomy. Whenever preservation of the rhomboids, latissimus dorsi, deltoid, and trapezius muscles is possible, scapular prosthetic reconstruction is associated with better functional results and superior cosmesis than humeral suspension. Although the rotator cuff is damaged, patients can usually compensate extremely well by using the preserved joints and the contralateral upper limb.

REFERENCES

1. Bickels J, Wittig JC, Kollender Y, et al. Limb-sparing resections of the shoulder girdle. *J Am Coll Surg.* 2002;194(4):422–435.
2. Francis KC, Worcester JN. Radical resection for tumors of the shoulder with preservation of a functional extremity. *J Bone Joint Surg (Am).* 1962;44;1423–1430.
3. Guerra A, Capanna R, Biagini R, et al. Extra-articular resection of the shoulder (Tikhoff-Linberg). *Ital J Orthop Traumatol.* 1985;11(2):151–157.
4. Ham SJ, Hoekstra HJ, Eisma WH, et al. The Tikhoff-Linberg procedure in the treatment of sarcomas of the shoulder girdle. *J Surg Oncol.* 1993;53(2):71–77.
5. Kiss J, Sztrinkai G, Antal I, et al. Functional results and quality of life after shoulder girdle resections in musculoskeletal tumors. *J Shoulder Elbow Surg.* 2007;16(3):273–279.
6. Lewis MM. *Bone Tumor Surgery. Limb Sparing Techniques.* Philadelphia, PA: JB Lippincott; 1988.
7. Malawer MM. Tumors of the shoulder girdle: technique of resection and description of a surgical classification. *Orthop Clin N Am.* 1991;22:7–35.
8. Malawer MM, Springfield D, Eckardt JJ, et al. Shoulder girdle and proximal humerus. In: Simon MA, Springfield D, eds. *Surgery for Bone and Soft-Tissue Tumors.* Philadelphia, PA: Lippincott-Raven Publishers; 1998:299–321.
9. Malawer MM, Sugarbaker PH. *Musculoskeletal Cancer Surgery.* Dordrecht: Kluwer Academic Publishers, 2001.
10. Marcove RC. Neoplasms of the shoulder girdle. *Orthop Clin N Am.* 1975;6:541–552.
11. Mnaymneh WA, Temple HT, Malinin TI. Allograft reconstruction after resection of malignant tumors of the scapular. *Clin Orthop Relat Res.* 2002;(405):223–229.
12. O'Connor MI, Sim FH, Chao EY. Limb salvage for neoplasms of the shoulder girdle. Intermediate reconstructive and functional results. *J Bone Joint Surg Am.* 1996;78(12):1872–1888.
13. Papaioannou AN, Francis KC. Scapulectomy for the treatment of primary malignant tumors of the scapular. *Clin Orthop.* 1965;41:125.
14. Pritsch T, Bickels J, Wu CC, et al. Is scapular endoprosthesis functionally superior to humeral suspension? *Clin Orthop Relat Res.* 2007;456:188–195.
15. Voggenreiter G, Assenmacher S, Schmit-Neuerburg KP. Tikhoff-Linberg procedure for bone and soft tissue tumors of the shoulder girdle. *Arch Surg.* 1999;134(3):252–257.
16. Volpe CM, Pell M, Doerr RJ, et al. Radical scapulectomy with limb salvage for shoulder girdle soft tissue sarcoma. *Surg Oncol.* 1996;5(1):43–48.
17. Wittig JC, Bickels J, Kellar-Graney KL, et al. Osteosarcoma of the proximal humerus: long-term results with limb-sparing surgery. *Clin Orthop Relat Res.* 2002;(397):156–176.
18. Wittig JC, Bickels J, Kollender Y, et al. Palliative forequarter amputation for metastatic carcinoma to the shoulder girdle region: indications, preoperative evaluation, surgical technique, and results. *J Surg Oncol.* 2001;77(2):105–114.
19. Wittig JC, Bickels J, Wodajo F, et al. Constrained total scapular reconstruction after resection of a high-grade sarcoma. *Clin Orthop Relat Res.* 2002;(397):143–155.
20. Damron TA, Rock MG, O'Connor MI, et al. Functional laboratory assessment after oncologic shoulder joint resections. *Clin Orthop Relat Res.* 1998;348:124–134.
21. Schwab JH, Athanasian EA, Morris CD, et al. Function correlates with deltoid preservation in patients having scapular replacement. *Clin Orthop Relat Res.* 2006;452:225–230.
22. Asavamongkolkul A, Eckardt JJ, Eilber FR, et al. Endoprosthetic reconstruction for malignant upper extremity tumors. *Clin Orthop Relat Res.* 1999;(360):207–220.

28 Shoulder Arthrodesis

Mary I. O'Connor

Shoulder arthrodesis remains an excellent reconstructive procedure for appropriate patients. Patient selection, attention to surgical technique, and preoperative patient education to establish reasonable postoperative expectations are critical to a successful outcome.

INDICATIONS

- Is appropriate in patients with segmental bone loss following tumor resection and in selected nontumor patients. Just as the surgical plan for sarcoma resection is individualized for each patient based on the extent of tumor involvement of bone and soft tissues, selection of the reconstructive procedure must also be tailored to the individual patient based on the functional potential of the remaining bone and soft tissues as well as the patient's needs and desires.
- Shoulder arthrodesis following sarcoma resection is an excellent reconstructive choice for a young patient who desires a strong and stable shoulder girdle. Specifically, for young patients who require an extra-articular resection, (the proximal humerus and glenoid [Fig. 28.1A–C]), arthrodesis with use of an intercalary allograft supplemented with a vascularized fibular graft (Fig. 28.1P) is an excellent reconstructive option.
- Likewise, in the nontumor patient, arthrodesis may be an appropriate salvage operation after multiple failed arthroplasties or stabilization procedures and may also be a consideration in a patient with chronic infection or posttraumatic brachial plexus injury. Table 28.1 lists indications for consideration of shoulder arthrodesis.
- The goal of shoulder arthrodesis is to achieve a pain-free, stable shoulder girdle that optimizes upper extremity strength. Again, the functional needs and desires of the patient should strongly influence selection of the reconstructive method.

CONTRAINDICATIONS

- Arthrodesis is contraindicated if another reconstructive procedure can be performed that preserves or restores more function.
- In general, arthrodesis is contraindicated when postresection function of the deltoid and rotator cuff musculature is maintained and either the glenoid or proximal humerus can be preserved or adequately reconstructed. For example, isolated resection of the glenoid can be reconstructed with an allograft or custom implant.

TABLE 28.1 Indications for Shoulder Arthrodesis

- Loss of function of the deltoid muscle
- Loss of function of the rotator cuff muscles
- Loss of the glenoid
- Loss of the proximal humerus
- Prior infection

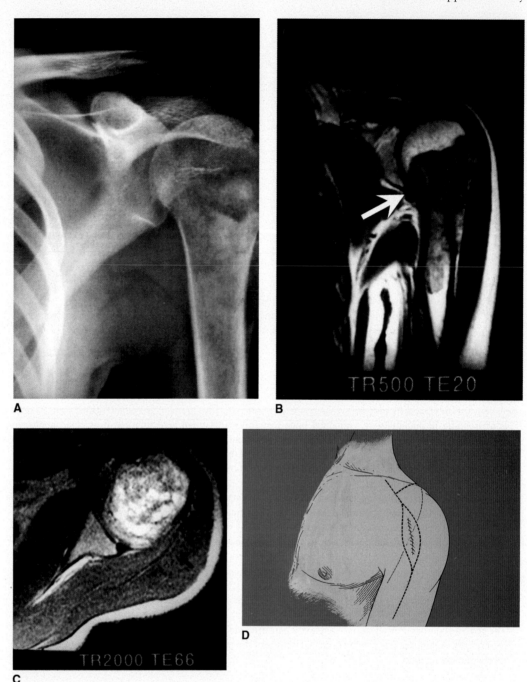

FIGURE 28.1

Wide resection of an osteosarcoma of the proximal humerus in a 15-year-old male patient. **A:** Plain radiographs of the proximal humerus showing mixed osteolytic and osteoblastic osteosarcoma. **B:** T1-weighted coronal magnetic resonance image of the proximal humerus showing intra-articular tumor extension after preoperative chemotherapy (*arrow*). **C:** T2-weighted axial images after preoperative chemotherapy. **D:** The incision begins at the midclavicle and courses laterally and distally to include the deltopectoral interval with elliptical excision of the prior biopsy site (if present). A second incision is made at a 90-degree angle from the first incision, beginning medial to the coracoid and coursing superiorly over the clavicle and then distally over the midline of the scapula. (Used Mayo Foundation for Medical Education and Research, with permission.)

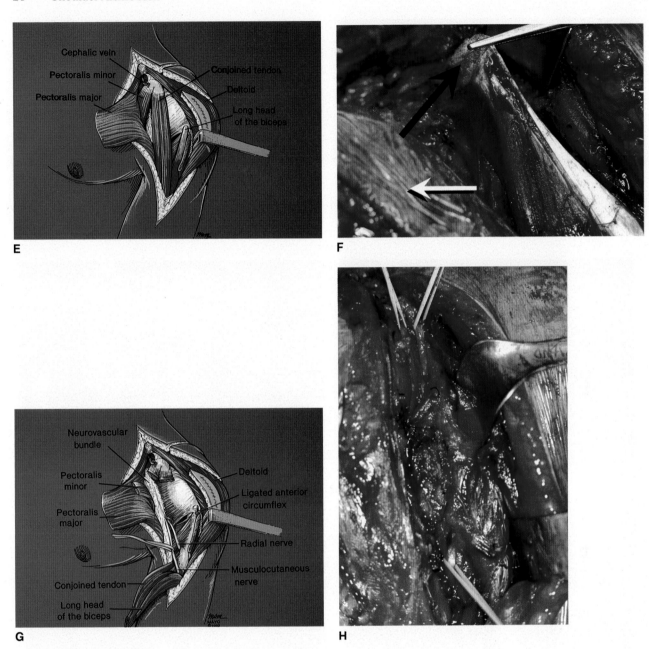

FIGURE 28.1 (*Continued*)

E: The pectoralis major tendon is divided from its humeral insertion; the underlying visible structure includes the conjoined tendon and long head of the biceps. (Used Mayo Foundation for Medical Education and Research, with permission.) **F:** Intraoperative photograph showing the elliptical skin incision around the prior biopsy site (*white arrow*). The pectoralis major tendon has been reflected, and the conjoined tendon is freed from coracoid (*black arrow*). **G:** After reflection of the long and short heads of the biceps and pectoralis minor, the neurovascular bundle is identified in the proximal aspect of the wound. The musculocutaneous nerve and radial nerve are identified. (Used Mayo Foundation for Medical Education and Research, with permission.) **H:** Intraoperative photograph showing a proximal loop around the anterior circumflex vessels and musculocutaneous nerve and a distal loop around the median nerve.

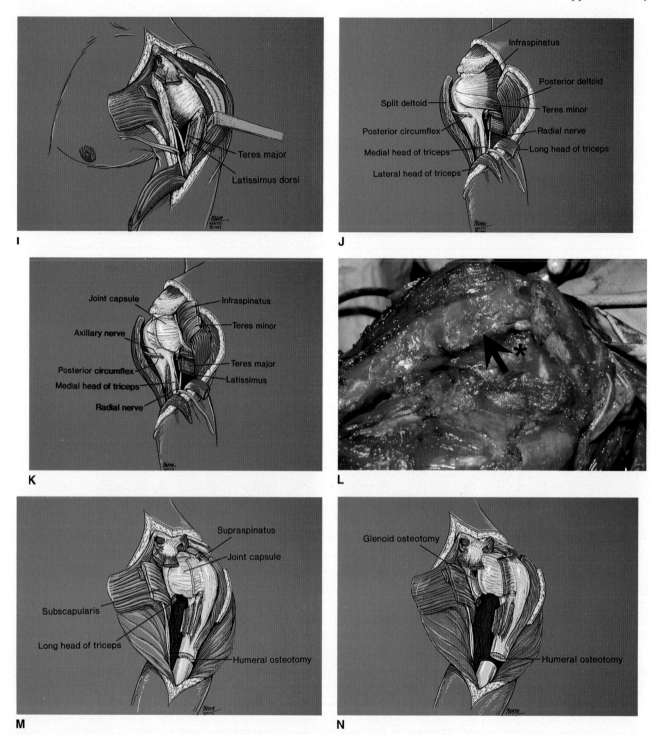

FIGURE 28.1 (*Continued*)

I: The broad insertion of the latissimus dorsi is divided from the humerus and just posterior to this is the insertion of the teres major. The radial nerve is identified and protected. (Used Mayo Foundation for Medical Education and Research, with permission.) **J:** The posterior dissection begins with the deltoid released from the acromion and scapular spine and divided along the posterior aspect of the biopsy site, and the posterior aspect of the rotator cuff musculature is identified. The posterior humeral circumflex vessels are ligated, the axillary nerve is transected (if necessary), the long head of the triceps is released from the inferior glenoid, and the lateral head of the triceps is released from the proximal humerus. The posterior humeral circumflex vessels and axillary nerve are located in the quadrangular space formed by the teres minor (superior), long head of the triceps (medial), teres major (inferior), and lateral head of the triceps (lateral). (Used Mayo Foundation for Medical Education and Research, with permission.) **K:** The infraspinatus and teres minor are divided to expose the posterior capsule of the shoulder joint. (Used Mayo Foundation for Medical Education and Research, with permission.) **L:** Intraoperative photograph showing division of the infraspinatus and teres minor (*arrow*), with exposure of underlying posterior capsule (*asterisk*). **M:** Attention is directed again anteriorly, and the supraspinatus and supscapsularis are transected to expose the anterior and superior joint capsule. (Used Mayo Foundation for Medical Education and Research, with permission.) **N:** Drawing of the anterior aspect of the glenoid osteotomy medial to the joint capsule. (Used Mayo Foundation for Medical Education and Research, with permission.)

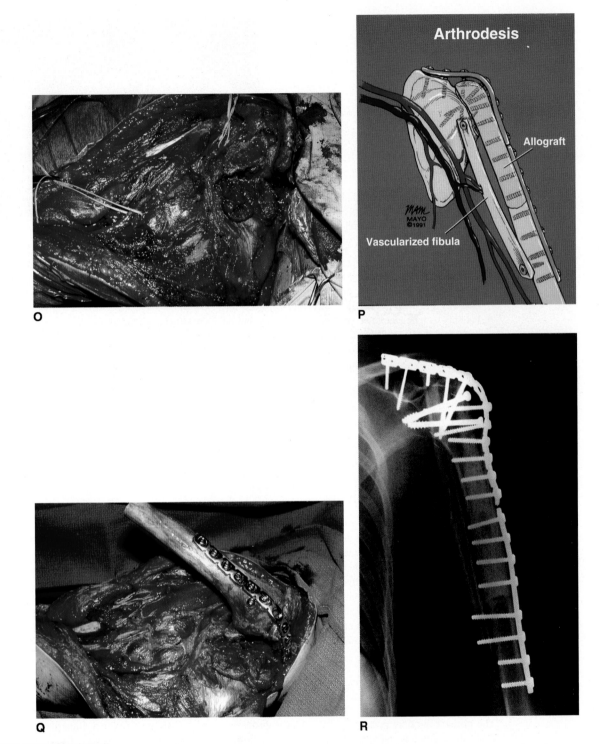

FIGURE 28.1 (*Continued*)

O: Intraoperative photograph of the posterior aspect of the glenoid osteotomy. Vessel loops identify the axillary nerve (proximally) and the radial nerve (distally). The distal humeral osteotomy is made, the marrow sampled for frozen-section analysis, and the specimen removed. **P:** Illustration of the reconstruction with an intercalary allograft bridging the remaining scapula and humerus (acromion and clavicle not illustrated) with vascularized fibular graft spanning from scapula to humerus. (Used Mayo Foundation for Medical Education and Research, with permission.) **Q:** Intraoperative photograph of intercalary allograft. The articular surface of the allograft is cut to match the glenoid osteotomy with the allograft in the desired position of arthrodesis. Contact is also made between the allograft and the denuded undersurface of the acromion. Large cannulated screws are first placed across the proximal allograft into the host glenoid and scapula. A pelvic reconstruction plate is then contoured and fixed from the scapular spine to the allograft. **R:** Postoperative radiograph. After placement of the pelvic reconstruction plate, the vascular anastomosis for the fibula is then performed, followed by placement of a second plate to fix the distal allograft to the host residual humeral diaphysis and screws to fix the vascularized fibular graft. Supplemental cancellous bone graft is placed at both the proximal and distal osteotomy junctions. Note cement augmentation of allograft intramedullary canal and near-complete spanning of allograft with fixation. Ideally, there is overlap of the plate fixation.

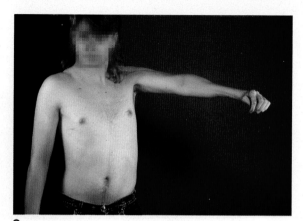

FIGURE 28.1 (*Continued*)

S: At 3 years after surgery, the patient is disease free, with a solid arthrodesis and active abduction and forward flexion of 85 degrees.   **S**

- With resection of only the proximal humerus, reconstructive options include an allograft-prosthetic composite, proximal humeral replacement implant, osteoarticular graft, or fibular graft (vascularized or nonvascularized), as described elsewhere in this volume.
- Patients with degenerative shoulder arthropathy and nonreconstructable rotator cuff disease may be candidates for reverse total shoulder arthroplasty.
- Specific contraindications for shoulder arthrodesis include lack of active scapulothoracic motion.
- Patients at high risk of nonunion such as elderly patients or those with neuropathic arthropathy are poor candidates.
- Because of postoperative functional limitations, bilateral shoulder arthrodeses should not be performed.

PREOPERATIVE PREPARATION

Preoperative preparation for shoulder arthrodesis should proceed in a logical fashion (Table 28.2).

Position of Arthrodesis

Before surgery, the targeted position of arthrodesis should be determined. While there is lack of consensus on the ideal position for fusion (Table 28.3), the surgeon should ensure that the patient's hand can reach his or her mouth without excessive winging of the scapula, which may promote chronic postoperative periscapular pain. The hand should also be able to reach the contralateral shoulder and axilla as well as the front zipper on pants. In general, the position of arthrodesis is an abduction range of 15 to 45 degrees, forward flexion range of 10 to 35 degrees, and internal rotation range of 20 to 60 degrees (1–4,7,9,10).

The position of rotation may influence the ability to perform certain tasks. Cofield and Briggs (11) noted that a patient who desires to write or type may prefer more internal rotation. They noted that lifting and dressing could be accomplished more often when the amount of internal rotation of the forearm above the horizontal plane was <21 degrees.

SURGICAL TECHNIQUE

The primary surgical principle of shoulder arthrodesis is to position the proximal humerus both underneath the acromion and against the glenoid to maximize the bony surface for fusion. The opposed bony surfaces are decorticated to produce cancellous-to-cancellous bone surfaces. Stabilization is performed with internal fixation using plates and screws. External compression has also been used successfully for shoulder arthrodesis in a small series reported by Schroder and Frandsen (12) but is not discussed in this chapter.

The specific surgical technique must be individualized to each patient. When appropriate, technical aspects unique to either a primary arthrodesis (sufficient host bone is available for contact of host humerus against host glenoid) or an intercalary arthrodesis (segmental allograft is required to bridge a defect between the remaining host humerus and host glenoid) (Fig. 28.1) are reviewed.

Positioning

The patient is placed supine in a beach chair position. The entire upper extremity and shoulder girdle are prepared. The surgeon should be able to access the scapula for plate fixation along the scapular spine. Furthermore,

TABLE 28.2   Preoperative Preparation for Shoulder Arthrodesis

Patient issues

    Confirm that the patient's goals and expectation are appropriate

    Determine that the patient has a thorough understanding of the procedure's complexity, risks, and postoperative functional limitations

    Ensure patient understanding of the potential for persistent postoperative pain

    Determine the patient's postoperative desired functional activities

    Confirm active scapulothoracic motion

Bone considerations

    Determine bone that is available for fusion; consider computed tomography particularly for evaluation of glenoid bone if routine radiographs are not conclusive

    Assess that bone at the planned fusion site is viable; magnetic resonance imaging or bone scintigraphy may be helpful.

    Determine the type of supplemental bone graft needed

        If segmental graft is required for intercalary fusion, obtain appropriate size, accounting for graft contact with both glenoid and undersurface of acromion as well as diaphyseal junction with host bone; typically, graft would be a proximal humeral allograft. Graft may have humeral head that is slightly larger than host bone to optimize the bone surface area of allograft for fusion.

        Determine if supplemental vascularized fibular graft is needed

            Routinely used for intercalary allograft arthrodesis

            Consider in patients with compromised bone viability (e.g., a patient with failed arthroplasty)

    Determine position of arthrodesis that is most likely to optimize the patient's functional needs

Soft tissue considerations

    Confirm that the patient has active scapulothoracic motion

    Determine that tissue is adequate for muscular coverage of reconstruction

    Determine that skin is adequate for wound closure

Equipment needs

    Intraoperative fluoroscopy (potentially)

    Internal fixation plates and screws, including malleable plates

    Cannulated screws

Postoperative needsv

    Determine need for shoulder spica cast or brace

TABLE 28.3   Suggested Position of Arthrodesis

Source, Year	Abduction (degrees)	Forward Flexion (degrees)	Internal Rotation (degrees)
Rowe, 1974 (1)	15–20	25–30	40–50
Hawkins and Neer, 1987 (2)	25–40[a]	20–30	25–30
Jonsson et al., 1989 (3)	20–30	20–30	20–30[b]
Richards and Kostuik, 1991 (4)	30[c]	30	30
Groh et al., 1997 (5)	10–15	10–15	40–60
Mah and Hall (pediatrics), 1990 (6)	45	45	45
Cheng and Gebhardt, 1991 (7)	60[d]	35	20–30
O'Connor et al., 1996 (8)	30[c]	30	20–30

[a]Relative to medial border of the scapula.
[b]Never more than 40 degrees.
[c]Clinical position of the arm relative to the side of the body.
[d]Relative to lateral border of the scapula.

the location of the mouth underneath the surgical drapes should be identified; while determining the position of arthrodesis, the surgeon verifies that the patient's hand can reach his or her mouth without excessive scapular winging. Surgery can also be performed with the patient in a lateral position; I favor the supine beach chair position to facilitate appropriate positioning of the arthrodesis.

Landmarks

Anatomic landmarks include the scapular spine, acromion, clavicle, coracoid process, and, underneath the operative drapes, the patient's mouth.

Surgical Incision

The method of arthrodesis influences the location and extent of the surgical incision. For arthrodesis performed for a nontumor condition in which host humerus is fused to host acromion and host glenoid, the extent of surgical exposure is less than that required for sarcoma resection and arthrodesis with an intercalary bone graft and vascularized fibula graft. For such nontumor reconstructions, the incision can be made beginning at the medial aspect of the scapular spine and coursing lateralward over the spine, then anteriorly over the acromion, and finally extending distally along the anterolateral aspect of the upper arm toward the deltoid tuberosity.

In patients who have undergone sarcoma resection, the surgical exposure is typically quite extensive. The incision may begin at the midclavicular region and course laterally and distalward in the deltopectoral interval. Prior open biopsy sites are elliptically excised and, if possible, prior needle biopsy tracks also elliptically excised. To obtain exposure of the scapular spine, a second incision can be made at 90 degrees from the first incision, beginning medial to the coracoid and coursing superiorly over the clavicle and then distally over the midline of the scapula. Figure 28.1D illustrates a typical incision with elliptical excision of the prior open biopsy tract. Such an incision permits more extensive exposure for mobilization and rotation of the latissimus dorsi as soft tissue coverage of the arthrodesis if required. For extra-articular resection of the proximal humerus, typical surgical steps include division of the pectoralis major tendon from its humeral insertion (Fig. 28.1E), which then exposes the underlying conjoined tendon and long head of the biceps. The conjoined tendon is divided from the coracoid (Fig. 28.1F); the long head of the biceps is cut and the pectoralis major tendon divided from its humeral insertion site, exposing the neurovascular bundle in the proximal aspect of the wound. The anterior humeral circumflex vessels are ligated and the musculocutaneous nerve and radial nerve identified (Fig. 28.1G,H). The broad insertion of the latissimus dorsi is divided from the humerus followed by the insertion of the teres minor while the radial nerve is protected (Fig. 28.1I). The surgeon then directs attention posteriorly and releases the deltoid from the acromion and scapular spine with distal division to permit, if necessary, elliptical excision of a prior open biopsy site (Fig. 28.1J). This exposes the posterior aspect of the rotator cuff; the posterior humeral circumflex vessels are ligated and the axillary nerve is transected. The posterior humeral circumflex vessels and axillary nerve are located in the quadrangular space formed by the teres minor (superior), long head of the triceps (medial), teres major (inferior), and lateral head of the triceps (lateral). The long head of the triceps is released from the inferior glenoid, and the lateral head of the triceps is released from the proximal humerus. The infraspinatus and teres minor are divided to expose the posterior capsule of the shoulder joint (Fig. 28.1K,L). Attention is directed again anteriorly, and the supraspinatus and subscapularis are transected to expose the anterior and superior joint capsule (Fig. 28.1M), and the glenoid osteotomy is made medial to the joint capsule for the extra-articular resection (Fig. 28.1N,O). The resection is completed with the distal humeral osteotomy (Fig. 28.1P), and the humeral marrow is sampled for frozen-section analysis.

Reconstructive Technique

For nontumor conditions, sufficient bone typically exists for a primary arthrodesis of host bone to host bone. The bony surfaces for arthrodesis are decorticated with good contact of the humerus against the glenoid and underneath the acromion in the desired position of fusion. Maximum bone contact area should be achieved to optimize fusion. Percutaneous-type cancellous screws may be used for initial fixation. The guide pins are placed and the position of arthrodesis verified. Cannulated screws are then placed over the guide pins to achieve initial compression and fixation. Typically, two screws are used; these should be placed anterior and posterior to the position of the subsequent plate. A 4.5-mm pelvic reconstruction plate is contoured to cover the scapular spine and acromion and the lateral proximal humerus. The medial aspect of the plate must be well fixed to the scapula; typically, two 6.5-mm cancellous screws placed through the plate into the neck of the scapula provide secure fixation of the plate to the scapula. Similar screws are placed across the acromion into the proximal humerus and across the proximal humerus into the glenoid to further secure the arthrodesis surfaces. The horizontal screws through the plate and across the proximal humerus into the glenoid should compress the humeral head into the glenoid. Cortical screws can be used to fix the plate to the humeral diaphysis and scapular spine. In general, cancellous screws are used in the midsection of the plate where the screws can achieve fixation to the scapular neck and through the proximal humerus to the glenoid, and cortical screws are used for the peripheral plate screw holes. Supplemental bone graft is added to the fusion site. If the quality of fixation with this plate is questionable, a second plate can be applied obliquely across the posterior aspect of the scapula, then laterally and somewhat distally to the proximal humeral metadiaphyseal region. This second plate increases bending and torsional stiffness compared with use of a single plate (13).

In cases with segmental bone loss (Fig. 28.1O), a primary arthrodesis is not possible. An intercalary allograft is used, often supplemented with a vascularized fibula graft (Fig. 28.1P). To increase resistance to fracture, the medullary canal of the allograft can be filled with antibiotic-impregnated bone cement (14). The graft is fashioned for fusion by osteotomizing the medial surface of the humeral articular surface to sit flush against the host glenoid in the desired position. The proximal aspect of the allograft is decorticated to have good contact against the undersurface of the host acromion. Fixation of the proximal humeral allograft is performed as described above (Fig. 28.1Q,R). The allograft diaphysis is then fixed to the host humeral diaphysis with a plate. If the intercalary allograft is short, then the initial plate may be contoured to extend from the scapular spine, across the lateral allograft, and distally past the allograft–host bone diaphyseal junction. More commonly, the intercalary allograft is of sufficient length that a separate plate to fix the diaphyseal junction is used. Because of the stress riser that exists between these two plates, a third plate can be added to traverse the region between the end of the proximal plate and the beginning of the distal plate.

Once fixation of the intercalary allograft is secure, a vascularized fibular graft can be added for supplemental fixation. Such a graft hypertrophies and provides greater strength to the arthrodesis mass. The proximal aspect of the fibula is placed against the anterior aspect of the glenoid and the distal aspect of the fibula to host bone just past the allograft–host bone diaphyseal junction. The fibula is secured with screws.

Soft Tissue Coverage

Adequate soft tissue coverage of the arthrodesis site and fixation is important to minimize the risks of infection and painful hardware. In a primary arthrodesis, the deltoid covers most of the plate; some of the plate along the scapular spine may be without muscle coverage. In an arthrodesis with an intercalary allograft, a portion of the deltoid may have been resected as part of the oncologic procedure, and there may be insufficient muscle for adequate soft tissue coverage. In such a situation, rotation of the ipsilateral latissimus dorsi muscle is performed to provide good soft tissue coverage.

PEARLS AND PITFALLS

- Optimize host bone surface by adequate decortication of the humerus, glenoid, and acromion while trying to minimize weakening of the bone.
- Temporarily fix the arthrodesis with Steinman pins and critically assess the position of the fusion before final fixation. Make sure that the hand can reach the mouth and that there does not appear to be excessive scapular winging.
- Use a pelvic reconstructive plate for fixation across the scapula to the proximal humerus rather than a standard dynamic compression plate. The pelvic reconstructive plate has a lower profile along the scapular spine.
- Ensure good fixation of the plate to the scapula by placing at least one but preferably two screws into the stronger bone of the scapular neck. The bone of the scapular body is thinner and does not provide the same degree of fixation as screws into the scapular neck.
- Avoid using a short plate. In a primary arthrodesis, make sure the plate is of sufficient length to extend along the scapular spine and humeral diaphysis with at least four cortical screws into the humeral diaphysis. In an arthrodesis with an intercalary allograft, the same degree of fixation should be attempted.
- In arthrodesis with an intercalary allograft, if two separate plates are required for fixation of the graft, make sure a third plate is added to span the junction to minimize the risk of stress fracture.
- For fixation of an intercalary allograft to host humeral bone, use standard plates because these are well covered by muscle.
- Ensure as much muscle coverage of the fixation hardware as possible to minimize the risk of subsequent discomfort related to prominent hardware.
- If a postoperative shoulder spica cast is to be applied, consider making a bivalved cast preoperatively to facilitate its application at the conclusion of the procedure.

POSTOPERATIVE MANAGEMENT

For primary arthrodesis, a sling is used for comfort for a few weeks. Range-of-motion exercises can be started the day after surgery. For arthrodesis with an intercalary allograft, a shoulder spica cast is applied for 8 to 12 weeks to immobilize the reconstructive site during the initial healing period. After the cast is removed, the patient is given a sling for comfort and started on range-of-motion exercises.

COMPLICATIONS

Complications following shoulder arthrodesis include nonunion, periarthrodesis fracture, infection, malunion, pain related to prominent hardware, and chronic pain. Rates vary depending on the complexity of the procedure. In patients undergoing limb salvage for neoplasm, 8 of 21 patients (38%) who had reconstruction with an arthrodesis had a postoperative complication that required major surgical intervention (15). Despite this high rate of complications, all limbs remain salvaged. In nontumor patients, complication rates are lower. However, for arthrodesis of the shoulder after septic arthritis, complication rates may be higher. Wick et al. (16) reported nonunion in 3 of 15 patients and persistent infection in 2 of 15 patients at mean follow-up of 8 years.

Nonunion

In nontumor patients, primary arthrodesis union rates are generally high, and the occasional nonunion heals with a secondary bone grafting procedure. Cofield and Briggs (11) reported union in 68 of 71 primary fusions and concluded that complex methods of internal fixation were not required for a primary arthrodesis. Other authors favor plating (17), with Kostuik and Schatzker (18) reporting 100% union using a double-plate technique. In pediatric patients, union rates are high for primary arthrodesis performed with various fixation techniques (19–21). In tumor patients, it is more difficult to assess initial fusion rates because of the higher rate of complications.

Malpositioning of Extremity

Malposition can limit function and result in pain due to traction on brachial plexus. Groh et al. (5) reported good results in corrective osteotomy in nine patients with substantial improvement in pain and function.

Postoperative Soft Tissue Problems

With time and muscle atrophy, discomfort can develop as a result of prominent hardware. This is not uncommon. Various reports detail hardware removal: in 6 of 18 patients with screws and plate fixation (20), in 5 of 8 patients fused with screws and pelvic reconstructive plates (22), and in 17 of 71 patients fused without plate fixation (11).

Infection

Infection is an unusual complication in primary arthrodesis performed for nonseptic conditions (11,18,20). Following tumor resection and reconstruction with an intercalary allograft and vascularized fibula, Fuchs et al. (15) reported removal of 2 of 13 intercalary allografts for infection, with salvage performed by the addition of a second vascularized fibula.

Postoperative Fracture

Shoulder arthrodesis puts additional stress on adjacent bones, and fracture of the limb can occur, particularly distal to the fixation. Various reports detail fracture occurrence in nontumor patients: in none of 11 patients (23), in 2 of 18 patients (20), in 3 of 27 patients (19), and in 8 of 71 patients (11). Fuchs et al. (15) reported 2 of 13 fractures of the intercalary allograft used in the arthrodesis procedure.

Chronic Pain

The incidence and severity of pain following shoulder arthrodesis are generally low. Severe pain is uncommon. Mild pain is common (11,20). Cofield and Briggs (11) noted a trend toward more pain in shoulders fused in more than 45 degrees of abduction. Following arthrodesis after tumor resection, 11 of 14 patients reported no pain, and 3 used intermittent anti-inflammatory medications (15).

RESULTS

Functional results are satisfactory after shoulder arthrodesis (Fig.28.1S). Function is not, however, normal. For patients who undergo arthrodesis for paralytic conditions, function is typically improved (19,21). For nontumor patients, Dimmen and Madsen (20) reported a mean American Shoulder and Elbow Surgeons score of 59, with a range of 15 to 95 (maximum score is 100), highlighting the variability in functional outcomes. Cofield and Briggs (11) noted that approximately 30% of patients had impairment of personal hygiene and toilet needs or use of eating utensils in the fused extremity. Richards and Kostuik (4) found that nearly all patients could perform work with the fused extremity at waist level. In tumor patients, Fuchs et al. (15) noted that the greatest functional limitation was with lifting an object to an overhead shelf and found no difference in function for patients who had a primary limb salvage arthrodesis compared with those who had a salvage arthrodesis performed after failure of a different primary limb salvage reconstructive technique. Finally, Damron et al. (24,25) found that in patients with an intercalary allograft arthrodesis, elbow flexion, elbow extension, and supination strength were less in the operated extremity than in the contralateral normal extremity, most likely because of resection of the long head of the biceps and the origin of the long head of the triceps (24,25).

Patient satisfaction following arthrodesis is generally good. In a series of 18 patients (20), 15 were satisfied with their fusion, and 3 would not or probably would not choose an arthrodesis if given the choice again. In a large series of 66 patients (11), 82% felt the fusion benefited them and 18% felt the fusion did not improve their condition or made it worse. A careful preoperative discussion with patients regarding the variability in clinical outcomes is appropriate prior to surgery.

CONCLUSIONS

Despite the risk of complications and functional compromise, shoulder arthrodesis remains an important surgical procedure. In nontumor patients, arthrodesis is generally a salvage procedure. In tumor patients, limb salvage with shoulder arthrodesis is far superior to loss of the upper extremity. Arthrodesis can provide stability to the shoulder girdle to optimize distal upper extremity function and remains a preferred outcome compared to a flail shoulder.

REFERENCES

1. Rowe CR. Re-evaluation of the position of the arm in arthrodesis of the shoulder in the adult. *J Bone Joint Surg Am.* 1974;56:913–922.
2. Hawkins RJ, Neer CS II. A functional analysis of shoulder fusions. *Clin Orthop Relat Res.* 1987;223:65–76.
3. Jonsson E, Lidgren L, Rydholm U. Position of shoulder arthrodesis measured with Moire photography. *Clin Orthop Relat Res.* 1989;238:117–121.
4. Richards R, Kostuik JP. Shoulder arthrodesis: indications and techniques. In: Watson, MS, ed. *Surgical Disorders of the Shoulder.* Edinburgh: Churchill Livingstone; 1991:443–457.
5. Groh GI, Williams GR, Jarman RN, et al. Treatment of complications of shoulder arthrodesis. *J Bone Joint Surg Am.* 1997;79:881–887.
6. Mah JY, Hall JE. Arthrodesis of the shoulder in children. *J Bone Joint Surg Am.* 1990;72:582–586.
7. Cheng EY, Gebhardt MC. Allograft reconstructions of the shoulder after bone tumor resections. *Orthop Clin North Am.* 1991;22:37–48.
8. O'Connor MI, Sim FH, Chao EY. Limb salvage for neoplasms of the shoulder girdle: Intermediate reconstructive and functional results. *J Bone Joint Surg Am.* 1996;78:1872–1888.
9. Clare DJ, Wirth MA, Groh GI, et al. Shoulder arthrodesis. *J Bone Joint Surg Am.* 2001;83-A:593–600.
10. Safran O, Iannotti JP. Arthrodesis of the shoulder. *J Am Acad Orthop Surg.* 2006;14:145–153.
11. Cofield RH, Briggs BT. Glenohumeral arthrodesis: operative and long-term functional results. *J Bone Joint Surg Am.* 1979;61:668–677.
12. Schroder HA, Frandsen PA. External compression arthrodesis of the shoulder joint. *Acta Orthop Scand.* 1983;54:592–595.
13. Miller BS, Harper WP, Gillies RM, et al. Biomechanical analysis of five fixation techniques used in glenohumeral arthrodesis. *ANZ J Surg.* 2003;73:1015–1017.
14. DeGroot H, Donati D, Di Liddo M, et al. The use of cement in osteoarticular allografts for proximal humeral bone tumors. *Clin Orthop Relat Res.* 2004;427:190–197.
15. Fuchs B, O'Connor MI, Padgett DJ, et al. Arthrodesis of the shoulder after tumor resection. *Clin Orthop Relat Res.* 2005;436:202–207.
16. Wick M, Muller EJ, Ambacher T, et al. Arthrodesis of the shoulder after septic arthritis: long-term results. *J Bone Joint Surg Br.* 2003;85:666–670.
17. Ruhmann O, Kirsch L, Buch S, et al. Primary stability of shoulder arthrodesis using cannulated cancellous screws. *J Shoulder Elbow Surg.* 2005;14:51–59.
18. Kostuik JP, Schatzker J. Shoulder arthrodesis: A. O. technique. In: Bateman JE, Welsh RP, eds. *Surgery of the Shoulder.* Philadelphia, PA: B. C. Decker Inc.; 1984:207–210.
19. Chammas M, Goubier JN, Coulet B, et al. Glenohumeral arthrodesis in upper and total brachial plexus palsy: a comparison of functional results. *J Bone Joint Surg Br.* 2004;86:692–695.
20. Dimmen S, Madsen JE. Long-term outcome of shoulder arthrodesis performed with plate fixation: 18 patients examined after 3–15 years. *Acta Orthop.* 2007;78:827–833.
21. Pruitt DL, Hulsey RE, Fink B, et al. Shoulder arthrodesis in pediatric patients. *J Pediatr Orthop.* 1992;12:640–645.
22. Diaz JA, Cohen SB, Warren RF, et al. Arthrodesis as a salvage procedure for recurrent instability of the shoulder. *J Shoulder Elbow Surg.* 2003;12:237–241.
23. Richards RR, Sherman RM, Hudson AR, et al. Shoulder arthrodesis using a pelvic-reconstruction plate: A report of eleven cases. *J Bone Joint Surg Am.* 1988;70:416–421.
24. Damron TA, Rock MG, O'Connor MI, et al. Distal upper extremity function following proximal humeral resection and reconstruction for tumors: contralateral comparison. *Ann Surg Oncol.* 1997;4:237–246.
25. Damron TA, Rock MG, O'Connor MI, et al. Functional laboratory assessment after oncologic shoulder joint resections. *Clin Orthop Relat Res.* 1998;348:124–134.

29 Proximal Humeral Osteoarticular Allograft

D. Luis Muscolo, Miguel A. Ayerza, and Luis A. Aponte-Tinao

The proximal humerus is one of the primary sites of tumors in the upper extremity and is the fourth most common site for osteosarcoma, chondrosarcoma, and Ewing sarcoma. Several techniques have been described for replacement of the proximal humerus that include prostheses, osteoarticular allografts, or a combination.

Osteoarticular allografts are utilized for reconstruction of one side of the joint after tumor resection and do not sacrifice the uninvolved side of the joint. They have the possibility of attaching soft tissues. Although osteoarticular allografts are an optimal material to reconstruct skeletal defects, biomechanically and biologically related complications including bone graft fractures and resorption, cartilage degeneration, joint instability, and delayed bone union or nonunion still occur. These biomechanically related complications can be grouped into two main categories, (a) related to geometric matching between the allograft and the host defect and (b) the stability achieved during surgery of the allograft-host bone and soft tissue junction sites.

INDICATIONS

- The procedure is appropriate for the treatment of a massive osteoarticular defect after tumor resection or massive traumatic bone loss.
- The major neurovascular bundle must be free of tumor (Figs. 29.1 and 29.2).

CONTRAINDICATIONS

- Patients in whom preoperative imaging studies demonstrate evidence of intra-articular (glenohumeral) compromise of the tumor.
- Inadequate host soft tissue to reconstruct the joint.
- Patients with glenohumeral osteoarthritis.

PREOPERATIVE PREPARATION ALLOGRAFT SELECTION

Fresh-frozen allografts are obtained and stored according to a technique that has been previously described (1). Poor anatomical matching of both size and shape between the host defect and the graft can significantly alter joint kinematics and load distribution, leading to bone resorption or joint degeneration. To improve accuracy in size matching between the donor and the host, we developed measurable parameters based on CT scans of the proximal humerus. The allograft is selected on the basis of a comparison of these measures of potential allografts available at the bone bank with those of the host.

TECHNIQUE

- All operations are performed in a clean-air enclosure with vertical airflow.
- After administration of adequate regional and/or general anesthesia, the patient is placed in the semiupright "beach-chair position," with the hips and knees flexed and all osseous prominences well padded.

317

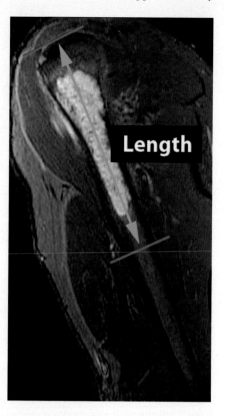

FIGURE 29.1

Anteroposterior radiograph of a proximal humerus showing
tumor extension and ossification in the surrounding soft tissues.

- The head is secured in a neutral position, and the entire upper extremity is prepared and draped to the level of the midclavicle. An extended deltopectoral approach is done that can be extended distally if more surgical exposure is needed (Fig. 29.3).
- The cephalic vein is mobilized with the deltoid muscle and retracted laterally. The biopsy tract is left in continuity with the specimen.
- Usually due to compromise from the tumor, a biceps tenotomy is performed. The conjoined tendon is not released from the coracoid. The subscapularis tendon is released off of the lesser tuberosity, just medial to the long head of the biceps, in order to allow atraumatic dislocation of the humeral head with gentle external rotation and extension of the arm.

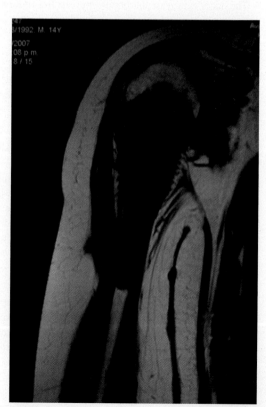

FIGURE 29.2

A coronal magnetic resonance image that illustrates
a sarcoma in the proximal humeral metaphysis with
extension to the humeral diaphysis.

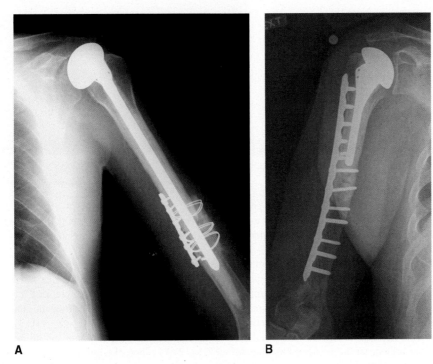

A   **B**

FIGURE 29.3

Intraoperative photograph that shows the extended deltopectoral approach that is employed.

- If there is an extraosseous tumor component, a cuff of normal muscle must be excised. It is preferable to dissect out the axillary nerve and protect it with a vessel loop to confirm its location and thereby diminish the risk of a nerve injury. The capsule is then released completely around the humeral neck. Then the infraspinatus, supraspinatus, and teres minor tendons are released off of the greater tuberosity, and the tendons are tagged. The deltoid is then dissected free from the humeral shaft after the rotator cuff tendons are released, as well as the teres major, latissimus dorsi, and the pectoralis major tendons if necessary.
- The humeral osteotomy is marked at the appropriate location as determined on the basis of the preoperative imaging studies (Fig. 29.4). All remaining soft tissues at the level of the transection are cleared.

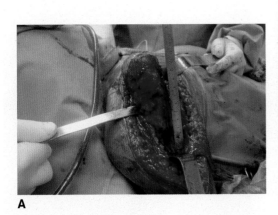

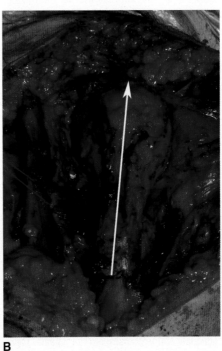

A   **B**

FIGURE 29.4

Intraoperative photograph marking the level of humeral osteotomy.

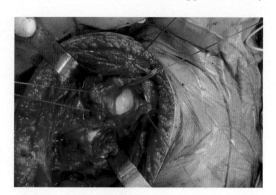

FIGURE 29.5

Intraoperative radiograph made after the proximal humerus is passed off the operative field, showing the osteoarticular defect.

The osteotomy is performed perpendicular to the long axis of the humerus. Following the osteotomy, the proximal humerus is then passed off the operative field revealing the remaining osseous defect within the patient (Fig. 29.5).

- Simultaneous with or subsequent to the tumor resection, the allograft specimen is prepared on the back table. The graft is taken out of the plastic packaging and placed directly in a warm normal saline solution. After being thawed, the donor bone is cut to the proper length and soft tissue structures are prepared for implantation. It is crucial during the joint reconstruction to have adequate soft tissue structures from the donor in order to repair them to corresponding host tissues (Fig. 29.6).
- The proximal humerus allograft is inspected to confirm that the size is appropriate and no degenerative changes are present on the humeral articular surface (Fig. 29.7). Then, the insertion of an allograft segment tailored to fit the bone defect is performed. Before the allograft bone is secured to the remaining host humerus, the shoulder joint reconstruction is performed. However, the plate can be secured to the allograft to help manage the graft during soft tissue reconstruction.
- First, we repair the posterior capsule suturing autologous capsular tissues to the capsular tissues provided by the allograft with a number-1 nonabsorbable suture (Fig. 29.8). After the posterior capsular tissues are secured, the supraspinatus, infraspinatus, and teres minor tendons are repaired suturing autologous tendon tissues to the allograft tendon tissues (Fig. 29.9).
- Finally, the anterior capsule and the subscapularis tendon are repaired similarly as done with the posterior capsule and the rotator cuff (Fig. 29.10). The rotator interval is repaired (Fig. 29.11) and if the intra-articular biceps tendon was sectioned due to tumor compromise, the tendon can be tenodesed in the bicipital groove. Fitting the osteotomy between the host humerus and allograft in close apposition is a crucial step. When cortical bone is avascular, as in the allograft, absolute stability is required and offers the best condition and chance for healing. The diaphyseal osteotomy is stabilized by internal fixation with an anterior short locking compression plate and, in order to minimize the risk of fracture, an additional lateral locking compression plate is placed to extend the entire length of the allograft (Figs. 29.12 and 29.13).

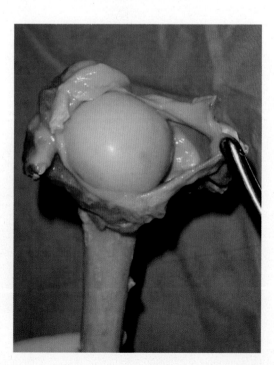

FIGURE 29.6

Intraoperative photograph that shows that the allograft has adequate soft tissue structures (capsule, rotator cuff) in order to repair them to the corresponding host tissues.

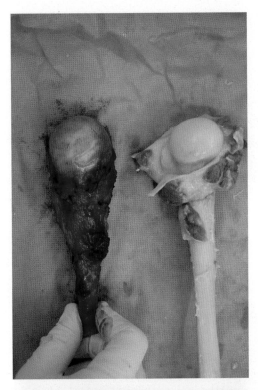

FIGURE 29.7

Intraoperative photograph after resection of the tumor that shows how the proximal humerus allograft is inspected to confirm that the size is appropriate and no degenerative changes are present along the humeral head.

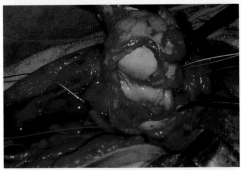

FIGURE 29.8

Intraoperative photograph made when the posterior capsule is repaired.

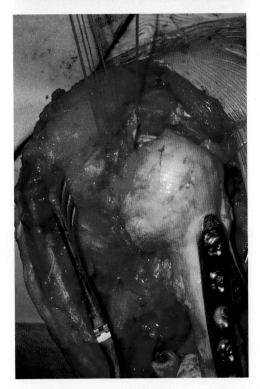

FIGURE 29.9

Intraoperative photograph made when the supraspinatus, infraspinatus, and teres minor tendons are repaired suturing autologous tendon tissues to the allograft tendon tissues.

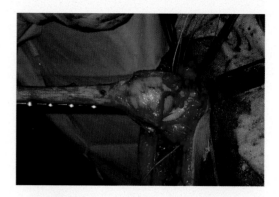

FIGURE 29.10

Intraoperative photograph made when the anterior
capsule and the subscapularis tendon are repaired.

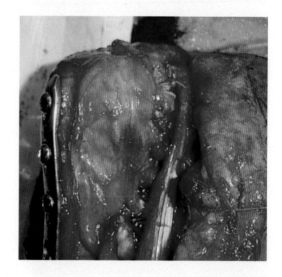

FIGURE 29.11

Intraoperative photograph made after the rotator
interval is repaired.

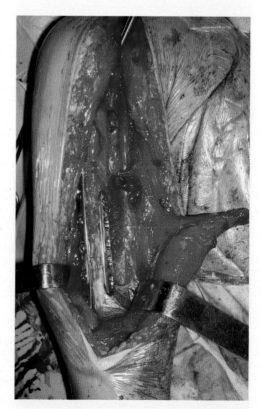

FIGURE 29.12

Intraoperative photograph showing the osteotomy
between the host and allograft in close apposition with
adequate compression after internal fixation with the
anterior short plate and how an additional lateral plate is
placed in order to cover the entire length of the allograft.

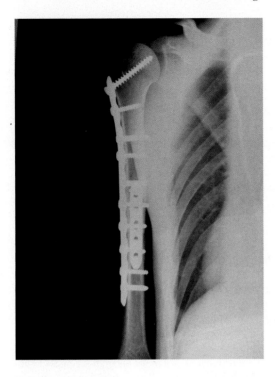

FIGURE 29.13
Anteroposterior radiograph made showing adequate articular position.

- Two suction drains are inserted and, after lavage of the wound with saline solution, a meticulous suture repair of the intermuscular septum between the anterior deltoid and the pectoralis major muscles is done. A layered closure of the subcutaneous tissues and skin is then performed.

POSTOPERATIVE MANAGEMENT

A shoulder immobilizer is worn for 4 weeks while pendulum-type exercises are performed. After the first 4 weeks, a sling is used and supine active-assisted range-of-motion exercises are initiated. Active-assisted elevation can begin at 8 weeks, but resistive exercises are delayed until 12 weeks. The patient is encouraged to begin active forward flexion beginning at 8 weeks as comfort allows.

PEARLS AND PITFALLS

- The procedure is best performed by an orthopedic oncologic or adult reconstruction surgical team with experience in shoulder reconstructive or sports medicine surgery.
- All previous biopsy sites and all potentially contaminated tissues should be removed en bloc with the underlying specimen.
- Poor anatomic matching of the size and shape between the host defect and the allograft will significantly alter joint kinematics and load transmission leading to potential bone resorption, fracture or joint degeneration.
- Reconstruction of the tendons, ligaments, and joint capsule must be meticulous and precise since the longevity of these grafts are related, in part, to the joint stability obtained during the procedure.
- Uniform cortical contact, compression of the osteotomy gap, and rotational stability are better when internal fixation with double plates and screws is used.
- To obtain a solid allograft construct, the internal fixation should span as much of the allograft as possible.
- Locking compression plates are now used for the majority of our patients to obtain greater mechanical stability of the reconstruction.

COMPLICATIONS

Although osteoarticular allografts are an ideal material for biologic reconstruction of skeletal defects, biomechanically and biologically related complications including allograft fractures and resorption, cartilage degeneration, joint instability, and delayed union or nonunion still occur (1,2). Reconstruction of the ligaments, tendons, and joint capsule must be meticulous and precise since the longevity of these grafts is related, in part, to the stability of the joint obtained during surgery.

RESULTS

Osteoarticular allografts in the upper limb are used less frequently than are other types of osteoarticular allografts (1,2). The benefit of this form of reconstruction compared with prosthetic reconstruction is that the attachment of the remaining deltoid muscle and rotator cuff tendons to the soft tissue of the allograft provides better potential for healing and function of the soft tissues. Gebhardt et al. (3) reported that 12 (60%) of 20 patients managed with proximal humeral allografts had a satisfactory result. O'Connor et al. (4) reported 57 patients who had different limb-salvage procedures for treatment of tumors of the shoulder girdle. They found that an osteoarticular allograft inserted after intra-articular resection of the proximal aspect of the humerus and preservation of the abductor mechanism provided function that was superior to that found after reconstruction with a proximal humeral replacement prosthesis. The prosthetic reconstructions produced symptomatic instability that led to a secondary arthrodesis in some patients. However, subchondral fracture and collapse of the osteoarticular allograft occurred in four of eight patients at the latest follow-up examination (average follow-up of 5.3 years). Getty and Peabody (5), in a study of 16 patients, reported that the Kaplan-Meier curve showed a 5-year survival rate of the allografts of 68%; however, the functional limitations as well as high rate of complications led those authors to abandon the routine use of osteoarticular allografts for proximal humeral reconstruction. Winkelmann et al. (6) analyzed 45 patients with three different reconstructive procedures after resection of primary tumors of the proximal humerus (11 osteoarticular allograft, 15 clavicula pro humero operation and 19 tumor prosthesis). Although they suggest the use of a tumor prosthesis in limb-salvage procedures for the proximal humerus, they found that cumulative survival rates and the functional results for the three reconstructive procedures were similar. In a recent report (7) of 31 patients with osteoarticular allografts of the proximal humerus, 23 of the allograft medullary canals were filled with cement and showed a survival of 78% at 5 years. Although the authors concluded that this technique modification is a reliable reconstructive option after proximal humerus resection, the cementation of the intramedullary canal of the allograft precludes a subsequent conventional hemiarthroplasty in the case of subchondral fracture or collapse of the allograft articular surface. Advances in operative techniques acquired in recent years in relation to allograft selection, joint stability, and allograft fixation may improve longevity and functional results of this reconstructive procedure.

REFERENCES

1. Muscolo DL, Ayerza M, Aponte-Tinao LA. Massive allograft used in orthopaedics oncology. *Orthop Clin North Am*. 2006;37:65–74.
2. Mankin HJ, Gebhardt MC, Jennings LC, et al. Long-term results of allograft replacement in the management of bone tumors. *Clin Orthop*. 1996;324:86–97.
3. Gebhardt MC, Roth YF, Mankin HJ. Osteoarticular allografts for reconstruction in the proximal part of the humerus after excision of a musculoskeletal tumor. *J Bone Joint Surg*. 1990;72A:334–345.
4. O'Connor MI, Sim FH, Chao EY. Limb salvage for neoplasms of the shoulder girdle. Intermediate reconstructive and functional results. *J Bone Joint Surg*. 1996;78A:1872–1888.
5. Getty PJ, Peabody TD. Complications and functional outcomes of reconstruction with an osteoarticular allograft after intra-articular resection of the proximal aspect of the humerus. *J Bone Joint Surg*. 1999;81A:1138–1146.
6. Rödl RW, Gosheger G, Gebert C, et al. Reconstruction of the proximal humerus after wide resection of tumours. *J Bone Joint Surg Br*. 2002;84(7):1004–1008.
7. DeGroot H, Donati D, Di Liddo M, et al. The use of cement in osteoarticular allografts for proximal humeral bone tumors. *Clin Orthop*. 2004;427:190–197.

30 Proximal Humeral Allograft Prosthetic Composites

Joaquin Sanchez-Sotelo

Reconstruction of the shoulder joint in the presence of massive bone loss may be performed with the combination of an allograft and a prosthesis (allograft prosthetic composite or APC) (1,2). Shoulder stability and function largely depend on the surrounding musculotendinous structures and the implant design used. Healing of the deltoid and rotator cuff tendons to the allograft is desirable. Reverse prosthesis designs may prove to play an important role when rotator cuff function cannot be reliably restored by other means. Alternatives to reconstruction with an APC include a tumor prosthesis, osteoarticular allografts, arthrodesis with or without vascularized autograft, Tikhoff-Linberg interscapulothoracic resection, and amputation.

INDICATIONS

Reconstruction of the proximal humerus with an APC is indicated in situations of massive loss of the proximal humerus secondary to

- Resection of tumors
- Implant failure
- Bone resection for deep infection
- Severe posttraumatic bone loss

Age and activity play some role in the choice of the reconstructive technique. Osteoarticular allografts are favored by some authors for the younger patients (3,4), whereas tumor prostheses, where the metal body of the prosthesis replaces the length of missing bone, usually are reserved for older patients with lower functional demands and life expectancy (5,6). For most patients, though, an APC represents the best alternative, as it provides restoration of bone stock and the potential for soft tissue healing to the allograft (2) but avoids problems secondary to allogeneic cartilage disintegration (4).

CONTRAINDICATIONS

The use of an APC may be contraindicated for the following reasons:

- Active deep infection
- Poor soft tissue envelope
- Inadequate remaining bone stock for secure fixation of the construct
- Oncologic contraindications for limb salvage surgery

PREOPERATIVE PLANNING

Preoperative planning is paramount to achieve a successful reconstruction when performing a shoulder APC. The preoperative evaluation and planning are different depending on the indication for reconstruction.

325

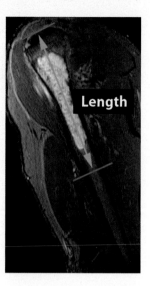

FIGURE 30.1

The length of the allograft used for reconstruction may be calculated preoperatively measuring the distance between the upper end of the humerus and the planned level of tumor resection on MRI.

Reconstruction After Tumor Resection

In patients with tumors requiring proximal humerus resection, radiographs should be complemented with magnetic resonance imaging (MRI) to determine a safe resection level to achieve negative margins if possible. An arteriogram may be useful when arterial involvement is suspected. The length of the allograft should match the length of the resected segment as measured on the MRI (Fig. 30.1) and intraoperatively. Radiographs with magnification markers also assist in the preoperative planning for the appropriate allograft size. The length of the allograft used will also depend on the implant used: when the reconstruction is performed with an anatomic hemiarthroplasty, the length of the graft should replicate the length of bone resected; nonanatomic reverse designs change the joint center of rotation to a more inferior position and may require a shorter allograft to avoid excessive overlengthening.

Failed Previous Reconstruction

When a proximal humerus APC is considered in patients for previous failed reconstructions, (failed osteoarticular allografts, failed shoulder replacements, resection after deep infection, large posttraumatic bone loss), the soft

FIGURE 30.2

Radiographs with magnification markers of the affected **(A)** and contralateral **(B)** humeri may be used to assist during preoperative planning for the size of the allograft.

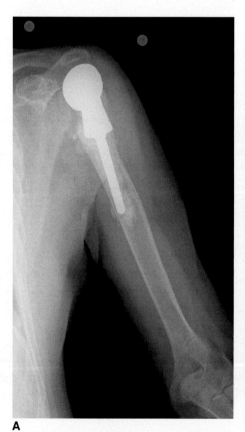

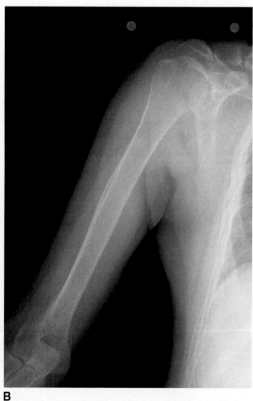

A   B

tissues around the shoulder will often present contractures or deficiencies, and the length of the allograft is largely determined intraoperatively based on ease of reduction, passive shoulder motion, soft tissue tension and balance, as well as the ability to perform a satisfactory soft tissue repair. Radiographs of the opposite intact humerus may be used for planning (Fig. 30.2), but intraoperative adjustments are needed to adapt to changes in the soft tissues.

TECHNIQUE

Principles

Proximal humeral reconstruction with an APC may be performed with different techniques depending on the size of the defect, cuff integrity, and surgeon preferences (Table 30.1; Fig. 30.3).

Implant Type and Fixation   Anatomic (nonreverse) implants are most commonly used for patients with a well-preserved rotator cuff, either after tumor resection or as revision of a previous reconstruction. Humeral head replacement (shoulder hemiarthroplasty) is selected for patients with no glenoid cartilage loss; otherwise, total shoulder arthroplasty should be considered. When an anatomic implant is used, a proximal humeral allograft with rotator cuff tendons attached to it should be used, so that the host rotator cuff can be repaired to the allograft tendons with multiple nonabsorbable sutures.

The design and length of the stem may change depending on the size of the defect and surgeon preferences. The humeral component needs to be fixed to the allograft with bone cement. If the length of the allograft needed is shorter than the length of the stem, the component is cemented into both the allograft and the native humerus (Fig. 30.3A). When the allograft length exceeds the length of a conventional primary stem, the author's preference is to just cement the standard stem into the allograft (Fig. 30.3B), but many surgeons prefer to bypass the graft-host junction with a long revision cemented stem providing additional intramedullary fixation.

When the integrity of the rotator cuff is severely compromised as a result of previous pathology or the need to remove it as part of a tumor resection, a reverse shoulder arthroplasty may be considered. Safe implantation of the uncemented glenoid component of a reverse prosthesis requires reasonable bone stock, which may be compromised in the revision setting. Reverse total shoulder arthroplasty may provide more stability and active elevation than an anatomic hemiarthroplasty in patients with severe cuff deficiency needing an APC. However, internal and external rotation may end up being more limited and the mid- and long-term complications and outcome are largely unknown.

Nonanatomic prostheses designed specifically to act as spacers are required when part or most of the glenoid needs to be removed as part of the tumor resection, not allowing a stable reconstruction with a hemiarthroplasty or the implantation of the glenoid component of a reverse prosthesis. These spacers

TABLE 30.1 Options for Proximal Humeral Reconstruction Using an APC	
Implant type	Anatomic hemiarthroplasty
	Reverse total shoulder arthroplasty
	Prosthetic spacer
Implant fixation	Cemented into allograft only
	Cemented into both allograft and host
Allograft-host junction	Transverse junction
	Step-cut junction
	Side extension of the graft on the host (strut-like)
	Intussusception allograft
Graft-host fixation	Plates and screws
	Cerclage wires
	Intramedullary fixation
	• Stem
	• Graft (intussusception)
	Combined
Biological augmentation	None
	Autograft
	Bone-graft substitutes

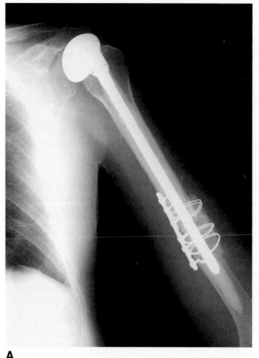

A

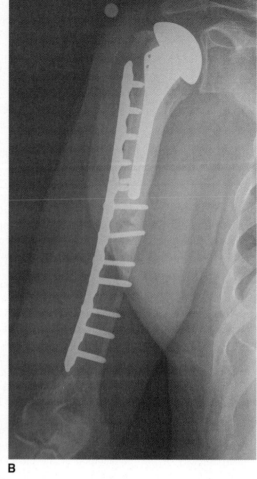

B

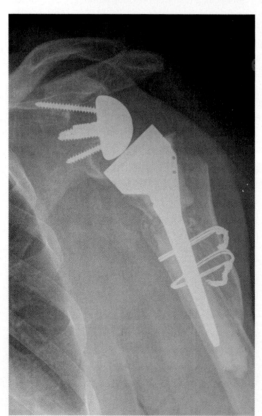

C

FIGURE 30.3

Different variations of an APC may be used depending on the length of the defect, the conditions of the rotator cuff, and patient preferences. **A:** Long cemented stem with or without supplementary fixation. **B:** Short cemented stem into long allograft and plate fixation. **C:** Lateral strut extension of the allograft with wire fixation.

provide suture holes for fixation of the proximal aspect of the implant to the scapula with transosseous nonabsorbable sutures.

Allograft-host Junction   A transverse junction is probably the easiest configuration. Attention should be paid to obtaining perfect matching and apposition between the graft and the host and to restoring adequate rotation by marking the host before resection and the graft before preparation and using reliable landmarks. A step-cut or chevron junction is attractive because it provides a larger contact surface between the graft and the host for healing and may also be more inherently stable. However, it makes it more difficult to obtain perfect apposition and to restore the correct rotation.

Side-to-side allograft-bone contact is very attractive in terms of promoting healing. When the graft diameter is considerably larger than the host diameter, it is sometimes possible to fashion the graft so that there is a lateral and distal strut-like extension for side-to-side apposition (Fig. 30.3C). However, when the sizes of the graft and host are very similar, or the graft is smaller, it is difficult to match and align the graft and the host without fracturing the lateral extension of the graft. Intussusception of the allograft inside the host can be extremely useful in the revision setting if the remaining distal humerus is enlarged allowing insertion of the allograft inside the medullary canal of the host, which provides both stability and a large contact surface for healing.

Graft-host Fixation   A plate and screws usually provide the most stable graft-host fixation. Locking-compression plates are ideal in this situation, as compression at the junction may be first applied using the compression holes of the plate and locking screws allow unicortical fixation where the humeral stem is in the way. The plate should span the allograft-host junction and overlap with at least part of the stem in order to protect the graft from fracture. The location of the plate is dictated by the surgical approach used for resection or removal of the previous reconstruction and by the length of remaining host bone. Most of these reconstructions are performed through a deltopectoral approach extended distally into Henry's approach by splitting the brachialis. An anterior or anterolateral plate is easily applied through this exposure. When the remaining distal bone segment is very short and does not allow insertion of at least three screws, consideration should be given to use of two parallel posteromedial and posterolateral plates as used for fixation of distal humerus fractures. This allows use of long screws into the articular portion of the distal humerus.

Cerclage wires or cables are used when the allograft is fashioned with a strut extension and may also be considered with step-cut junctions. Cables provide stronger fixation than wires, but they may be associated with debris generation. Wire fixation generally provides adequate stability. The main concern with cerclage fixation of the humerus is the potential for iatrogenic injury to the radial nerve, which should be identified and protected during cable or wire passage and tightening.

Long stems bypassing the host-graft junction and allografts intussuscepted in the native medullary canal provide intramedullary fixation. Depending on the stability of the construct, intramedullary fixation may be used alone or supplemented with a plate, strut, or cerclage fixation.

Biological Augmentation   Nonunion at the graft-host junction is one of the potential complications of APC reconstruction. Iliac crest autograft may be considered in order to stimulate healing, but this adds potential morbidity in patients already undergoing a major procedure. Bone graft substitutes are more appealing, but their efficacy for this particular application has not been studied. When a long-stemmed prosthesis is used, the reamings obtained from the distal native humerus may be used as autograft as well.

Preferred Techniques

Anatomic Hemiarthroplasty APC   A careful tumor resection or removal of a previous failed prosthesis is a critical first step prior to reconstruction with an APC. Special care should be taken to protect the neurovascular structures. In tumor cases, the resected specimen is confirmed to be free of tumor at its margin and measured to determine the length of the allograft needed (Fig. 30.4).

The proximal humeral allograft is prepared on a back table outside the operative field. It is helpful to prepare the graft for implantation of the prosthesis before performing the distal osteotomy, so that the whole graft can be held and supported while the instrumentation is used. Depending on the prosthetic system selected, the humeral neck osteotomy is performed using a cutting guide or freehanded at the anatomic neck level. The prosthetic humeral head size is initially selected to match the resected humeral head size, but in the revision setting, the final humeral head implant is not selected until the shoulder soft tissue balance is complete.

The allograft canal is reamed and broached for implantation of a cemented stem. Whenever possible, the author's preference is to use an anatomic design with a short stem cemented only into the allograft (Fig. 30.3). Care is taken to achieve a good cementing technique by using a cement restrictor, vacuum mixing the cement, cleaning the canal of debris, and using a cement gun and pressurization. Antibiotic powder is mixed with the cement routinely (1 g of vancomycin and 1.2 g of tobramycin per 40 g of polymethylmethacrylate).

We use a transverse osteotomy for most reconstructions. Rotational landmarks are selected and marked in the allograft and the host. A marking pen or electrocautery is used to mark a vertical reference line. On the lower third of the humerus, the lateral ridge for insertion of the lateral intermuscular septum is a useful landmark. On the upper two thirds, the lateral aspect of the bicipital groove continues distally into the anterior apex of the humerus and may be used to judge rotation. A saw is used to perform the distal osteotomy on the graft so that it will match the host avoiding varus, valgus, flexion, or extension. A burr may be used to fine-tune the graft-host junction so that there is less than 1 mm of gap anteriorly, posteriorly, medially, and laterally.

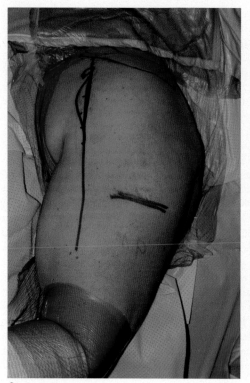

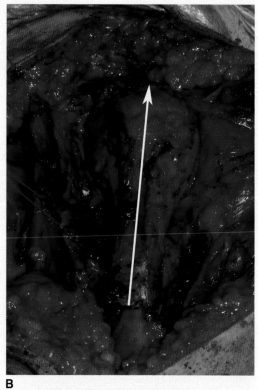

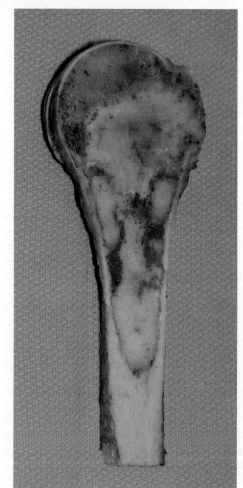

FIGURE 30.4

A: Most humeral APCs are performed through a long deltopectoral approach. **B:** Careful deep exposure allows removal of previous reconstructions or tumor resection. **C:** The resected specimen assists in determining the exact length of the allograft needed.

The junction is then reduced and fixed with a locking compression plate (Fig. 30.5). The plate should be long enough to allow insertion of at least three screws into the native humerus distally and to overlap with at least part of the stem proximally. Otherwise, the graft may be placed at an increased risk of fracture where it

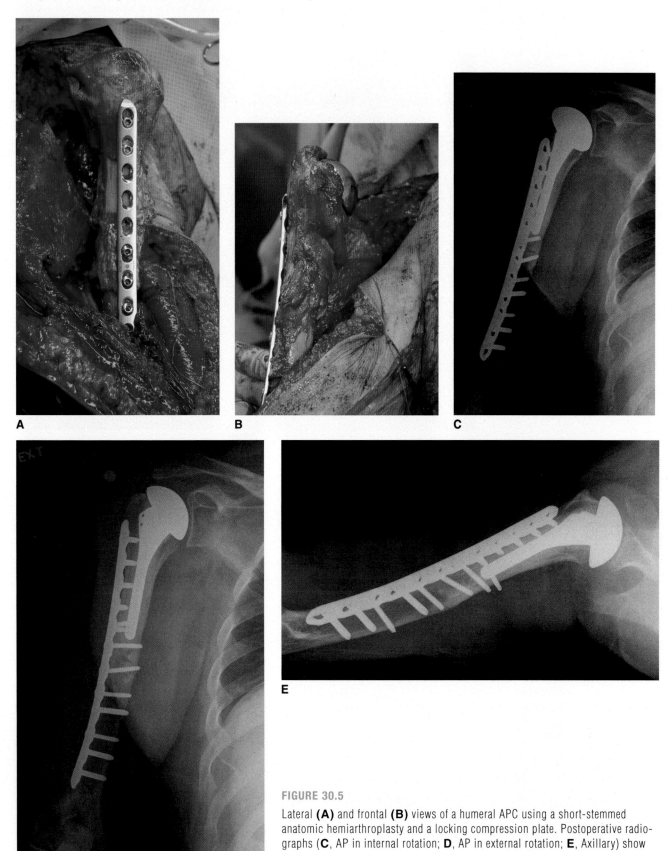

FIGURE 30.5

Lateral **(A)** and frontal **(B)** views of a humeral APC using a short-stemmed anatomic hemiarthroplasty and a locking compression plate. Postoperative radiographs (**C**, AP in internal rotation; **D**, AP in external rotation; **E**, Axillary) show adequate length restoration, good cementing technique, and adequate compression at the host-graft transverse junction.

is not protected by either the stem proximally or the plate distally. The plate may be slightly undercontoured and fixed first with two nonlocking screws in the compression mode proximal and distal to the junction. Once compression is achieved, the rest of the holes may be filled with locking screws. Locking screws are especially attractive proximally, where bicortical fixation may not be possible at the level of the stem. Demineralized bone matrix or other osteoinductive material may then be placed at the host-graft junction.

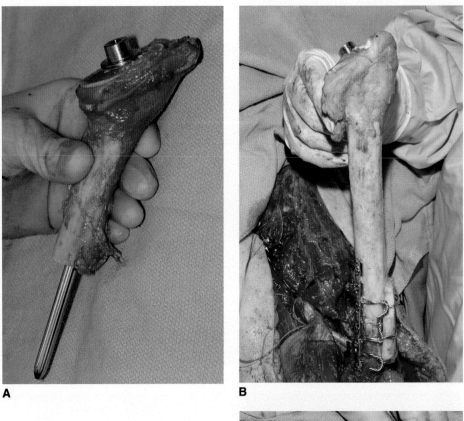

A

B

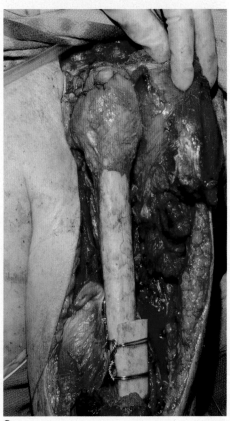

FIGURE 30.6

A: A long-stemmed prosthesis has been cemented into the allograft. **B:** The junction is stabilized by cementing the stem into the native humerus and supplementing the fixation with a plate and an allograft strut. **C:** The rotator cuff tendons of the graft and the host are repaired with multiple interrupted nonabsorbable sutures. Sutures are seen.

C

When a longer cemented stem is used to bypass the graft-host junction, the author's preference is to cement the component in two stages. The stem is first cemented into the allograft on the back table, taking care to remove cement of the lower 1 cm of the intramedullary canal of the graft to facilitate healing (Fig. 30.6A). The APC is cemented into the host as a separate second stage, which allows avoidance of cement interposition at the host-graft junction and better control of the overall positioning of the reconstruction. Additional fixation with a plate and/or strut may be added as needed depending on the strength of the reconstruction and bone quality (Fig. 30.6B).

The patient's native cuff is then repaired to the allograft cuff with multiple heavy nonabsorbable sutures (Fig. 30.6C). The posterior sutures for repair of the teres minor, infraspinatus and posterior aspect of the supraspinatus may be placed and tagged first. The proximal humerus is then reduced, all the posterior sutures are tied, and the anterior supraspinatus and subscapularis are repaired next. The deltoid and pectoralis are repaired to the allograft as well, and the rest of the closure is routine.

Reverse Total Shoulder Arthroplasty APC   Reconstruction of the proximal humerus with a reverse prosthesis APC may provide improved function in patients with severe rotator cuff deficiency (Fig. 30.7). The glenoid component should be implanted prior to reconstruction of the proximal humerus, as glenoid exposure is easier with the resected humerus out of the way (Fig. 30.8). The glenoid component should be placed flush with the inferior margin of the glenoid to avoid notching. Controversy remains about the use of a

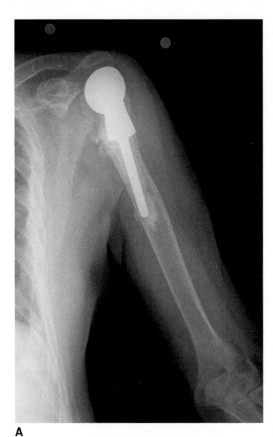

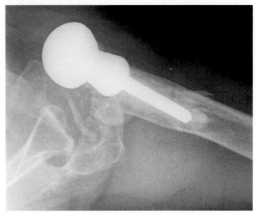

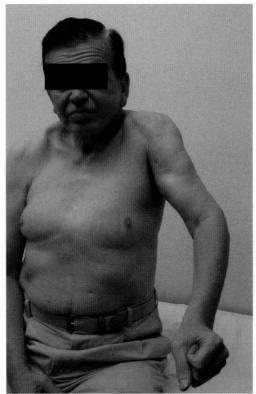

FIGURE 30.7

Anteroposterior **(A)** and axillary **(B)** radiographs showing anterior dislocation and severe bone loss in a patient with very limited active motion and antero-superior escape **(C)** after failed reconstruction using a tumor prosthesis.

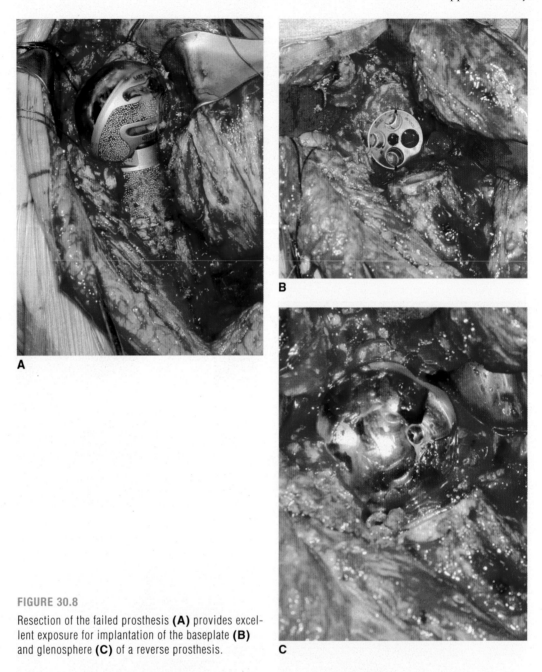

FIGURE 30.8

Resection of the failed prosthesis **(A)** provides excellent exposure for implantation of the baseplate **(B)** and glenosphere **(C)** of a reverse prosthesis.

glenoid component with a medial or lateral center of rotation for any type of reconstruction using a reverse prosthesis. We tend to use a larger glenosphere if possible to provide better range of motion before impingement.

Preparation of the humerus is similar to what was described for anatomic hemiarthroplasty. The instrumentation for preparation of the reverse prosthesis is used to prepare the allograft (Fig. 30.9). Controversy remains about the ideal version for implantation of a reverse prosthesis. Our preference is to cement these stems in approximately 20 to 30 degrees of retroversion. Reverse prosthesis stems are longer than some of the short anatomic stems, and they frequently need to be cemented into both the graft and the host. Fixation may then be supplemented with a plate and/or strut (Fig. 30.10).

Judging adequate soft tissue tension is one of the most difficult parts of this procedure. A tighter joint provides better deltoid tensioning and decreases the risk of dislocation. However, excessive soft tissue tension may lead to brachial plexopathy, delayed acromial stress fractures, or soft tissue–related discomfort. The author judges soft tissue tension based on the ease of joint reduction, the tension on the conjoined tendon, and intraoperative passive range of motion.

Any remaining rotator cuff is repaired if possible. Repair of the teres minor and supraspinatus may result in better active external rotation. When the posterior cuff cannot be repaired, consideration may be given to performing a latissimus dorsi transfer in order to achieve better active external rotation. Repair of any remaining subscapularis may decrease the risk of dislocation.

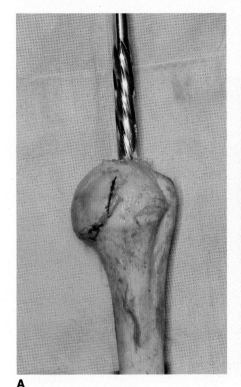

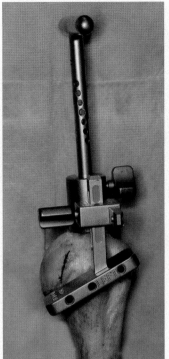

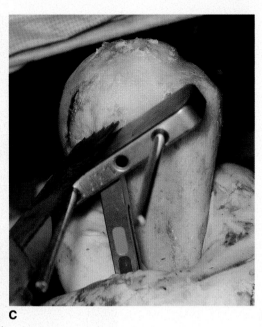

A   **B**   **C**

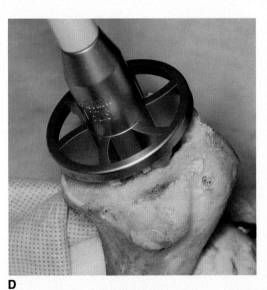

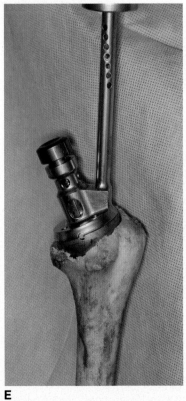

D   **E**

FIGURE 30.9

The allograft is prepared on the back table for insertion of the humeral component. **A:** Canal reaming. **B:** Osteotomy guide. **C:** Proximal humeral osteotomy. **D:** Proximal reaming. **E:** Trial humeral component.

PEARLS AND PITFALLS

There are a few important points to remember when reconstructing the shoulder with a humeral APC:

- Oncologic considerations always take precedence over reconstruction preferences.
- Identification and protection of neurovascular structures are extremely important for patient outcome.
- When an APC is considered for the treatment of failed previous reconstructions, always rule out an associated deep periprosthetic infection.

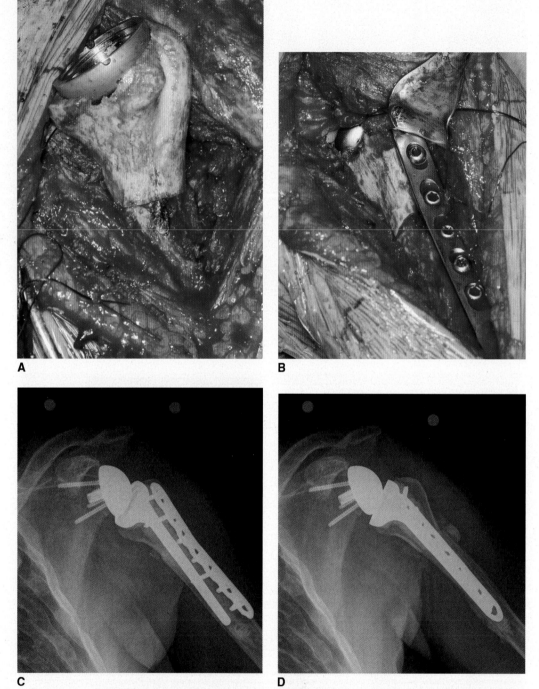

FIGURE 30.10

A: Careful restoration of length and rotation are critical for a successful reconstruction. **B:** The joint is reduced after plate fixation, and soft tissue tension is carefully assessed. **C,D:** Radiographs taken in internal and external rotation show adequate contact and compression between the graft and the host.

- Consideration should be given to adding antibiotics to the cement routinely to decrease the risk of deep periprosthetic infection.
- Preparation and fixation of the host-graft junction are critical in order to obtain optimal bone contact and a stable fixation.
- Adequate soft tissue repair and tension are required to achieve good stability and function.

POSTOPERATIVE MANAGEMENT

APCs require careful postoperative protection and rehabilitation. Joint stability and healing of the soft tissues and allograft-host junction take precedence over motion. After surgery, the upper extremity is placed in a shoulder immobilizer and the physical therapy program is tailored to intraoperative assessments of range of motion within safe limits not to endanger the reconstruction.

When an adequate soft tissue repair is possible, our preference is to start passive shoulder range of motion exercises in elevation and external rotation the first postoperative day. Most patients are allowed elevation to 120 degrees and external rotation to 20 degrees during the first 2 weeks and are advanced as tolerated over the following month. At 6 weeks, we discontinue use of the shoulder immobilizer and start a program of active-assisted range of motion exercises adding internal rotation. Isometrics are started at 10 weeks and resistive strengthening exercises with elastic rubber bands are added at 12 weeks. Patients are not allowed lifting more than 5 lb for the first 6 months or until there is evidence of healing at the host-graft junction.

A few changes are introduced to this general rehabilitation plan when the reconstruction is performed using a reverse prosthesis. Active-assisted motion may be initiated earlier (2 to 3 weeks) if there was no rotator cuff to repair. Fewer gains in rotation are to be expected, and the physical therapy program should be centered on elevation and deltoid strengthening.

COMPLICATIONS

The main complications of this procedure include deep infection, nerve injury, nonunion at the graft-host junction, shoulder instability, stiffness, and mechanical failure of the reconstruction. Deep infection may be treated occasionally with chronic suppression, especially in patients with low expected survival but often requires removal of all foreign material and delayed reimplantation. Nonunion at the graft-host junction may be salvaged with revision internal fixation and bone grafting, but it may lead to failure of the reconstruction requiring revision surgery. Mechanical failure of the humeral implant is rare in the absence of nonunion, but mechanical failure of reverse glenoid component should be expected to occur in some patients.

RESULTS

There is relatively little published information about the results of APC reconstructions of the proximal humerus, and most reports refer to the use of this technique after tumor resection as opposed to salvage of a failed arthroplasty. Initial reports on graft-prosthetic composites included isolated cases using either autograft (7) or autoclaved autograft (8).

Black et al. (1) reported on six consecutive patients who underwent reconstruction using a proximal humerus APC after resection of a malignant tumor. A long cemented anatomic hemiarthroplasty fixed to the distal humerus with two interlocking screws was combined with fresh frozen humeral allografts with intact soft tissue attachments. The junction was fashioned with matching chevron osteotomies and no supplemental fixation was used. At a mean follow-up of 5 years, one patient required bone grafting and cable plating for nonunion and a second patient required revision for mechanical failure. Three patients reported subjective instability. The mean DASH score was 68.5 points and the mean shoulder score was 59. There were no details provided about range of motion.

Dudkiewicz et al. (9) reported on 11 patients with osteosarcoma of the proximal humerus treated by resection and reconstruction using a structural allograft and a long shoulder hemiarthroplasty. Complications included superficial infection and graft-host nonunion requiring bone autografting.

We recently reviewed the Mayo Clinic experience after shoulder reconstruction for bone tumors using anatomic shoulder prostheses (11). Twenty-five patients were reconstructed with an APC. There was a low rate of objective satisfactory results but a high rate of subjective patient satisfaction. Complications included instability, nonunion, and loosening among others. Nonunion was less common with cemented distal humeral fixation than with press-fit or plate fixation.

There is limited information about the use of reverse shoulder arthroplasty combined with a proximal humerus structural graft. De Wilde et al. (10) reported on four proximal humerus reconstructions using a reverse prosthesis and radiated proximal humerus autograft. Mean active forward abduction and flexion improved to 175 degrees (range, 160 to 180 degrees) and 169 degrees (range, 135 to 180 degrees), respectively Musculoskeletal Tumor Society (MSTS) ability scores ranged between 90% and 97%, and Constant scores improved to an average 91%. There were no complications.

SUMMARY

Proximal humerus APCs represent an excellent reconstructive option for patients with severe bone loss in the setting of tumor resection or failure of previous reconstructive efforts. Careful preoperative planning and execution of the different surgical steps are critical for the success of these complex reconstructive procedures. An anatomic hemiarthroplasty is used most frequently, but reverse arthroplasty is gaining popularity for patients with no remaining functional rotator cuff. Attention should be paid to adequate restoration of length, rotation, and soft tissue tension, as well as to obtaining satisfactory bone contact and adequate stability at the graft-host junction.

REFERENCES

1. Black AW, Szabo RM, Titelman RM. Treatment of malignant tumors of the proximal humerus with allograft-prosthesis composite reconstruction. *J Shoulder Elbow Surg.* 2007;16(5):525–533.
2. De Wilde LF, Plasschaert FS, Audenaert EA, et al. Functional recovery after a reverse prosthesis for reconstruction of the proximal humerus in tumor surgery. *Clin Orthop Relat Res.* 2005;430:156–162.
3. Dudkiewicz I, Velkes S, Oran A, et al. Composite grafts in the treatment of osteosarcoma of the proximal humerus. *Cell Tissue Bank.* 2003;4:37–41.
4. Fuhrmann RA, Roth A, Venbrocks RA. Salvage of the upper extremity in cases of tumorous destruction of the proximal humerus. *J Cancer Res Clin Oncol.* 2000;126:337–344.
5. Gebhardt MC, Roth YF, Mankin HJ. Osteoarticular allografts for reconstruction in the proximal part of the humerus after excision of a musculoskeletal tumor. *J Bone Joint Surg Am.* 1990;72:334–345.
6. Getty PJ, Peabody TD. Complications and functional outcomes of reconstruction with an osteoarticular allograft after intra-articular resection of the proximal aspect of the humerus. *J Bone Joint Surg Am.* 1999;81:1138–1146.
7. Gitelis S, Piasecki P. Allograft prosthetic composite arthroplasty for osteosarcoma and other aggressive bone tumors. *Clin Orthop Relat Res.* 1991;270:197–201.
8. Harrington KD, Johnston JO, Kaufer HN, et al. Limb salvage and prosthetic joint reconstruction for low-grade and selected high-grade sarcomas of bone after wide resection and replacement by autoclaved autogeneic grafts. *Clin Orthop Relat Res.* 1986;211:180–214.
9. Imbriglia JE, Neer CS, Dick HM. Resection of the proximal one-half of the humerus in a child for chondrosarcoma. Preservation of function using a fibular graft and Neer prosthesis. *J Bone Joint Surg Am.* 1978;60:262–264.
10. O'Connor MI, Sim FH, Chao EY. Limb salvage for neoplasms of the shoulder girdle. Intermediate reconstructive and functional results. *J Bone Joint Surg Am.* 1996;78:1872–1888.
11. Veillete C, Cil A, Sanchez-Sotelo J, et al. Reconstruction of the proximal humerus for bone neoplasm using an anatomic shoulder prosthesis, in AAOS (ed) 75th Annual Meeting of the American Academy of Orthopedic Surgeons, 2008.

31 Intercalary Prosthesis in Reconstruction of Humeral Defects

Timothy A. Damron

Intercalary prostheses were designed for replacement of segmental defects in diaphyseal bone. They are most commonly used for humeral defects, although they are available for other sites on a custom basis. Although the initial design of the humeral intercalary prosthesis employed a male-female taper junction, the latest design is that of a modified lap joint.

INDICATIONS

Indications for the intercalary humeral prosthesis involve both the location of the bone lesion and the underlying diagnosis, the latter of which relates to expected survival. It is recommended that the tumor or segmental defect be in the location as defined by all of the criteria listed below. Furthermore, it is strongly recommended that these prostheses be limited to patients with limited life expectancy. Patients should generally have an estimated survival of at least 4 to 6 weeks to be able to live long enough to benefit from this procedure. Anticipated survival beyond a few years would suggest that consideration should be given to a more biological reconstruction that would have the potential to last longer.

- *Location within bone* (ALL criteria advisable)
  - Segmental diaphyseal humeral defects 4 cm or greater
    - Rationale: The minimum size of the body portion of these prostheses is 5 cm. Often, even for 4-cm defects, the bone edges require some trimming back to solid margins, resulting in a 5-cm defect. Care should be taken not to overlengthen the arm by inserting a body section larger than the original defect, as this may result in neuropraxia.
  - Defect within middle third of humerus
    - Rationale: Middle third defects are more likely to have intact bone proximal and distal to accept a cemented intramedullary stem.
  - Five centimeter or more of intact remaining proximal and distal medullary canal
    - Rationale: Minimum off-the-shelf stem sizes are 5 cm. While standard stems may be trimmed to shorter lengths, this may compromise fixation.
    - Alternatives: For shorter defects, adequate treatment may be able to be achieved by shortening and internal fixation or by cementation of the defect with spanning internal fixation using either intramedullary nailing or plate and screw fixation.
- *Limited life expectancy* (EITHER/OR)
  - Disseminated malignancy (metastatic disease or myeloma)
    - Rationale: Patients with disseminated disease have limited life expectancy and are less likely to outlive the prosthesis before complications such as aseptic loosening occur, as suggested by the premature

TABLE 31.1 Contraindications		
Category	**Contraindication**	**Alternative Surgical Treatment**
Location	Defects <4 cm	Shortening and internal fixation
	Defects of proximal third	ORIF vs. proximal humeral endoprosthesis
	Defects of distal third	ORIF vs. distal humeral endoprosthesis
Life expectancy	Nonmetastatic primary bone or soft tissue sarcoma[a]	Intercalary diaphyseal allograft or autograft with internal fixation

[a]Relative contraindication.

high rate of loosening observed with the latest version of this device at relatively short duration of follow-up.[2]

○ OR solitary metastatic carcinoma undergoing resection (renal or thyroid carcinoma)

  ❑ Rationale: In these patients, life expectancy is unknown but often still limited. If they become long-term survivors, the reconstruction may require conversion to a potentially more long-lasting solution such as an intercalary allograft or vascularized fibular autograft with appropriate fixation.

CONTRAINDICATIONS

Contraindications also involve the location of the tumor and the patient's life expectancy. Normal life expectancy should be considered a relative contraindication to the use of this device (Table 31.1). For patients who are anticipated to live for longer than a few years, consideration should be given to a more biological reconstruction, such as an intercalary diaphyseal allograft or autograft with spanning internal fixation. When allograft is not available or is not acceptable to the patient, vascularized fibular grafts have been used to reconstruct such deficits.

PREOPERATIVE PLANNING

● Confirm diagnosis
  ○ Preoperative metastatic workup to search for likely primary and identify extent of disease
    ❑ Total body bone scan
    ❑ Computerized tomography of chest/abdomen/pelvis
  ○ Serum protein electrophoresis and urine protein electrophoresis to evaluate for multiple myeloma
  ○ Establish diagnosis of humeral lesion with tissue before proceeding with treatment
    ❑ Preoperative needle biopsy
    ❑ Intraoperative needle or open biopsy with frozen section
● Assess extent of bone defect and remaining proximal and distal bone
  ○ Plain biplanar radiographs of entire humerus
  ○ Consider MRI or CT to assess extent of defect
● Entertain alternative means of operative management
  ○ Consider alternatives to spacer
    ❑ Internal fixation with bone cement or allograft to fill defect
    ❑ Proximal or distal endoprosthetic device if closer to one end of humerus
  ○ Decide upon a backup plan
● Ensure all equipment will be available
  ○ Primary plan: spacer implants, trials, insertion equipment, straight reamers, reamer driver, antibiotic loaded bone cement (author utilizes a pre-mixed Tobramycin containing PMMA), insertion tool of choice for bone cement (author utilizes a Toomey syringe)
  ○ Backup plan(s): internal fixation implants and insertion equipment, allograft, other prostheses (such as proximal humeral replacement for more proximal lesions or a total elbow distal humeral replacement for more distal lesions)
● Consider pre-operative embolization
  ○ Consider for vascular malignances (renal carcinoma, thyroid carcinoma, myeloma) if intralesional procedure planned
  ○ Not absolutely necessary if wide en bloc resection planned

TECHNIQUE

Positioning

Typically, the patient is positioned supine with the arm on an armboard in order to facilitate stability after resection of the involved segment. The author prefers a Jackson table or other equivalent vascular imaging table without metallic bars on the side that may impede fluoroscopic imaging. The patient may also be positioned far enough to the opposite side of the imaging table that no armboard is needed.

Landmarks

The landmarks of the shoulder, including the acromion, distal clavicle, coracoid, arm, and elbow should be identified and marked to facilitate accurate placement of the surgical incision.

Surgical Incision

For most cases, an anterior approach to the humerus is preferred. Exceptional situations would include simultaneous resection of a soft tissue sarcoma involving the bone where the location of the tumor itself or the presence and position of a biopsy tract that requires excision along with the tumor necessitates a medial, lateral, or posterior approach (also see "Contraindications" section). The surgical incision is longitudinal and extending in line with the coracoid proximally to the anterolateral distal arm just at the medial aspect of the mobile wad. The extent of the incision may be limited to the region of planned resection alone. More extensive exposure is needed for en bloc resections and less extensive for intralesional procedures.

Surgical Approach

Proceed along lateral aspect of biceps tendon, splitting the brachialis muscle fibers longitudinally through their midportion. Proximally, the deltoid may be retracted laterally typically with the cephalic vein. Stay lateral to the biceps tendon, lateral ridge of biceps groove, and insertion of the pectoralis major. Beware of the anterior humeral circumflex humeral vessels at the inferior border of the infraspinatus in the proximal aspect of the wound. Distally, be aware of the lateral antebrachial cutaneous nerve as it arises from beneath the mobile wad laterally.

Bone Resection

When continuity of bone remains, before any resection is done, the anterior aspect of the cortex particularly on the proximal bone should be marked for orientation purposes during the cementing of the prosthesis later. For cases in which an en bloc resection with clear margins is indicated, fluoroscopic imaging is useful to define the sites of planned resection. For cases being approached in an intralesional fashion, the lesional tissue is removed and then the bone at the edges of the defect should be trimmed back to an intact rim of bone when feasible. When one or both edges of the lesion border on leaving <5 cm of intramedullary canal left, partial defects in the rim of remaining cortical bone may be accepted in lieu of further shortening, but consideration should be given to prophylactic cerclage cabling to prevent fracture and extension away from the defect.

Canal Preparation

Straight reamers are typically used to prepare the canals proximally and distally. Alternatively, flexible reamers may be used, but smaller reamer diameters are necessary, sometimes beginning with 6 mm. Overreaming by at least 1 mm and preferably 2 mm beyond the diameter of the stem to be placed is desirable in order to allow for adequate cement mantle.

Trialing

Body size selection is estimated either from the original defect size with the added bone resection or from the size of the resected bone in the case of en bloc resection (Fig. 31.1). A minimum of 5 cm body size must be utilized to overlengthening the limb. Intramedullary stem lengths may be estimated from the depth of penetration of the intramedullary reamers. Combination body/stem trials are then inserted within the medullary canals, and the body portions are approximated. At this point, soft tissue tension and limb length must be assessed to avoid overlengthening.

Insertion and Cementing

The intramedullary canals are prepared with irrigation and brushing and then packed with a sponge or tampon device to optimize the field for cementing. Typically, two batches of cement are mixed since cement restrictors are not utilized. It is desirable in this instance to fill as much of the canal as possible with bone cement to

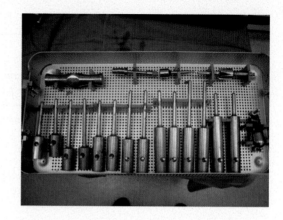

FIGURE 31.1

Trial components are available in an array of body sizes and stem lengths.

minimize risk of fracture in unprotected bone proximally or distally. Retrograde cementing of antibiotic-loaded bone cement within both the proximal and distal canals simultaneously is then done. Typically, these canals are not large enough to accept the tip of a standard intramedullary cement gun, so the author prefers to fill a Toomey syringe with cement in a fairly liquid state before allowing the cement to become doughy and then introducing the cement into the canals.

Final Positioning

Positioning of the components is crucial, which is the reason both should be done with a single mixing of cement (Fig. 31.2). After reducing both components in approximately the correct position, excess cement at the base is removed. The lap joints are then reduced with care taken to ensure that the set screws, which are located 180 degrees apart in the prosthesis, are positioned directly medially and laterally so they are accessible (Fig. 31.3). Both set screws should be threaded in by hand before tightening either all the way (Fig. 31.4). Final fluoroscopic views should be carefully inspected for periprosthetic fractures to cement extrusion.

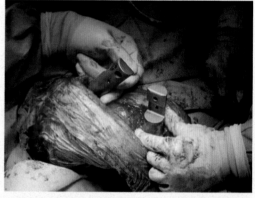

FIGURE 31.2

Care must be taken during insertion of the two humeral components to ensure that the lap joints are oriented correctly.

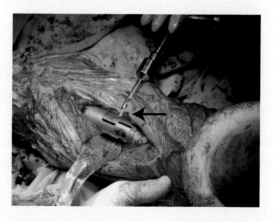

FIGURE 31.3

Before the cement has hardened completely, the components should be reduced, rotational alignment of the arm must be assessed, and access to both screws, which are placed 180 degrees apart (arrow), must be ensured.

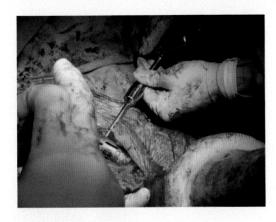

FIGURE 31.4

Final tightening of the set screws is done using the torque-limiting screwdriver.

PEARLS AND PITFALLS

- Restrict usage to patients with > 4 cm central 1/3 humeral defects who have limited life expectancy.
- Be wary of over-resection that results in less than 5 cm of remaining intramedullary canal proximal or distal.
- Avoid over-lengthening that may result in neurologic defecits.

Positioning of components is crucial in order to allow access to both medial and lateral set screws 180 degrees apart.

POSTOPERATIVE MANAGEMENT

Patients may move as tolerated without restrictions and are encouraged to do so beginning on the first postoperative day (Fig. 31.5). Wound care is routine.

Complications

The problems of neuropraxia have been attributed to the need for overdistraction with the first-generation male-female taper junction design. Rotational instability at the junction and disengagement have also been reported exclusively with the earlier design. The occurrence of periprosthetic fractures has been attributed to the more

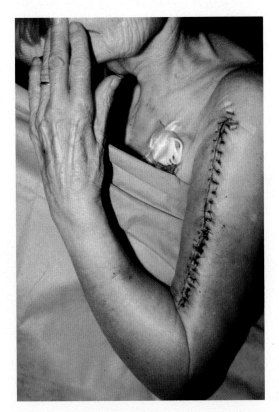

FIGURE 31.5

Patients are encouraged to use the upper extremity beginning on the first postoperative day, as shown for this patient.

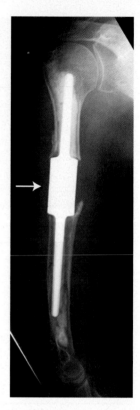

FIGURE 31.6

Circumferential radiolucencies (arrow) are evident around the distal stem of this intercalary humeral spacer.

limited selection of stem lengths available with the earlier design, possibly leaving too much of the bone unprotected (2,3). The finding of symptomatic aseptic loosening in over one fourth of the newer design prostheses despite the short median follow-up (20 months) underscores the need to reserve the use of these devices to patients with limited life expectancy (Fig. 31.6) (3) (Table 31.2).

RESULTS

Biomechanical testing has demonstrated the second-generation lap joint humeral intercalary prosthesis to provide biomechanically superior strength when compared to other alternatives for a segmental defect. Utilizing a segmental 5-cm defect middiaphyseal model in fresh frozen cadaver humeri, cemented intercalary humeral spacers were compared to locked antegrade humeral nails with cement and locked antegrade humeral nails with allograft. In torsional testing, the spacer prostheses provided significantly higher peak torque and stiffness than the two alternatives (4).

Two clinical reports describe the results with the intercalary humeral spacer prostheses in patients (2, 3). The original Mayo male-female taper design prostheses were the subject of the first review of 17 patients with disseminated malignancy in whom the spacers had been implanted (3) (Fig. 31.7). Metastatic carcinoma made

TABLE 31.2 Complications			
Complication	**Overall (%, _N_ = 32)**	**First Generation (%, _N_ = 21)**	**Second Generation (%, _N_ = 11)**
Neuropraxia	9	14	0
Rotational instability/disengagement	6	10	0
Pathologic post-op periprosthetic fracture	6	10	0
Intraoperative periprosthetic fracture	3	5	0
Aseptic loosening	16	10	27
Mean duration of clinical follow-up (months)	NA	20.3	19.2

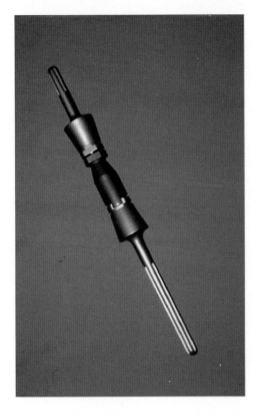

FIGURE 31.7

The first-generation intercalary humeral spacer prosthesis utilized a male-female Morse taper junction that required overdistraction in order to reduce. The arrows indicate the two sites of male-female junctions adjoining a modular body segment to the proximal and distal intramedullary stem components.

up the majority of the lesions, with breast and renal cancer being the two most common primaries. These were accompanied by lesions due to myeloma, lymphoma, and less common entities.

Results in this first report showed pain relief in 88% but complications in at least 29% of patients overall. The most common complications were attributed to limitations of the original design.

Hence, in the latest design employing a modified lap joint junction, modifications were made to compensate for earlier limitations (2) (Fig. 31.8). In addition to the modified junction, a wider array of stem lengths was made available. In the latest report comparing the first- and second-generation spacer prostheses, 21 patients with the original male-female taper design were compared to 11 patients with the newer design. Results showed that there was a significant improvement from preoperatively to postoperatively in both groups for average MSTS total scores and pain scores. There was no significant difference in overall scores or any of the individual components between the two groups.

At median 20-month follow-up, implant survival rate was 94% (30/32), 100% in the patients with the latest design prosthesis and 90.5% in the earlier patients (Fig. 31.9). Currently, only the modified lap joint configuration is available from the original manufacturer. Newer devices that have been introduced by other companies also include this concept in their design, but there are have been no reports to date in the literature on those devices.

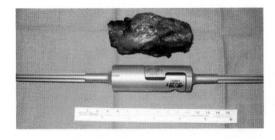

FIGURE 31.8

The second-generation intercalary humeral spacer utilizes a modified lap joint junction, which is secured with set screws separated 180 degrees.

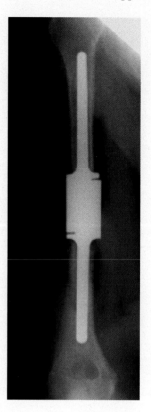

FIGURE 31.9

A well-fixed intercalary humeral spacer device is shown.

REFERENCES

1. Chin HC, Frassica FJ, Hein TJ, et al. Metastatic diaphyseal fractures of the shaft of the humerus. The structural strength evaluation of a new method of treatment with a segmental defect prosthesis. *Clin Orthop Rel Res*. 1989;248:231–239.
2. Damron TA, Leerapun T, Hugate R, et al. Does the second-generation intercalary humeral spacer improve on the first? *Clin Orthop Rel Res*. 2008;466(6):1309–1317.
3. Damron TA, Sim FH, Shives TC. Intercalary humeral spacers in the treatment of destructive diaphyseal humeral pathologic bone lesions. *Clin Orthop Rel Res*. 1996;324:233–243.
4. Henry JC, Damron TA, Weiner MM, et al. Biomechanical analysis of humeral diaphyseal segmental defect fixation. *Clin Orthop Rel Res*. 2002;396:231–239.

32 Total Humeral Reconstruction

Kristy L. Weber

Total humeral reconstruction is a rare procedure with limited indications. Its use is generally confined to the oncologic patient, and other indications are not extensively discussed here. When performed in the ideal clinical scenario, local control can be achieved while preserving maximal function. Although most tumors that involve the distal humerus are treated palliatively with radiation and limited surgery, extensive lesions can lead to severe pain and loss of function. A limb-sparing total humeral resection and reconstruction allows the patient to avoid a disfiguring amputation of the upper extremity and maintain elbow, wrist, and hand function. This chapter outlines total humeral reconstructions using either a prosthesis or an allograft.

INDICATIONS

- (Most common) Primary malignant bone tumor of the humeral diaphysis that extends too close to the shoulder and elbow to effectively use a diaphyseal intercalary spacer (Chapter 31), a proximal humeral reconstruction (Chapter 29), or a distal humeral reconstruction (Chapter 32) (Fig. 32.1)
- In a patient with a reasonable expected lifespan, painful metastasis to the humerus that cannot be reconstructed or stabilized with a simpler, more functional reconstruction
- Pathologic fracture through a primary malignant bone tumor of the humerus where adequate margins can still be achieved with total humeral resection
- Solitary extensive metastasis to the humerus where the procedure would be done to theoretically provide the patient a longer survival (controversial)
- Primary soft tissue sarcoma that extensively involves the upper arm/humerus but spares the neurovascular bundle
- Failed prior stabilization (retrograde flexible nails, anterograde humeral nail) or reconstruction for oncologic/nononcologic reasons (proximal/distal humeral prosthesis, allograft or combination) (Fig. 32.2)

CONTRAINDICATIONS

- Prior infected shoulder/humeral/elbow reconstruction (although in specific cases, an antibiotic spacer and intravenous antibiotics could be justified to clear an infection prior to reconstruction)
- Primary sarcoma with widespread metastasis or metastatic carcinoma to the upper arm/humerus in a patient with a limited lifespan or extensive co-morbidities/operative risk (Fig. 32.3)

PREOPERATIVE PREPARATION

Patient Expectations

A total humeral resection and reconstruction is an extensive surgery often used to avoid a forequarter amputation. Although it is a limb salvage procedure, the patient should be aware of the potential complications (specifically infection and nerve injury) as well as the expected postoperative shoulder function. Generally, patients will have painless shoulder and elbow motion that allows completion of most basic activities of daily living. However, the shoulder function will be limited to an active range of motion of approximately 30 degrees of motion in any plane and decreased lifting ability.

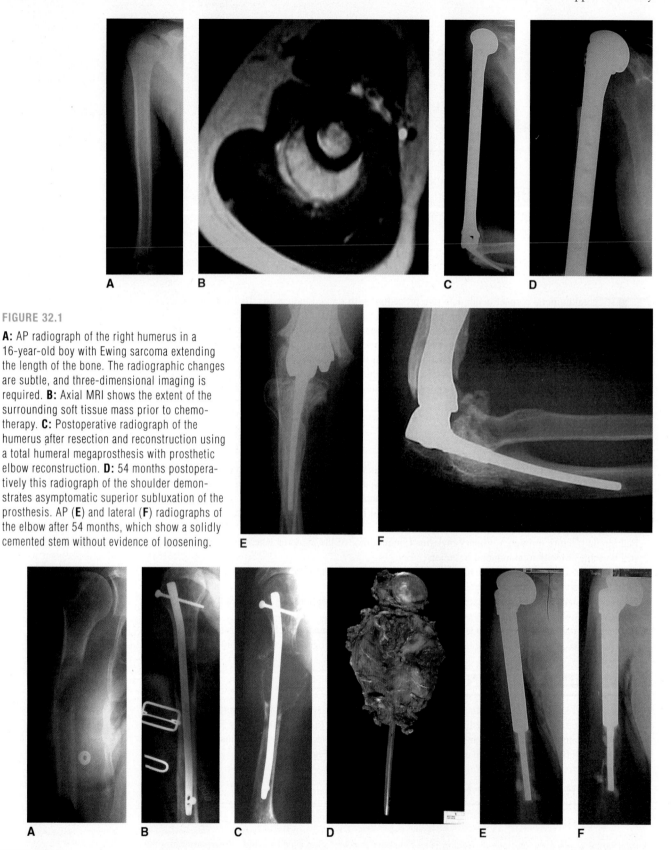

FIGURE 32.1

A: AP radiograph of the right humerus in a 16-year-old boy with Ewing sarcoma extending the length of the bone. The radiographic changes are subtle, and three-dimensional imaging is required. **B:** Axial MRI shows the extent of the surrounding soft tissue mass prior to chemotherapy. **C:** Postoperative radiograph of the humerus after resection and reconstruction using a total humeral megaprosthesis with prosthetic elbow reconstruction. **D:** 54 months postoperatively this radiograph of the shoulder demonstrates asymptomatic superior subluxation of the prosthesis. AP (**E**) and lateral (**F**) radiographs of the elbow after 54 months, which show a solidly cemented stem without evidence of loosening.

FIGURE 32.2

A: AP radiograph of a patient with metastatic renal cell carcinoma to the right humerus and a pathologic fracture. **B:** He was stabilized with a locked humeral rod without curettage of the lesion or radiation. **C:** Six months later a radiograph reveals progression of disease with impending failure of the stabilization. **D:** Gross specimen after resection of the tumor and intramedullary nail (preoperative embolization). **E:** AP radiograph after reconstruction with a proximal humeral megaprosthesis. The native distal humerus was maintained despite the continued presence of microscopic tumor cells so as to provide improved function of the elbow. **F:** Eleven months after surgery the disease progressed in the distal humerus, but the patient continued to have limited systemic disease.

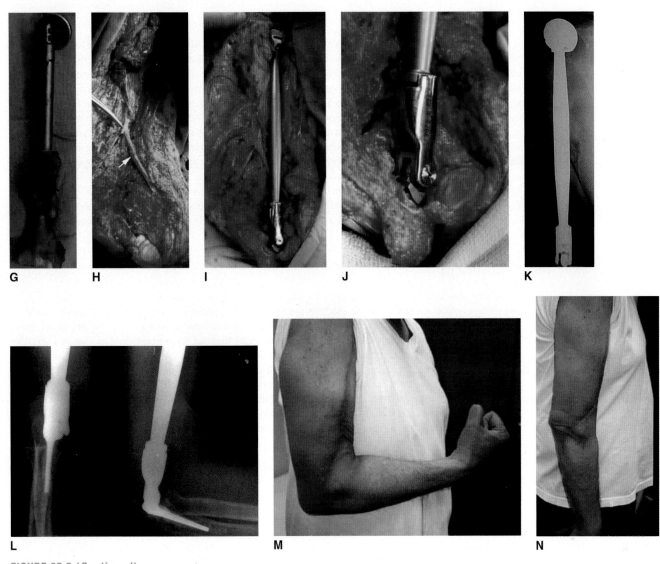

FIGURE 32.2 (*Continued*)

G: Gross specimen after removal of the entire humerus with the proximal humeral prosthesis. **H:** Intraoperative picture after resection revealing the radial nerve (see *arrow*). **I** and **J:** Intraoperative pictures of the entire prosthesis and elbow segment. **K:** AP radiograph of the humerus. **L:** AP and lateral radiographs of the right elbow postoperatively. **M** and **N:** Function of the elbow postoperatively. (Figures 32.2C and 32.2L from Weber KL, Lin PP, Yasko AW. Complex segmental elbow reconstruction after tumor resection. Clin Orthop Rel Res. 2003;415:31-44; with permission).

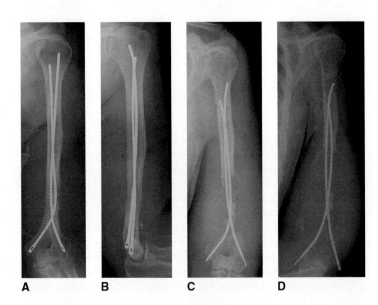

FIGURE 32.3

AP (**A**) and lateral (**B**) postoperative radiographs of the left humerus in a 53-year-old man with aggressive metastatic thyroid cancer treated with retrograde flexible nails for a distal humerus pathologic fracture. Six weeks (**C**) and twelve weeks (**D**) postoperatively, the tumor progressed locally causing severe pain and bone destruction. If this patient had a longer predicted lifespan, he would be a candidate for total humeral reconstruction.

Workup

A detailed history and physical examination are performed preoperatively with attention to pain, neurologic status, stage of tumor, expected lifespan, handedness, prior activity level, range of motion at the shoulder and elbow, use of the ipsilateral hand, presence of any signs/symptoms of infection, axillary lymphadenopathy, and presence of prior incisions/biopsy tracts. Plain radiographs of the humerus are obtained in two planes and include the shoulder and elbow. An MRI is necessary in patients with primary malignant bone tumors to assess the extent of disease in preparation for an adequate surgical margin. Specifically, the extent of tumor at the shoulder/elbow joints and amount of soft tissue extension in relation to the neurovascular structures are assessed. If tumor extends into the glenohumeral joint, an extra-articular resection may be required. Appropriate imaging of the chest, abdomen, and pelvis is performed to assess the stage of disease. Appropriate laboratory tests to include a complete blood count and electrolytes in patients on chemotherapy or who have medical comorbidities are indicated. If the patient has a highly vascular metastasis to the humerus (renal cell carcinoma, thyroid carcinoma), consideration should be given to preoperative embolization. If a large soft tissue defect is expected around the elbow or shoulder, a rotational or free flap might be necessary, so a preoperative plastic surgery consultation is prudent.

Equipment

A decision should be made as to the type of reconstruction to be used after humeral resection. If an allograft-prosthetic composite (APC) is to be used for the shoulder, an appropriate total humeral allograft should be appropriately sized and procured. The length of the allograft is important as well as a close match at the elbow joint. The proximal humerus is less critical for size matching than the distal humerus. The standard shoulder prosthesis to be placed in the proximal end of a total humeral allograft is templated. If a total humeral mega-prosthesis is used, the elbow stems should be templated for the proximal ulna. If an extra-articular resection is performed at the shoulder, the standard prosthetic humeral head may not fit well against the scapular neck. Instead, a spacer can be used that is fitted to the top of the prosthetic humeral body segment and attached with heavy suture to the scapula and clavicle. Methylmethacrylate is used to fix the elbow prosthesis into the ulna. If an olecranon osteotomy is performed, wire fixation is necessary. A shoulder immobilizer or spica cast is used postoperatively.

Anesthesia Considerations

General anesthesia with or without a regional block is used during the procedure. It is important, however, that the neurologic status of the arm can be assessed postoperatively. The patient should have a viable type and screen/cross for blood products. Patients who receive preoperative chemotherapy may be anemic, and there is no tourniquet option during the case.

TECHNIQUE

Positioning

The patient should be positioned supine on the operative table to facilitate the anterior incision and dissection around the medial epicondyle and ulnar nerve. The entire upper extremity is prepared and draped up to the neck. The endotracheal tube should be positioned toward the opposite arm. A urinary catheter is placed if the procedure is anticipated to last more than 2 hours. Intravenous antibiotics are given and redosed throughout the procedure as appropriate.

Resection

An anterior approach to the shoulder and humerus is made with the incision starting posterior to the clavicle and extending midway between the coracoid process and the lateral acromion process (just lateral to the deltopectoral approach), taking into account prior incisions or excising previous open biopsy scars. Raise wide medial and lateral flaps and proceed in the deltopectoral interval. If the cephalic vein is maintained, it is retracted medially with the pectoralis or laterally with the deltoid. The remainder of the incision follows the lateral aspect of the biceps toward the elbow and then curves either medially or laterally depending on the location of the tumor. The author usually ends the incision medially along the elbow and proximal ulna to facilitate the reconstruction in this area and protect the ulnar nerve. When removing primary malignant bone tumors or metastasis where a wide or marginal margin is expected for local control, a cuff of normal tissue is left with the underlying tumor and humerus. If the deltoid cannot be adequately retracted laterally despite its insertional release from the humerus, it can be released proximally from the clavicle and acromion process and later reattached with heavy sutures through drill holes. The following muscles are released from the humerus leaving a cuff of tissue as necessary to achieve a margin: pectoralis, latissimus dorsi, teres major, medial and lateral triceps, and brachioradialis. The anterior humeral circumflex vessels are ligated and tied to facilitate the proximal exposure. This may cause some devascularization of the anterior deltoid, but it usually maintains viability with collateral flow. Avoid abduction of the arm in order to minimize stretch on the musculocutaneous nerve. If greater exposure is needed along the proximal humerus, the conjoined tendon (short head of the biceps and coracobrachialis) is released from the coracoid process leaving a cuff of tendon for later reattachment. The long head of the biceps is released from the superior glenoid and tagged for later reattachment to surrounding tissues at resting length. The biceps is retracted medially and the brachialis is split, leaving a cuff of muscle with the underlying tumor. Care should be taken to dissect and protect the medial neurovascular bundle. The radial and axillary nerves dive posteriorly at the level of the humeral neck and should be carefully dissected and protected. The axillary nerve exits through the quadrangular space inferior to the subscapularis. The radial nerve should also be protected at the spiral groove where it is in close contact with the posterior humerus.

Next, the humerus can be disarticulated at either the elbow or the shoulder. At the shoulder, the subscapularis is released from the humerus and tagged. The long head of the triceps is released posteriorly. The remaining rotator cuff (supraspinatus, infraspinatus, teres minor) and joint capsule are released and tagged with a cuff of tendon depending on their proximity to the tumor. If the coracoacromial ligament is maintained, it will help prevent superior subluxation of the humeral prosthesis. The proximal humerus is gently brought anteriorly, and the axillary nerve and posterior humeral circumflex vessels are dissected. *If an extra-articular resection is required at the shoulder, the capsule should not be violated. The subscapularis is transected just lateral to the coracoid process. The glenoid is dissected medially and cut just medial to the capsular insertion (lateral to the coracoid process).* Distally, the radial, median, and ulnar nerves are dissected and protected at the level of the elbow. The ulnar nerve is carefully released from the ulnar groove at the medial epicondyle. The brachioradialis, flexor (medial epicondyle), and extensor (lateral epicondyle) tendons of the forearm are released from the distal humerus and tagged. The insertion of the triceps is maintained on the posterior aspect of the olecranon, and the biceps insertion is maintained on the proximal radius. The elbow capsule is transected anteriorly for an intra-articular resection. The medial and lateral collateral ligaments are transected, and the humerus is lifted away, measured carefully, and sent to pathology for processing. The wound is irrigated with saline and hemostasis is obtained. After the humerus is removed, care is taken to avoid stretch on the neurovascular structures. New gowns, gloves, instruments, and drapes are used for the reconstruction in the case of a primary malignant bone tumor.

Reconstruction with Megaprosthesis/Total Elbow Replacement

A trial prosthesis is assembled based on the measurement of the resected humeral length. Attention is then directed to placement of the ulnar component of the elbow prosthesis. The triceps is subperiosteally elevated from the olecranon process with only the posterior portion remaining attached. The tip of the olecranon and coronoid process are removed with a sagittal saw to accommodate the ulnar prosthesis (protect the ulnar nerve). Remove the articular cartilage in the olecranon fossa and use a canal finder to open the medullary canal. Widen the medullary canal with a high speed burr if necessary. The proximal ulna is broached by hand (the direction of broaching is toward the radius). The trial ulnar component is placed along with the elbow hinge and trial humeral prosthesis. An appropriate-sized humeral head is chosen to fit well within the glenoid and allow as much soft tissue reconstruction as possible using any remaining rotator cuff tendons and capsule. At this point, the real modular components are opened and assembled. The ulnar canal is irrigated and dried. A narrow cement gun nozzle or large syringe is used to inject the cement, and the ulnar stem is placed in appropriate rotation. After the cement hardens and all excess is removed, the bushing and pin attachment is placed to connect the modular humeral prosthesis. The reconstruction is placed in approximately 30 to 40 degrees of retroversion at the shoulder. Supplemental support of the humeral head in the glenoid can be obtained by using a rolled mesh along the prosthetic neck or a gortex graft attached circumferentially to the labrum. The rotator cuff and capsule are attached to the holes in the prosthetic humeral head with heavy suture. *In the case of an extra-articular resection, a narrow longitudinal metal spacer is used instead of a round prosthetic humeral head. It is attached with heavy sutures from the holes in the spacer to drill holes in the remaining lateral scapula. When attached in this fashion, there is limited rotation available at the shoulder. In addition, this medializes the humerus, which may result in a prominent acromion process that can be trimmed as necessary for closure* (Figs. 32.4 and 32.5). The muscles previously detached from the humerus (latissimus dorsi, teres major, brachioradialis, flexor/extensor origins) can be wrapped around the prosthesis and sutured to each other. The conjoined tendon is reattached to the coracoid process if necessary. The long head of the biceps is tenodesed at resting length to the surrounding muscles. Deep drains are placed exiting closely in line with the incision. The deltoid and pectoralis are loosely closed together. The proximal deltoid is reattached to the clavicle and acromion if necessary via drill holes. A layered closure is completed and sterile dressings are applied. The patient is placed in a shoulder immobilizer with or without an abduction pillow prior to extubation. Young children can be placed in a shoulder spica cast to maintain immobilization at the shoulder.

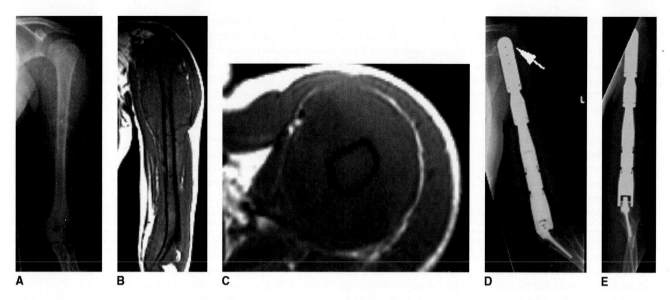

FIGURE 32.4

A: AP radiograph of the left humerus in a 12-year-old girl with osteosarcoma. Note the bone formation around the large proximal soft tissue mass after neoadjuvant chemotherapy. Coronal T1-weighted (**B**) and axial T1-weighted (**C**) MR images showing the extent of the tumor and surrounding soft tissue mass. The tumor invaded the glenohumeral joint and required an extra-articular resection at the shoulder. AP (**D**) and lateral (**E**) postoperative radiographs after resection and reconstruction with a total humeral megaprosthesis and prosthetic elbow replacement. Due to the extra-articular resection, a spacer was fashioned to the proximal humeral body segment (see *arrow*) and attached to the remaining scapula using heavy sutures through drill holes. She died of metastatic disease 3 years later.

Reconstruction with Allograft-Prosthetic Composite (Shoulder) and Osteoarticular Allograft (Elbow)

The fresh-frozen total humeral allograft is thawed in warm saline with or without antibiotics. A standard prosthesis is placed in the proximal end after an appropriate transection of the allograft articular surface. The position of the prosthesis should be 30 to 40 degrees retroverted at the shoulder. The canal is prepared with

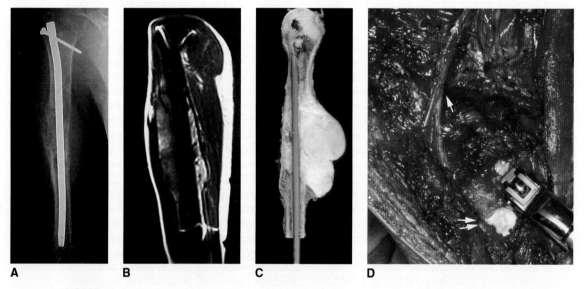

FIGURE 32.5

A: AP radiograph of the right humerus of a 28-year-old woman with osteosarcoma. She was initially misdiagnosed and stabilized with an intramedullary rod, therefore the entire humerus was contaminated. **B**: A T1-weighted MR image with contrast shows the extent of disease and surrounding soft tissue mass. The patient refused an amputation and had neoadjuvant chemotherapy followed by extra-articular total humeral resection and reconstruction. **C:** Gross picture of the involved humerus and intramedullary rod. **D:** Intraoperative view of the defect with the radial nerve exposed (see *arrow*). The radial head is also seen as the prosthesis is pulled out of the way (see *double arrows thicker*).

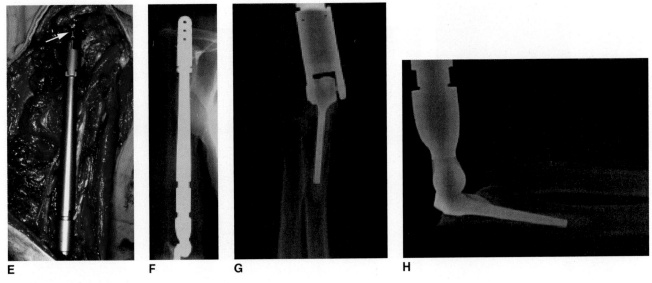

FIGURE 32.5 (*Continued*)

E: Intraoperative view with the total humeral megaprosthesis in place. Note the spacer component at the top of the prosthesis, which is attached to the remaining scapula in the case of an extra-articular resection (see *arrow*). The deltoid was resected and axillary nerve cut due to prior contamination. A latissimus dorsi rotational flap was used for soft tissue coverage. **F:** Postoperative radiograph of the humerus 4 years later shows subluxation of the prosthesis that was painful (inferior subluxation during daily activities). AP (**G**) and lateral (**H**) radiographs of the elbow after 4 years with no sign of loosening.

reamers and broaches to allow for a cement mantle. The rotator cuff tendons and capsule are maintained on the allograft for soft tissue reconstruction to any remaining host tendons and capsule. A cement restrictor does not need to be used if the surgeon prefers to fill the entire humeral allograft with cement to potentially increase resistance to fracture. The distal humeral allograft is fit into the olecranon fossa, which requires an olecranon osteotomy in some cases (Figs. 32.6 and 32.7). The collateral ligaments are balanced and repaired simultaneously from allograft to host ligament on the medial and lateral sides. If any of the ligamentous struc-

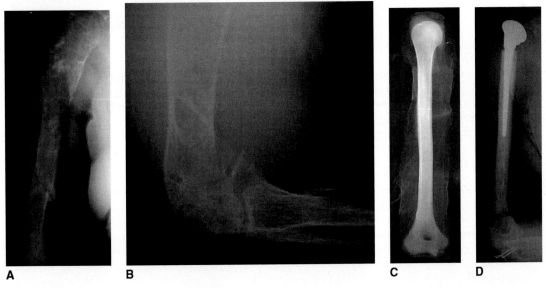

FIGURE 32.6

A: AP radiograph of the right humerus in a 58-year-old man with a grade 2 chondrosarcoma extending the entire length of the bone. **B:** A lateral radiograph of the elbow shows the distal extent of the tumor. **C:** A structural allograft was size matched to fit exactly at the native elbow joint. **D:** A total humeral resection was performed followed by an allograft-prosthetic composite reconstruction at the shoulder and osteoarticular allograft at the elbow. This is the initial postoperative radiograph in 1996. Note that the humeral prosthesis was placed into the diaphysis of the allograft because the allograft was too long. Cement was placed throughout the entire allograft.

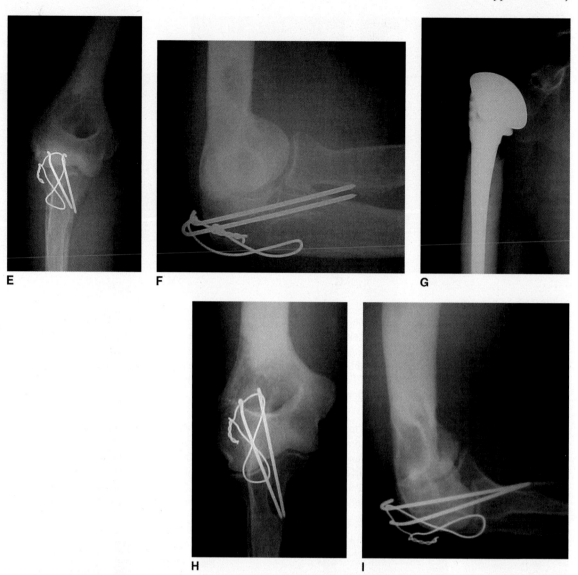

FIGURE 32.6 (Continued)

AP (**E**) and lateral (**F**) postoperative radiographs of the elbow showing the excellent match of the allograft to the native joint. Note that an olecranon osteotomy was performed and repaired with a tension band wire technique. **G:** AP radiograph of the shoulder 5 years after surgery with no loosening and only minimal superior subluxation. AP (**H**) and lateral (**I**) radiographs of the elbow after 5 years with a healed osteotomy and no evidence of degenerative changes.

tures are missing or deficient, attachment of the remaining ligament can be done via drill holes into the bone. Any remaining elbow capsule is repaired as well. If an olecranon osteotomy is performed, it is repaired with a tension band wiring technique. The elbow is put through a gentle range of motion intraoperatively along with testing to varus and valgus stress to assess the soft tissue reconstruction. Postoperatively, the patient is placed into a hinged elbow brace along with immobilization of the shoulder. Gentle passive- and active-assisted elbow range of motion is started immediately. Active range of motion and strengthening are started at 6 weeks.

PEARLS AND PITFALLS

- The indications for a total humeral megaprosthesis are few. Be sure there is not a simpler, more functional reconstruction available that still achieves adequate margins.
- If using a total humeral allograft, match the diameter and length with the host, especially at the elbow joint. Be sure that all ligamentous, tendinous, and capsular attachments remain with the allograft for optimal soft tissue reconstruction.

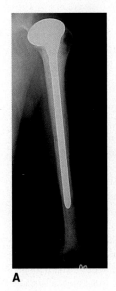 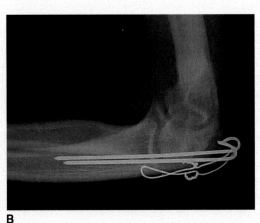 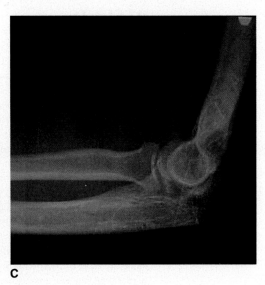

A   **B**   **C**

FIGURE 32.7

A: A postoperative AP radiograph of the left humerus in a patient with osteosarcoma who was reconstructed with an allograft-prosthetic composite at the shoulder and osteoarticular allograft with olecranon osteotomy at the elbow. Note that the shoulder prosthesis is cemented into the allograft. The rotator cuff tendons on the allograft are reattached to the remaining native rotator cuff tendons for an improved repair. **B:** A lateral radiograph of the elbow immediately postoperatively shows the olecranon osteotomy fixed with a tension band wire technique. **C:** A lateral radiograph of the elbow 29 months from surgery after the painful hardware was removed. (Figures 32.7A and 32.7C from Weber KL, Lin PP, Yasko AW. Complex segmental elbow reconstruction after tumor resection. Clin Orthop Rel Res. 2003;415:31-44; with permission).

- Do not allow any undue stretch on the neurovascular structures during resection or reconstruction.
- Use rotational or free flaps for soft tissue defects to minimize the chance of deep infection.

POSTOPERATIVE MANAGEMENT

Intravenous antibiotics are given according to standard protocols. Blood transfusions and electrolyte replacements are given as needed. The patient's shoulder should be immobilized until there is adequate healing of the proximal soft tissue reconstruction. The author prefers 6 weeks in an immobilizer followed by 6 weeks in a simple sling. During the first 6 weeks, the patient can do passive- and active-assisted elbow range of motion exercises as well as normal exercises to strengthen and stretch the wrist and hand. After the shoulder is removed from all immobilization, the patient starts passive shoulder range of motion exercises to regain maximal motion before starting to strengthen the shoulder muscles. The patient is often discharged on postoperative day No. 2. The author prefers that any wound drains be discontinued prior to discharge. If the patient needs postoperative chemotherapy, it is recommended that the incision be allowed to heal first (generally 2 weeks).

COMPLICATIONS

The most common complications after total humeral reconstruction are infection and neurologic injury. Other complications including dislocation or instability of the elbow (after osteoarticular reconstruction) or upper extremity deep venous thrombosis are rare (1,2).

Infection

The deep infection rate for patients with total humeral reconstruction varies from 0% to 9%, although no prosthesis in these series required removal (3,4,2). There was an 11% superficial infection rate in one of the series (4). In the series that involved only elbow prosthetic or allograft reconstruction after tumor resection, there is a 0% to 11% overall infection rate (1,5).

Neurologic Injury

The radial and ulnar nerves are most at risk for injury during a total humeral resection and reconstruction. The majority of injuries are temporary palsies and occur in 8% to 56% of cases (2,3,4). In series that involve isolated elbow reconstruction after tumor resection, the incidence is 11% to 25% (1–3). Traction on the nerves during the procedure is the most likely cause and should be avoided.

RESULTS

The early prosthetic elbow reconstructions were performed for complex fractures of the elbow, degenerative or rheumatoid arthritis, or severe bone loss. These were standard prostheses used in cases that did not involve a segmental tumor resection. However, these initial results led the way for more complex, segmental prosthetic elbow reconstructions to be used after tumor resection.

There are few series in the literature that document the results of total humeral resection and reconstruction. The majority of series focus on prosthetic or allograft elbow reconstruction without involvement of the entire humerus (1,5). The largest series of total humeral reconstruction reports on 12 patients along with 11 additional patients with isolated segmental elbow reconstruction (2). In this series, 15 patients had a primary malignancy, 8 had metastasis or multiple myeloma, and 10 (43%) presented with a pathologic humeral fracture. For the entire series, 74% had local control of their disease at mean follow-up of 34 months. Six patients developed a soft tissue recurrence treated with amputation in two patients and local resection in four patients. Of the 12 patients with a total humeral reconstruction, 7 had a megaprosthesis with prosthetic elbow reconstruction and 5 had humeral allograft reconstruction with an APC at the shoulder and an osteoarticular allograft at the elbow. Of the five patients with osteoarticular elbow reconstruction, two had an olecranon osteotomy fixed with a tension-band technique. The Musculoskeletal Tumor Society (MSTS) score was 70% in patients with a total humeral reconstruction compared to 83% for patients with a segmental elbow reconstruction. The patients with a total humeral reconstruction had decreased range of motion and strength at the shoulder but normal manual dexterity and an elbow arc of motion of 66 to 135 (mean 111) degrees. Eleven of the twelve patients had marked improvement in pain postoperatively. There was stable allograft resorption in two of five patients but no varus or valgus instability at the elbow. One of the two patients with an olecranon osteotomy required removal of painful wires. One of seven patients had osteolysis around the ulnar component of a megaprosthesis (2). Another series that included nine patients with total humeral megaprostheses after tumor resection reported an average of 32 degrees of active shoulder motion in any plane and an elbow arc of motion of 55 to 125 (mean 90) degrees (4). Finally, there was one series that included six children with total humeral reconstruction using expandable megaprostheses (3). There were no infections or prosthetic revisions, but one patient required a forequarter amputation for continued postoperative pain.

REFERENCES

1. Kharrazi FD, Busfield BT, Khorshad DS, et al. Osteoarticular and total elbow allograft reconstruction with severe bone loss. *Clin Orthop Relat Res.* 2008;466:205–209.
2. Weber KL, Lin, PP, Yasko AW. Complex segmental elbow reconstruction after tumor resection. *Clin Orthop Relat Res.* 2003;415:1–14.
3. Ayoub KS, Fiorenza RJ, Grimer RM, et al. Extensible endoprostheses of the humerus after resection of bone tumours. *J Bone Joint Surg Br.* 1999;81:495–500.
4. Ross AC, Sneath RS, Scales JT. Endoprosthetic replacement of the humerus and elbow joint. *J Bone Joint Surg Br.* 1987;69:652–655.
5. Athwal GS, Chin PY, Adams, et al. Coonrad-Morrey total elbow arthroplasty for tumours of the distal humerus and elbow. *J Bone Joint Surg Br.* 2005;87:1369–1374.

33 Shoulder/Humerus: Surgical Treatment for Metastatic Bone Disease

Kristy L. Weber

The previous chapters have focused on the resection of primary bone tumors and reconstruction of the defect or on the issues related to complex revision surgery about the shoulder and humerus. This section is focused on the treatment of patients with metastatic bone disease (MBD) of the humerus, which is the second most common long bone where this occurs. The goals of surgical treatment in patients with MBD are to (a) provide pain relief and (b) restore function. The surgical treatment is palliative rather than curative, and every effort should be made to provide the most durable reconstruction possible so that the terminally ill patient does not have failure of the reconstruction. It should be assumed that the reconstruction will be load-bearing, as pathologic fractures may not heal even with radiation. The surgical concepts often vary from those employed for patients with traumatic humerus fractures. Patients with MBD are at risk for disease progression and resultant continued bone loss, thus necessitating a different approach to surgical fixation.

INDICATIONS

Patient Requirements

- Has a destructive lesion in the humerus with an actual or impending fracture
- Able to tolerate surgery and anesthesia given comorbidities
- Anticipated life span that will make risk/benefit profile worthwhile

Prophylactic Fixation

- High risk of fracture (osteolytic lesion, cortical destruction, histology not responsive to radiation/chemotherapy)
- If patient requires stable upper extremity for weight bearing (i.e., requires crutches or walker due to lower extremity disease) or for bed-to-chair transfers

Fixation of Pathologic Fracture

- Fracture has low chance of healing
- Patient in substantial pain uncontrolled by medication or radiation
- Internal fixation (intramedullary nail) requires unaffected bone at proximal and distal ends of implant to allow durable fixation

Resection of Proximal or Distal Humerus

- No substantial bone remaining in which to anchor internal fixation
- High likelihood of failure of internal fixation
- Solitary metastasis (controversial)

SPECIFIC ANATOMIC CONSIDERATIONS/INDICATIONS

Anatomic Considerations for Fixation/Reconstruction—Proximal Humerus

- Resection and reconstruction with megaprosthesis—when there is not adequate bone for stable fixation with an intramedullary nail
- Locked intramedullary nail extending throughout humerus—if there is adequate proximal and distal bone for fixation

Anatomic Considerations for Fixation/Reconstruction—Humeral Diaphysis

- Locked intramedullary nail extending through the humerus is the most commonly used procedure.
- Intercalary spacer when increased, local control is warranted despite the risk of resection—used with extensive diaphyseal bone loss but intact proximal and distal segments

Anatomic Considerations for Fixation/Reconstruction—Distal Humerus

- Crossed flexible nails inserted from humeral condyles ± methylmethacrylate supplementation—when entire humerus requires some intramedullary support
- Dual plate fixation ± methylmethacrylate supplementation—when a stable construct is required and there are no additional proximal lesions
- Resection and reconstruction with segmental elbow replacement—when there is not adequate bone for distal internal fixation.

CONTRAINDICATIONS

- Patient with limited life span (anticipated length of life does not justify the risks of surgical procedure)
- Small metastatic lesions that have not fractured (especially those that are radiosensitive)
- Minimally displaced fracture that can be easily managed in a sling or clamshell brace (i.e., multiple myeloma often heals with appropriate systemic therapy)
- Extensive comorbidities (pulmonary metastasis) prevent safe general or regional anesthesia

Nonsurgical options for treatment include functional bracing, external beam radiation, bisphosphonates, and radiofrequency ablation.

PREOPERATIVE PREPARATION

Patients with a destructive humeral lesion over the age of 40 years are most likely to have metastatic disease, which is the subject of this chapter. It is important, however, that the workup confirms this diagnosis as primary bone sarcomas occur in the humerus and would be treated quite differently in anticipation of a possible cure (1).

History

- Pain—severity, anatomic location, timing (rest, activity-related, night), radiation of pain, medication requirements, interventions that relieve pain (ice, heat, NSAIDS, sling), duration (days, weeks, months),

and progression (improving, worsening). Pain from a malignancy is often persistent, progressive, and present at rest/night.
- Neurologic symptoms—paresthesias, numbness in the extremity
- Constitutional symptoms—fatigue, loss of appetite, weight loss, fevers, chills
- Symptoms related to common cancers that metastasize to bone—shortness of breath/dyspnea/pleuritic pain/hemoptysis (lung), hematuria/flank pain (kidney), breast mass/pain (breast), urinary frequency/pain (prostate), heat/cold intolerance (thyroid), and change in bowel habits/bleeding (colorectal)
- Recent history related to arm—trauma to arm, appearance of lumps/masses, and new/changed skin lesions
- Personal medical/social/family history—history of cancer (even if remote), prior radiation/chemotherapy, dates of most recent tests (mammogram, colonoscopy, prostate examination, pap smear), smoking history, exposure to chemicals (asbestos), and family history of cancers (breast, colon, etc.)

Physical Examination

- Evaluate for soft tissue masses, tenderness, swelling, decreased range of motion, and neurovascular compromise of arm/shoulder/elbow
- Evaluate for regional lymphadenopathy
- Complete blood count
  - Anemia—advanced metastatic disease, multiple myeloma
  - Leukocytosis—leukemia
- ESR-erythrocyte sedimentation rate/C-reactive protein (elevated with advanced cancer or infection)
- Chemistry panel
  - Hypercalcemia—advanced metastatic disease
  - Abnormal calcium/phosphorus—metabolic bone disease (osteomalacia, hyperparathyroidism, rickets)
  - Elevated alkaline phosphatase—Paget disease
- Urinalysis
  - Microscopic hematuria—renal cell carcinoma
- Protein electrophoresis/Immunofixation
  - Serum/urine studies abnormal in multiple myeloma
- Cancer markers
  - Tests for specific anatomic locations of primary disease (thyroid function tests, prostate specific antigen, CA-125, carcinoembryonic antigen)

Imaging

- Plain radiographs
  - Obtain in two planes
  - Image entire humerus to include shoulder/elbow
  - Lytic (lung, kidney, thyroid, colorectal, myeloma, lymphoma) versus mixed (breast) versus blastic (prostate) lesions
  - Assess cortical involvement and size of lesion
  - Assess quality of uninvolved bone
  - Three-dimensional imaging of the metastatic lesion is not usually necessary
- Computed tomography (CT)
  - Useful for staging disease (chest/abdomen/pelvic CT)
  - Can assess cortical integrity better than plain radiographs (but usually not necessary)
- Magnetic resonance imaging
  - Not usually necessary in the humerus for metastatic disease
- Technetium bone scan
  - Useful for staging studies to assess additional sites of bone metastasis
  - False-negative results in multiple myeloma

Biopsy

- If the surgeon is not 100% confident that the humeral lesion is a metastasis, a biopsy (needle or open) should be performed
- If the patient has known cancer and metastasis to multiple sites including bones, then no biopsy is necessary and treatment can proceed

Management of Comorbidities

Patients with metastatic disease often have multiple comorbidities due to the cancer or their age including hypercalcemia, impending fractures, cervical spine metastasis with potential instability, primary or metastatic lung cancer, and medical problems (hypertension, diabetes, coronary artery disease, peripheral vascular disease).

- Consult with anesthesiology, internal medicine, oncology, and/or cardiology services as needed preoperatively
- If there are known spine metastasis or neck pain, cervical spine imaging is suggested before intubation
- Obtain appropriate preoperative laboratory studies, and type and screen/cross for intraoperative blood products

Embolization

- Consider preoperative embolization for patients with hypervascular metastasis (renal cell carcinoma, thyroid carcinoma, multiple myeloma) if a tourniquet cannot be used. This can be done the day prior to the procedure or the morning of the procedure for optimal results (2).
- As contrast dye is used for the embolization procedure, check for Basal urea and nitrogen/creatinine and discuss with the interventional radiologist if the results are abnormal. This is especially important for patients with metastatic renal cell carcinoma as they frequently have only one functioning kidney.

Equipment Needs

- Intraoperative fluoroscopy (if internal fixation is planned)
- Intramedullary nail versus proximal humeral megaprosthesis versus intercalary spacer versus intramedullary flexible nails versus segmental distal humeral/elbow replacement versus plates/screws
- Methylmethacrylate
- Postoperative sling/immobilizer

Considerations in the Operating Room

- Position and draping
  - For proximal humeral prosthetic reconstruction or antegrade intramedullary nail placement, consider a beach chair position with the patient's head padded and secured
  - For distal humeral reconstruction or retrograde flexible crossed nails, consider a lateral position on a beanbag
  - The patient should be prepped and draped with the entire arm free up to the neck. The patient should be positioned with the arm slightly off the table and secured if fluoroscopy is to be used.
- Preoperative antibiotics should be given as per routine
- Urinary catheter—depending on the length of the planned procedure, expected blood loss, and comorbidities

TECHNIQUE

Proximal Humerus

1. Proximal humeral resection/reconstruction with megaprosthesis (Figs. 33.1 and 33.2)

An anterior approach to the shoulder and humerus is used. Landmarks (coracoid process, acromion, clavicle) should be outlined prior to the incision. The incision is lateral to the true deltopectoral interval as it extends proximally to the superior aspect of the shoulder midway between the coracoid and the lateral aspect of the acromion process. Distally follow the lateral aspect of the biceps as far as necessary toward the elbow, depending on the length of planned humeral resection. The fact that the resection is being performed for metastatic disease means that a wide margin is usually not necessary (radiation is added postoperatively if an intralesional resection is performed). Often the surgeon will want to preserve tissue to improve function, which may lead to positive margins. If a truly wide resection is performed, however, it precludes the need for postoperative radiation and minimizes the chance of local recurrence. The following description presumes that there is a purely *intraosseous* destructive lesion in the proximal humerus and can be modified depending on the anatomic location and extent of any associated soft tissue mass. In general, involvement of the glenoid with metastatic disease is rare, and this section focuses on resection and reconstruction of only the proximal humerus with placement of a humeral head only without a glenoid component.

Develop wide medial and lateral subcutaneous flaps. Expose the deltopectoral interval. If the cephalic vein is maintained, it can be retracted medially or laterally with the deltoid (author prefers laterally). The pectoralis insertion is identified on the humerus, released, and tagged with a cuff of tendon maintained. The deltoid is retracted laterally, and its insertion on the humerus is detached and tagged. Sometimes a portion

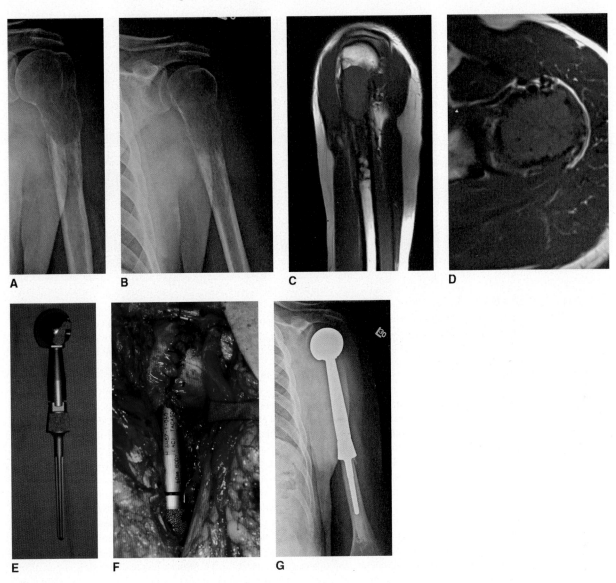

FIGURE 33.1

A: AP and **(B)** lateral radiographs of the left proximal humerus in a 35-year-old man with metastatic pheochromocytoma to a solitary site in the humerus. There is an osteolytic lesion in the metaphysis and upper diaphysis involving the cortex. **C:** Sagittal T1-weighted and **(D)** axial T1-weighted MR images of the proximal humerus lesion demonstrate the extensive nature of the lesion. Given the solitary site of disease and relative resistance to chemotherapy and radiation, the patient's primary tumor was removed followed by resection of the proximal humeral metastasis. **E:** Reconstruction was performed using a proximal humeral megaprosthesis. Note the porous-coated segment adjacent to the host humeral bone. Note the holes in the head of the prosthesis used to reattach the rotator cuff muscles. **F:** Intraoperative view showing the soft tissue reconstruction completely covering the prosthetic head and neck. **G:** Postoperative radiograph after 5 months. Note that the prosthetic head is well located in the glenoid with no subluxation.

of this attachment can be maintained for shorter humeral resections. For patients with an extensive proximal soft tissue mass, the deltoid can be released from the clavicle and acromion as far as the lateral acromion to increase exposure. The anterior humeral circumflex vessels are ligated and tied. This may cause some devascularization of the anterior deltoid, but it usually maintains viability with collateral flow. The conjoined tendon (short head of the biceps and coracobrachialis) originates at the coracoid process and is gently retracted medially. Do not abduct the arm or this will pull the axillary sheath toward the coracoid process. The musculocutaneous nerve is most likely to be injured if dissection occurs in this position. If additional exposure is necessary, the short head of the biceps and coracobrachialis are detached with a cuff of tendon and tagged. If the coracoacromial ligament can be maintained, it will help prevent superior subluxation of the humeral prosthesis. The teres major and latissimus dorsi are released from the humerus and tagged. The subscapularis is released from the humerus and tagged. Beware the axillary nerve as it exits through the quadrangular space inferior to the subscapularis. The long head of the biceps is identified and released distal to its origin on the glenoid and tagged.

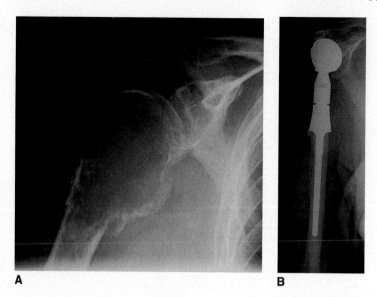

FIGURE 33.2

A: An AP radiograph of the right shoulder in a 65-year-old woman with metastatic melanoma that completely destroys the humeral head and neck. There is no option for intramedullary fixation in this case, so a resection and prosthetic reconstruction was performed. **B:** An AP radiograph of the right humerus 30 months postoperatively with the prosthesis in good position.

The planned transaction of the humerus is marked and circumferential subperiosteal dissection is performed at this level. Maintain as much biceps and brachialis as possible in the setting of metastatic disease. Identify and protect the radial nerve within the spiral groove. At this point, the remaining proximal dissection can be completed (shoulder capsule, rotator cuff) or the humerus can be cut and elevated from the wound (author prefers the latter). Prior to humeral transection, the anterior cortex should be marked with an osteotome and marking pen to allow appropriate rotational placement of the prosthesis. Next, the triceps are released posteriorly. Proximally, the supraspinatus, infraspinatus, and teres minor are released as close as possible to the greater tuberosity and tagged with long sutures as they will retract. The shoulder joint capsule is incised as close as possible to the humeral head and neck to facilitate a stable soft tissue reconstruction. The proximal humerus is then delivered from the wound with careful dissection of the axillary nerve and posterior humeral circumflex vessels posteriorly. A distal marrow margin can be checked by frozen section if a wide resection is planned.

New gowns, gloves, instruments, and drapes can be used for the reconstruction, although it is not strictly necessary when dealing with metastatic disease. The distal humeral canal is reamed to allow placement of a cemented humeral stem (author prefers 2 mm overream). The longest available stem should be used to protect the remainder of the humeral diaphysis from additional metastasis. A planer reamer is used to facilitate a tight fit of the prosthesis to the distal humerus. The canal is irrigated and dried. The modular proximal humeral trial component is assembled to replace the resection length. The humeral head is sized and selected for appropriate fit within the remaining glenoid. The trial is placed to be sure there is no tension on the neurovascular structures. It is better to be slightly short rather than too long. The real assembled prosthesis is then cemented into the distal humerus with the humeral head in 30 to 40 degrees of retroversion.

The soft tissue reconstruction is performed to cover the exposed prosthesis and maximize shoulder function (Fig. 33.1F). After the wound is irrigated, supplemental support of the humeral head against the glenoid can be achieved by using a mesh rolled into a tube, wrapped around the neck of the prosthesis, and sewed into the anterior and posterior labrum. Other options include a mesh or gortex graft to cover the entire prosthetic head with circumferential attachment to the labrum. Most proximal humeral prostheses have holes/grooves within the humeral head to allow reattachment of the capsule or rotator cuff tendons. Depending on how much of these structures remain, they can be reattached with large sutures or tapes. If a large abduction pillow is planned as part of the postoperative immobilization, the soft tissue reconstruction should be done with the arm in the appropriate amount of abduction. Deep drains are placed. The long head of the biceps tendon is reattached to the short head of the biceps at resting length. The muscles previously detached from the humerus (latissimus dorsi, teres major, distal deltoid) can be reattached to each other around the prosthesis or sutured around the prosthesis itself. Proximally, the deltoid origin and conjoined tendons are reattached if necessary. The deltopectoral interval is loosely closed. The remaining layered closure is performed and the skin closure should be performed knowing that radiation may be used postoperatively.

Prior to extubation, the patient's arm should be sterilely dressed and placed in an immobilizer with or without an abduction pillow. Depending on the patient's medical condition, he/she can often be discharged on postoperative day 2. There is not good evidence available to suggest how long intravenous postoperative

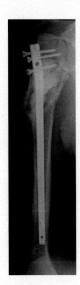

FIGURE 33.3

Postoperative radiograph of the right humerus in a 65-year-old man with metastatic renal cell carcinoma. For this proximal lesion, intramedullary fixation was used with extra proximal screws and methylmethacrylate for additional fixation.

antibiotics should be given in patients with large prosthetic reconstructions after tumor resection, so the surgeon should review the literature and use his/her judgment. The postoperative rehabilitation varies widely in the literature. Physical therapy is usually started in the immediate postoperative period focused on elbow, wrist, and hand motion. Shoulder motion is initially avoided. Generally, a period of at least 6 weeks in a shoulder immobilizer is used to allow the soft tissue reconstruction to heal (author prefers 6 weeks of a strict immobilizer followed by 6 weeks in a sling with minimal shoulder motion). After the period of immobilization is over, physical therapy is instituted to regain passive shoulder motion followed by active shoulder motion and strengthening.

2. Locked intramedullary nail (Fig. 33.3)

Placement of a locked humeral intramedullary nail in a patient with an impending or actual proximal humeral fracture secondary to metastatic disease requires enough bone present in the humeral head and neck to achieve satisfactory fixation with the nail and interlocking screws. Nail systems are available with the option of placing up to four proximal screws at various angles to maximize fixation.

The patient is semireclined in a beach chair position on a radiolucent table with the affected shoulder and arm positioned slightly off the table to facilitate intraoperative fluoroscopic views. An anterolateral incision is made from the tip of the acromion and extended distally 2 to 3 cm. Extending the incision ≥5 cm puts the axillary nerve at risk for injury. The lateral deltoid is split in line with the skin incision to expose the subdeltoid bursa, and the supraspinatus is incised in line with its fibers. The entrance point for the humeral nail is just medial to the greater tuberosity (some nail systems allow for a central insertion directly through the humeral head articular surface). Fluoroscopic guidance is used throughout the case. After an entrance hole is made with an awl or a Steinman pin, a guide wire is placed along the length of the humerus while the fracture (if present) is reduced. Measurement of the length of the humerus is performed and an appropriate size reamed or unreamed nail is placed (the author prefers to ream 1 mm over the nail size and place the largest nail possible). There are both solid and hollow right/left nails available from different manufacturers. The nail should extend along the entire length of the humerus. For proximal lesions, up to four screws are placed to achieve maximal stabilization. These can be locking or nonlocking screws, but care should be taken when drilling the far cortex to avoid penetration of the glenohumeral joint or damage to the axillary nerve as it courses around the humeral neck. The fixation can be augmented with methylmethacrylate and/or washers, but this requires a larger surgical incision to place the cement. In cases of actual fractures, one to two distal interlocking screws are also placed to achieve rotational stability (the author stably locks impending fractures as well). To avoid neurovascular damage in the distal arm, a 2 to 4 cm incision is made longitudinally over the anterior interlocking holes with careful dissection of the deep structures until bone can be directly visualized. Fluoroscopic views are used to check the position of the hardware before irrigation of the wounds and closure. A sling is used for comfort. The patient can start gentle range of motion exercises on postoperative day 1 and progress as tolerated. If there is a fracture, heavy lifting or whole body weight bearing should be minimized initially. Postoperative radiation is used to treat the entire length of the nail (POD 10–14).

Humeral Diaphysis

1. Locked intramedullary nail (Figs. 33.4–33.6)

The procedure is that described above for proximal humeral lesions/fractures except that >2 proximal interlocking screws are not usually necessary.

2. Humeral intercalary spacer

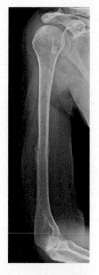

FIGURE 33.4

An AP radiograph of the right humerus in a 63-year-old woman with widely metastatic breast cancer. She has a pathologic nondisplaced diaphyseal fracture and substantial pain despite prior radiation to this site. Because she has extensive lower extremity metastasis, she decided on intramedullary fixation of the humerus fracture so that she could bear weight on her right arm.

FIGURE 33.5

A: An AP radiograph of the right humerus in a 49-year-old man with metastatic thyroid cancer. There are multiple osteolytic lesions throughout the bone. **B:** Given the vascular nature of thyroid cancer, the lesions were embolized preoperatively. **C:** A postoperative radiograph after stabilization of the impending fractures with an intramedullary locked humeral nail. A nondisplaced fracture through the mid-diaphyseal lesion occurred during the procedure.

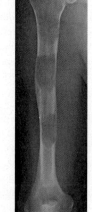 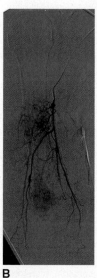 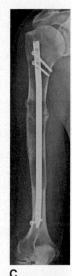

A   B   C

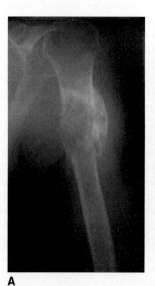 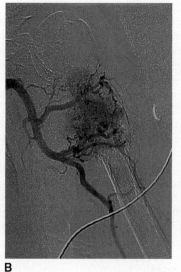 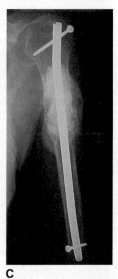

A   B   C

FIGURE 33.6

A: An AP radiograph of the left humerus in a 55-year-old man with metastatic renal cell carcinoma and a pathologic fracture. **B:** Renal metastasis can be extremely vascular and preoperative embolization is often warranted. **C:** Postoperative radiograph after curettage and cementation of the lesion and stabilization with an intramedullary locked humeral nail (the nail was placed prior to the cement).

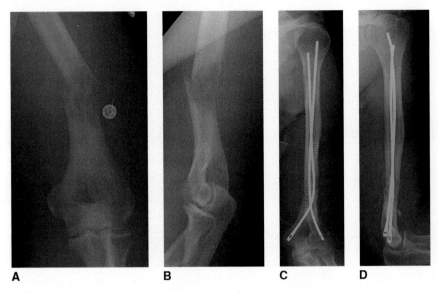

FIGURE 33.7

AP (**A**) and lateral (**B**) radiographs of the left distal humerus in a 53-year-old man with metastatic poorly differentiated papillary thyroid cancer and a pathologic fracture. The patient was treated with flexible Enders nails inserted from the medial and lateral humeral condyles. The lesion was initially curetted and later cemented after the hardware was placed. AP (**C**) and lateral (**D**) postoperative radiographs show the nails extending into the humeral neck to help stabilize the entire bone. The patient received postoperative radiation to the entire humerus.

For specific cases of solitary bone metastasis occurring in the mid-diaphysis, a resection may be indicated, which would allow placement of this spacer (3). The author has used this device several times for resection of diaphyseal renal cell carcinoma metastasis, which allows local control for relatively radioresistant lesions. It can also be used for salvage in cases when a lesion (such as renal cell carcinoma) has progressed extensively around the diaphysis of a humeral nail. The technique is described in Chapter 32 by T. Damron.

Distal Humerus

- Crossed flexible nails (Fig. 33.7)

The benefits of using flexible crossed nails are that (a) they are inserted distally to stabilize lesions that are too distal for anterograde humeral nail, and (b) some stabilization of the entire humerus is achieved. This technique can be attempted in a closed fashion with the use of postoperative radiation of the entire humerus to achieve disease control. In most cases, however, an open exposure of the lesion or fracture is performed with curettage of the lesion, placement of the flexible nails, reduction of the fracture, and cementation of the osteolytic area. For stable fixation, it is important to use the widest diameter of nails possible, but this occasionally leads to an intraoperative fracture through the metastatic lesion. Flexible nail sizes range from 3.0 to 4.5 mm in diameter. Care must be taken to avoid damage to the ulnar nerve when placing the medial flexible nail. The nails are inserted through a minimal incision (5 to 10 mm) over the medial and lateral epicondyles. Fluoroscopic guidance is used to confirm the length of the nails. The surgical approach to the distal humeral lesion in cases of open procedures can be done with the patient lateral or prone on the operating table. A triceps splitting approach is used most frequently to expose the lesion. If there is no fracture, or if the fracture fixation is supplemented with methylmethacrylate, the patient can begin early motion of the elbow postoperatively and commence gradual strengthening as tolerated.

- Dual plate fixation (Figs. 33.8 and 33.9)

This reconstructive technique can be used for distal humeral metastasis to stabilize the elbow, but its limitations include the possibility of pathologic humeral fracture proximal to the reconstruction. The patient is positioned prone or lateral on the operating table and the entire extremity is prepared. A triceps splitting approach is made to the posterior supracondylar humerus. The ulnar nerve is isolated and protected along the medial condyle. The metastatic lesion is exposed and curetted to remove all gross disease. A reduction is achieved in the case of fracture using K-wires for provisional fixation. The osteolytic defect can be filled with cement before or after the plates and screws are in place. An olecranon osteotomy has been described to improve visualization of the elbow joint, but this is usually not necessary. The plates are positioned posterolateral followed by medial, as the double plating technique strengthens the fixation. The plates are generally 3.5 mm distal humeral compression plates, although some surgeons prefer pelvic reconstruction plates. A combination of locking and nonlocking screws can be used. The posterolateral plate functions as a tension band during elbow flexion, and the medial

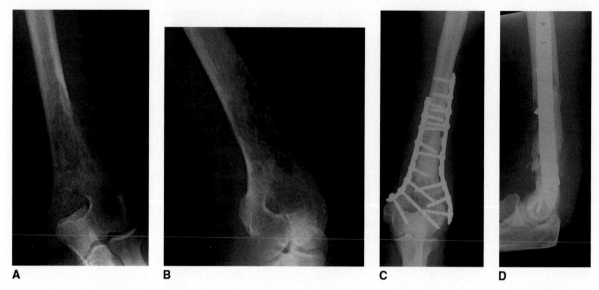

FIGURE 33.8

AP (**A**) and lateral (**B**) radiographs of the left distal humerus in a 70-year-old woman with metastatic uterine cancer and an impending fracture. It was felt to be too distal to achieve stable fixation with an anterograde nail, and she had no additional humeral lesions. Postoperative AP (**C**) and lateral (**D**) radiographs after double plating of the distal humerus impending fracture. The reconstruction was supplemented with methylmethacrylate.

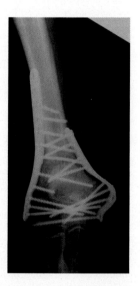

FIGURE 33.9

This is another postoperative example of a double plating technique in a patient with metastatic lung cancer. The most distal screws cross the condyles distal to the olecranon fossa.

plate supports the medial column of the distal humerus. The plates are stainless steel or titanium. Newer plates have tapered ends and limited contact to better preserve the periosteal blood supply of the bone. If the reconstruction is stable intraoperatively, an early return to function is preferred with range of motion exercises started on postoperative day 1. Postoperative radiation is used 10 to 14 days after the surgery to minimize the chance of local recurrence.

- Resection and reconstruction with segmental total elbow prosthesis (Fig. 33.10)

This is an aggressive approach for patients with MBD and is warranted in patients with severe bone loss in the distal humerus and condyles. As the implants are modular, they are fashioned to fit the amount of individual bone loss and resection. Please refer to the chapters by Weber and Morrey for specific details on complicated prosthetic reconstruction of the elbow (Chapters 35 and 34).

PEARLS AND PITFALLS

- Appropriate indications are paramount. Upper extremity pathologic fractures often heal with or without radiation. Patients who require upper extremity use for ambulation or have excessive pain from the lesion or fracture and who have a reasonable remaining life span may benefit from surgical stabilization of the humerus.

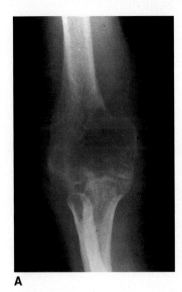
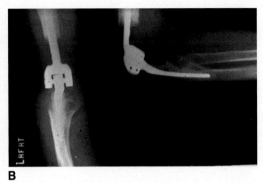

A   **B**

FIGURE 33.10

A: AP radiograph demonstrating extensive destruction of the distal humeral condyles from MBD. **B:** A resection of the distal humerus was performed with reconstruction using an early generation distal humeral prosthesis with total elbow replacement.

- A proximal humeral resection and reconstruction is performed for pain control or to achieve definitive local control, as shoulder function is limited postoperatively.
- Oncologic techniques should be used rather than basic fracture techniques. These include stabilization of the entire humerus, use of methylmethacrylate to supplement the fixation, and postoperative radiation of the entire bone. Tumor progression will cause failure of standard fixation. It is important to achieve durable, long-standing fixation for patients with MBD and limited life spans (1,4–6)
- Stably lock all humeral nails as patients can develop a postoperative fracture and fixation failure from disease progression around the nail (7).

POSTOPERATIVE MANAGEMENT

This has been addressed at the end of each technique section. In general, the patient can start immediate mobilization and return to function with intramedullary fixation or distal humeral reconstruction. The proximal humeral prosthetic reconstruction requires a period of immobilization (6 to 12 weeks) to allow healing of the soft tissue reconstruction and minimize superior subluxation of the humerus.

COMPLICATIONS

This chapter covers multiple procedures for patients with humeral bone metastasis. Most of the existing literature includes the treatment of primary malignancies of bone with MBD, and this makes it difficult to separate the results. Patients with MBD tend to be older than those with primary bone tumors and often do not require a wide resection of the tumor prior to reconstruction. The complications of patients with primary bone tumors and those with metastatic disease are, therefore, often different.

- Infection

The occurrence of infection after intramedullary fixation of humeral metastatic disease is negligible. There is a 0% to 5% infection rate after proximal humeral resection and prosthetic reconstruction in patients with all types of bone tumors (8–11). Cannon et al. reported two deep infections in 83 proximal humeral prosthetic reconstructions.

- Neurologic injury

The radial nerve is primarily at risk with upper extremity reconstructions for bone metastasis. The risk of nerve injury ranges from 0% to 12% after prosthetic reconstruction of the proximal humerus (8,9,12,13). Thai et al. (12) reported a 6% incidence of radial nerve palsy after intramedullary fixation for humeral metastasis.

- Subluxation of a proximal humeral megaprosthesis (Fig. 33.11)

Subluxation is not clearly defined when comparing studies of proximal humeral prosthetic reconstruction, although a range from 9% to 56% is noted (8,11–15). Overall, this complication is common and well tolerated,

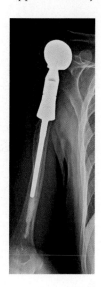

FIGURE 33.11

An AP radiograph of the right proximal humerus of a 33-year-old man who had resection of the proximal humerus for an extensive hemangioendothelioma of bone 5 years earlier. The patient has no pain, but he has limited shoulder motion to 30 to 40 degrees in most planes. Note the superior subluxation of the prosthesis that has occurred over time.

as most patients do not complain of pain. Cannon et al. (8) found 22 of 83 patients with superior migration of the prosthesis, which correlated with the length of follow-up. They noted there was no skin breakdown over the prosthesis, and only one patient had a revision for subluxation.

- Pain

There are few studies that report on this specific outcome after humeral reconstruction for bone metastasis. Thai et al. (12) reported that 8% of patients had residual pain after intramedullary humeral fixation, and 13% had continued pain after prosthetic reconstruction of the proximal humerus.

RESULTS

As described in the Complications section, it is difficult to separate the results of patients with humeral reconstruction or stabilization for metastasis from those treated for primary bone tumors. The surgical approach and goals in these two populations are different as is the expected postoperative life span. For patients with metastatic tumors to the proximal humerus and extensive bone destruction, an *intra-articular* resection with prosthetic reconstruction is performed, but a patient with a primary bone tumor might be indicated for an extra-articular resection in order to achieve an appropriate margin. Patients with bone metastasis often have a mean survival of approximately 12 months, depending on the primary site of disease (13,16).

Proximal humeral resection and prosthetic reconstruction are infrequently used for patients with MBD, as intramedullary fixation with methylmethacrylate is used whenever possible to maintain the glenohumeral joint. Overall, the goals of this reconstruction are pain relief and maintenance of elbow, wrist, and hand function. The postoperative shoulder function is uniformly quite poor with mean abduction and forward flexion approximately 45 degrees or less (8,9,11). Mean Musculoskeletal Tumor Society scores for function postoperatively range from 65 to 75 points (8,9,10,15). The overall loosening and revision rate ranges from 0% to 8%, and most patients die before these complications occur (8,9,12,15,17). Jeys et al. (17) reported an 84% 10-year survival of the prosthesis in 103 patients, but those with metastatic disease died much earlier than the nonmetastatic patients. Kumar et al. have the largest series of 100 proximal humeral prosthetic reconstructions, and they found no difference in functional outcome in patients whose axillary nerve was resected compared to those in whom it was maintained (9).

Thai et al. (12) reported on 96 patients with treatment of humeral bone metastasis using a variety of reconstructive techniques. Only 50% of the patients were alive at 8 months. The metastatic lesions were located in the proximal humerus in 47%, diaphysis in 42%, and distal humerus in 11% with 56% of patients presenting with pathologic fractures. Intramedullary fixation was used in 51 cases with or without methylmethacrylate, while a proximal humeral prosthetic reconstruction was used in 22 cases.

REFERENCES

1. Weber KL, Lewis VO, Randall L, et al. An approach to the management of the patient with metastatic bone disease. *Instr Course Lect Ser*. 2004;53:663–676.
2. Chatziioannou AN, Johnson ME, Penumaticos SG, et al. Preoperative embolization of bone metastases from renal cell carcinoma. *Eur J Radiol*. 2000;10:593–596.
3. Damron TA, Sim FH, Shives TC, et al. Intercalary spacers in the treatment of segmentally destructive diaphyseal humeral lesions in disseminated malignancies. *Clin Orthop*. 1996;324:233–243.
4. Frassica FJ, Frassica DA. Metastatic bone disease of the humerus. *J Am Acad Orthop Surg*. 2003;11:282–288.

5. Harrington KD, Sim FH, Enis JE, et al. Methylmethacrylate as an adjunct in internal fixation of pathologic fractures. *J Bone Joint Surg.* 1976;58(8):1047–1055.

6. Townsend P, Smalley S, Cozad S. Role of postoperative radiation therapy after stabilization of fractures caused by metastatic disease. *Int J Radiat Oncol Biol Phys.* 1995;31:43.

7. Yazawa Y, Frassica FJ, Chao EY, et al. Metastatic bone disease: a study of the surgical treatment of 166 pathologic humeral and femoral fractures. *Clin Orthop.* 1990;251:213–219.

8. Cannon CP, Paraliticci GU, Lin PP, et al. Functional outcome following endoprosthetic reconstruction of the proximal humerus. *Elsevier.* 2009;18:705–710.

9. Kumar D, Grimer RJ, Abudu A, et al. Endoprosthetic replacement of the proximal humerus. Long-term results. *J Bone Joint Surg Br.* 2003;85(5):717–722.

10. Naill RW, Gosheger G, Geber C, et al. Reconstruction of the proximal humerus after wide resection of tumors. *J Bone Joint Surg Br.* 2002;84-B:1004–1008.

11. Ross AC, Wilson JN, Scales JT. Endoprosthetic replacement of the proximal humerus. *J Bone Joint Surg Br.* 1987;69(4):656–661.

12. Thai DM, Kitagawa Y, Choong PF. Outcome of surgical management of bony metastases to the humerus and shoulder girdle: a retrospective analysis of 93 patients. *Inter Seminars Surg Oncol.* 2006;3:5.

13. Eckardt JJ, Kabo M, Kelly CM, et al. Endoprosthetic reconstruction for bone metastases. *Clin Orthop.* 2003;S254–S262.

14. Asavamongkolkul A, Eckardt JJ, Eilber FR, et al. Endoprosthetic reconstruction for malignant upper extremity tumors. *Clin Orthop Relat Res.* 1999;360:207–220.

15. Potter BK, Adams SC, Pitcher JD, et al. Proximal humerus reconstructions for tumors. *Clin Orthop Relat Res.* 2009;467:1035–1041.

16. Sugiura H, Yamada K, Sugiura T, et al. Predictors of survival in patients with bone metastasis of lung cancer. *Clin Orthop Relat Res.* 2008;466:729–736.

17. Jeys LM, Kulkarni A, Grimer RJ, et al. Endoprosthetic reconstruction for the treatment of musculoskeletal tumors of the appendicular skeleton and pelvis. J bone Joint Surg. 2008;90(6):1265–1271.

34 General Considerations: Elbow and Wrist

Kristy L. Weber

The elbow and wrist are uncommon areas for metastatic bone disease and primary bone or soft tissue sarcomas. Large series of limb salvage procedures in these areas are not available. For primary bone and soft tissue sarcomas, multidisciplinary treatment with surgical resection, radiation and/or chemotherapy is used to maximize local control. For metastatic disease, the goal is to maintain function of the upper extremity for activities of daily living, and each case is individualized as to the surgical and nonsurgical options. The following chapters review the use of allografts and metal prostheses around the elbow for oncologic and non-oncologic scenarios. Osteoarticular (OA) allografts for distal radius tumors are also reviewed, and options for treatment of metastatic disease around the elbow and wrist are outlined.

INDICATIONS

- Primary bone/soft tissue sarcomas that involve the elbow or wrist are indicated for wide resection (Figure 34-1).
- Reconstruction of the elbow can be performed with an OA allograft, alloprosthetic composite, or a megaprosthesis (Figure 34-2).
- Reconstruction of the wrist can be performed with an OA allograft to preserve motion or an allograft arthrodesis to avoid the complications at the joint surface.
- Metastatic disease about the elbow or wrist (with or without a pathologic fracture) is indicated for internal fixation and methylmethacrylate if enough bone remains to achieve a stable reconstruction.
- Modular elbow replacement can be used for solitary metastatic disease around the elbow or if there is massive bone loss that requires a prosthetic reconstruction.

CONTRAINDICATIONS

- Patients with primary bone/soft tissue sarcomas and involvement of the neurovascular bundle about the elbow or wrist are not indicated for limb salvage.
- Patients with growth of a primary sarcoma about the elbow or wrist on chemotherapy or radiation are not indicated for limb salvage.
- Patients with a nonfunctional hand or lack of motor function to flex the elbow are not indicated for elbow reconstruction.
- Patients with metastatic bone disease and a limited lifespan who can be treated with nonoperative modalities such as radiation and/or immobilization are not indicated for surgery.
- Patients with an active infection of the elbow or wrist are contraindicated for a prosthetic or allograft reconstruction.

IMAGING

Plain radiographs can document obvious bone destruction about the elbow and wrist. Obtain views of the entire humerus and forearm in case there are additional sites of disease that need to be managed. These plain films are used to size match and template allografts and prostheses. Magnetic resonance imaging best outlines the extent of the bone and soft tissue disease and the relationship to surrounding neurovascular structures. Other imaging modalities (CT and technetium bone scan) are used to stage patients for evaluation of possible additional sites of disease.

ANATOMIC CONSIDERATIONS

Elbow

The complexity around the elbow arises from the close proximity of the neurovascular structures, stabilizing ligaments, and muscle origins and insertions, all of which play a key role in normal function of the arm. The *brachial artery* lies between the biceps and brachialis in the distal arm. It enters the cubital fossa on the brachialis just lateral to the median nerve and then splits into the radial and ulnar arteries. The *radial artery* passes medial to the biceps tendon and runs down the forearm under the brachioradialis. The *ulnar artery* passes deep to the pronator teres, which separates it from the median nerve. It runs down the forearm on the radial side of the ulnar nerve. The *median nerve* is covered by the bicipital aponeurosis as it crosses the medial side of the cubital fossa. It travels between the two heads of the pronator teres and runs down the forearm on the deep surface of the flexor digitorum superficialis. The *ulnar nerve* crosses the elbow posteromedially in the ulnar groove of the medial epicondyle. It crosses to the anterior elbow between the two heads of the flexor carpi ulnaris and runs down the forearm on the anterior surface of the flexor digitorum profundus. The *radial nerve* is found between the brachialis and the brachioradialis and divides into the posterior interosseous nerve at the level of the elbow joint where it enters the supinator. It also divides into the superficial radial nerve which runs into the forearm under the brachioradialis. The *flexor* muscles of the forearm originate on the medial epicondyle of the distal humerus, and the *extensor* muscles of the forearm originate on the lateral epicondyle.

Wrist

The median nerve lies in the carpal tunnel on the volar surface of the carpus. The flexor retinaculum forms the roof over the nerve. The ulnar nerve runs down the forearm under the flexor carpi ulnaris, is ulnar to the artery, and is eventually enclosed in Guyon's canal at the wrist. The radial artery is radial to the flexor carpi radialis at the wrist and easily palpable.

SURGICAL CONSIDERATIONS

Most cases about the elbow can be performed with tourniquet control, thus embolization is not required. Fluoroscopy may be necessary for stabilization of pathologic fractures. For resection about the elbow, the patient is usually supine with the arm extended on a table or crossed over the chest, depending on which approach is used. For resection of the distal humerus followed by total elbow reconstruction with an allograft or a prosthesis, an anterior approach is generally used but might vary in exact location depending on the extraosseous extent of the tumor. Wide flaps are raised, and the neurovascular structures are protected throughout the case. If a constrained or modular prosthesis is used, the medial and lateral ligamentous structures are sacrificed. If an OA allograft is used, the ligamentous structures are saved if possible for appropriate tensioning to the allograft tissues. For stabilization of metastatic disease in the distal humerus, a posterior triceps-splitting approach is

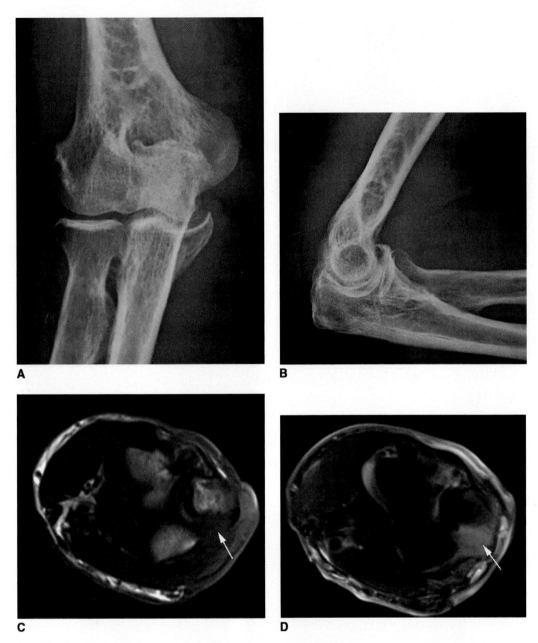

FIGURE 34.1

AP (**A**) and lateral (**B**) radiographs of the elbow in a 56-year-old man with a high-grade soft-tissue sarcoma involving the joint and no evidence of metastasis. T1-weighted (**C**) and T2-weighted (**D**) axial MR images show involvement of the ulna and joint by tumor (*arrows*). The patient had preoperative radiation followed by surgical resection and prosthetic elbow reconstruction.

expedient and allows placement of flexible nails, plates/screws, and methylmethacrylate without substantial risk to neurovascular structures. For tumors around the wrist, a dorsal incision is used but can be modified depending on the location of the tumor (Figure 34-3). The distal ulna remains intact with ligamentous attachments to the carpus. Often the pronator quadratus is taken as a margin over the volar extension of tumor. An OA allograft used to reconstruct the distal radius must be sized appropriately to avoid a mismatch that does not line up well with the native carpus.

COMPLICATIONS

Major complications associated with resection and reconstruction around the elbow include neurologic compromise, infection, allograft nonunion, prosthetic loosening, stiffness, and pain. The neurologic complications are usually traction-related and temporary. Aseptic loosening of an elbow prosthesis is less clinically relevant

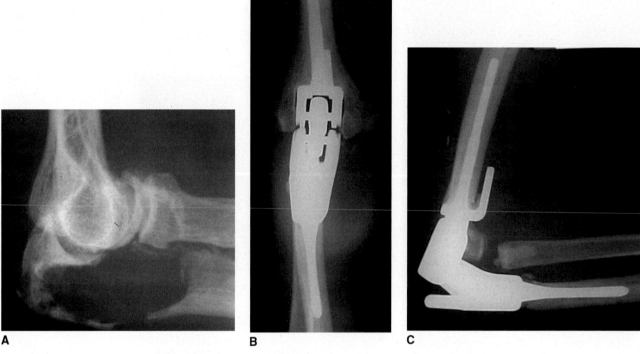

FIGURE 34.2

A: Lateral radiograph of the elbow in a 61-year-old man with multiple myeloma involving the proximal ulna and a pathologic fracture. There was a large surrounding soft tissue mass, and the patient had difficulty performing daily activities. He had no other symptomatic areas of disease. AP (**B**) and lateral (**C**) radiographs two years after prosthetic elbow reconstruction with a modular proximal ulnar component.

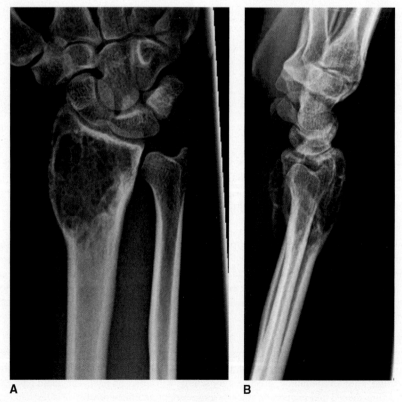

FIGURE 34.3

AP (**A**) and lateral (**B**) radiographs of a 32-year-old woman with a distal radius giant cell tumor. Coronal

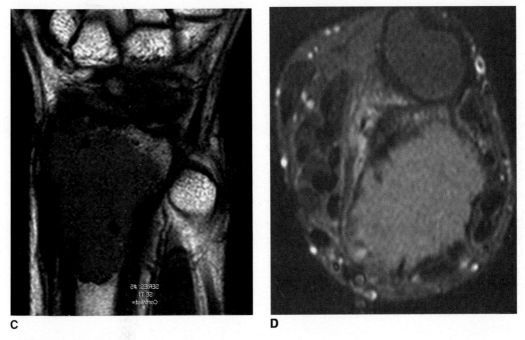

FIGURE 34.3 (*Continued*)

(**C**) and axial (**D**) MR images reveal expansion of the cortex. Some surgeons would treat this with intralesional curettage and others with resection and allograft reconstruction. (Figures 34.A, C, and D from Weber KL, Lin PP, Yasko AW. Complex segmental elbow reconstruction after tumor resection. Clin Orthop Rel Res. 2003;415:31-44).

than lower extremity prosthetic loosening given the lesser weightbearing demand on the arms. Complications that occur during resection and reconstruction about the wrist include rare neurologic deficits, stiffness, and pain. Known problems with OA allografts include joint degeneration, graft resorption, instability, nonunion, and fracture.

35 Massive Bone Loss About the Elbow

Bernard F. Morrey and Joaquin Sanchez-Sotelo

Because the elbow is a subcutaneous joint and vulnerable to trauma and infection and less so malignant conditions, massive loss of bone and soft tissue about the elbow is relatively common and constitutes a devastating problem (1). This probably represents the most challenging of all interventions about the elbow. The salvage treatment is either implant or nonimplant salvage (2–5).

INDICATIONS

- Bone loss proximal to the olecranon fossa or distal to the coronoid
- Motivated patient

CONTRAINDICATIONS

- Active or acute sepsis
- Prior sepsis with potential to be subacute (exclude with staged procedure)
- Absence of neural function of the hand
- Absence of potential to flex the elbow if reconstructed
- Deficiency of soft tissue coverage, until adequately addressed, if possible
- Inability of patient to cooperate

IMPLANT SALVAGE OPTIONS

The implant salvage option may be either a prosthetic or an allograft replacement. In fact, the most efficient way of managing massive bone loss at the elbow is an allograft prosthetic composite (APC). In recent years, we have refined our thought process and clinical experience and feel as though reliable APC options are now available even for the most devastating circumstances (5).

NONPROSTHETIC MANAGEMENT

The basic approach to nonprosthetic management is that of stabilizing the forearm referable to the humerus. This is often done in the acute setting using an external fixator with the intent to achieve a resection arthroplasty that may have some stability due to the scar tissue. This is usually indicated in instances of gross or refractory infection but the outcome is highly unpredictable and thus is truly the final salvage option (6).

RECONSTRUCTION OPTIONS

There are four forms of functional reconstruction: osteoarticular allograft, allograft augmentation, impaction grafting, and allograft prosthetic composite. We regularly employ two methods of reconstructing massive bone loss at the elbow: allograft augmentation, that is, the use of struts and APC. Impaction cancellous grafting is used when there is adequate circumferential albeit expanded, cortex available and is not discussed here (1,7).

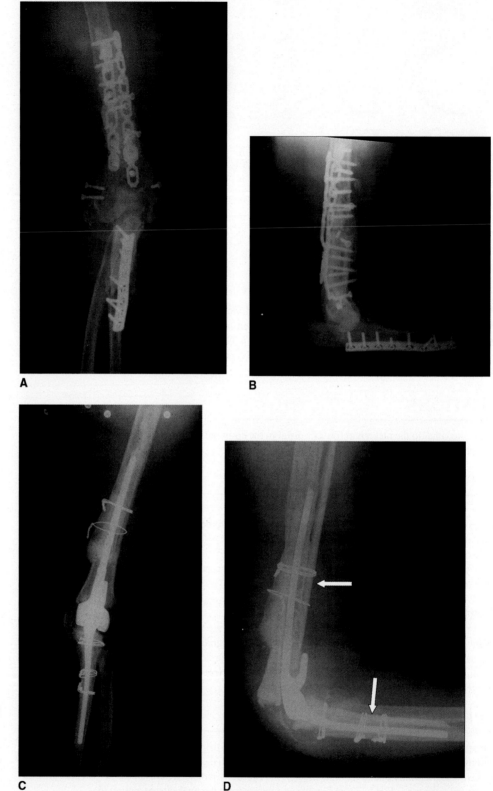

FIGURE 35.1

An osteoarticular allograft reconstruction of the elbow demonstrates neuropathic changes 10 years after insertion **(A,B)**. This was successfully revised with a linked Coonrad/Morrey implant and a Type 2 APC for both the humerus and the ulna **(C,D)**. (*Arrows* in **D** depict the strut of the APC.)

Osteoarticular Allograft

Osteoarticular allograft reconstruction of the elbow has not proven effective long-term due to the inevitable development of neuropathic degeneration (2) (Fig. 35.1).

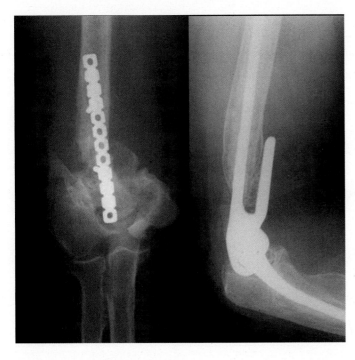

FIGURE 35.2

A patient with failed distal humeral fracture fixation but reasonable host bone is an ideal candidate for an allograft strut without the need for an APC.

Allograft Augmentation

INDICATIONS

- When the loss of bone is relatively mild or not so great as to preclude secure fixation of the implant into host bone
- To stabilize the flange of the prosthetic implant
- At the ulna in order to reconstruct an absent olecranon and to improve the extension strength of the triceps mechanism
- To bridge osseous defects that may have occurred at the time of implant revision

These have a very good rate of incorporation (8–10). Regardless, secure implant fixation into host bone is expected and required (Fig. 35.2).

Allograft Prosthetic Composite

This construct is used when there is a need to obtain implant fixation within a circumferential osseous construct, either at the distal humerus or at the proximal ulna (Fig. 35.3) (4).

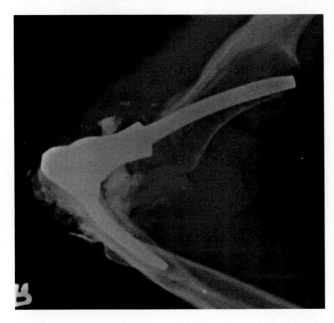

FIGURE 35.3

A patient with osteolysis to such an extent as to preclude fixation within the host bone. In this instance, secure prosthetic fixation within the allograft with the plan to then obtain healing between the allograft and the host is the desired option.

INDICATIONS

The most common underlying problems are a septic or nonseptic failed implant or a posttraumatic situation.

- Circumferential (loss of distal humerus, loss of proximal ulna, loss of both distal humerus and proximal ulna)
- Inability to stabilize with strut or impaction grafting
- Motivated patient
- Extremity required for function
- Significant pain
- Gross instability

CONTRAINDICATIONS

- Recent sepsis.
- Nonfunctional hand.
- Lack of motor power to flex the elbow.

Note: Loss of extension power can be compensated by gravity and is not an absolute contraindication.

- Simpler solutions exist (i.e. direct recementation and use of struts) (Fig. 35.4).

STRUT RECONSTRUCTION

Technique

Patient positioning   The patient is supine on the table. The arm is brought across the chest (Fig. 35.5A).

Incision
1. A posterior skin incision is employed in the majority of instances. As this is often a salvage procedure, prior incisions are followed.

2. Typically wide and thick subcutaneous tissue flaps are raised both medially and laterally but only to the extent needed for the reconstruction (Fig. 35.5B).

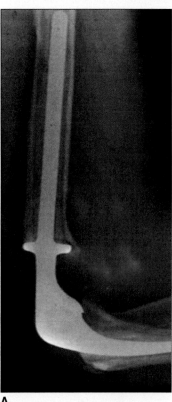 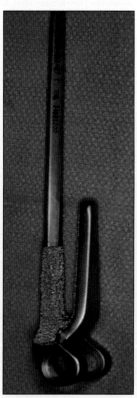 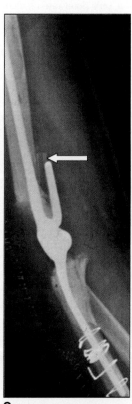

FIGURE 35.4

Failed custom device with loss of distal humeral bone (**A**). Easily reconstructed with recementation of a long flanged device with an anterior strut (arrow) (**B,C**).

A   B   C

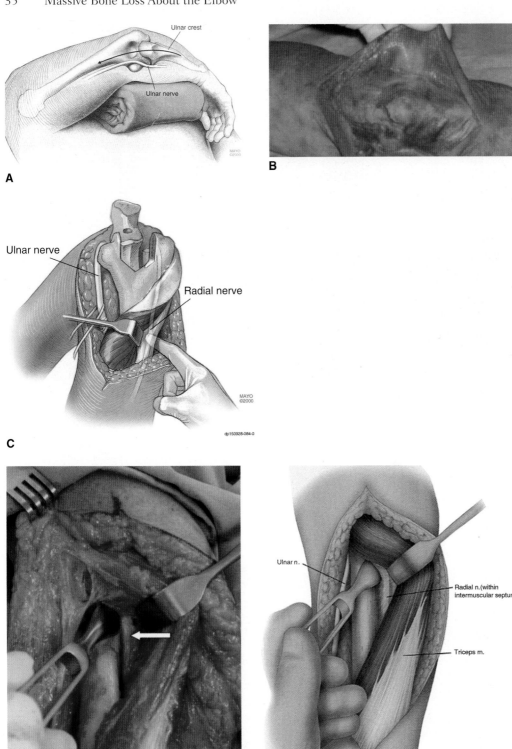

FIGURE 35.5

A: The patient is supine and the arm is brought across the chest. (Morrey BF, Morrey MC, eds. *Relevant surgical exposures, master technqiues in orthopaedic surgery.* Lippincott Williams & Wilkins, with permission.) **B:** Medial and lateral and subcutaneous flaps are elevated. These should be as thick as possible. (Morrey BF, Morrey MC, eds. *Relevant surgical exposures, master technqiues in orthopaedic surgery.* Lippincott Williams & Wilkins, with permission.) **C:** The ulnar nerve is always identified. The radial nerve is identified if the humerus is being revised. (By permission for Mayo Foundation for Medical Education and Research. All rights reserved.) **D:** The radial nerve must be addressed and protected. One technique is to elevate nerve from the humerus by release of the intermuscular septum. (Morrey BF, Morrey MC, eds. *Relevant surgical exposures, master technqiues in orthopaedic surgery.* Lippincott Williams & Wilkins, with permission.)

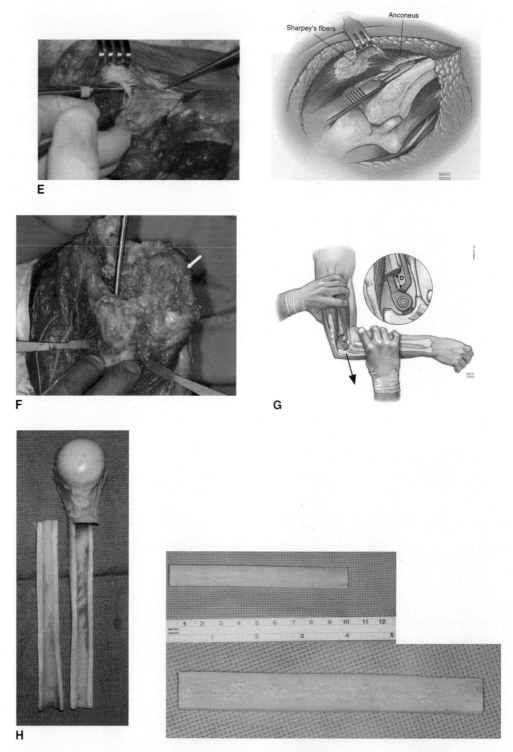

FIGURE 35.5 (*Continued*)

E: The triceps is reflected if the ulna is to be revised. This is done from medial to lateral leaving the anconeus in continuity with the triceps if possible. (Morrey BF, Morrey MC, eds. *Relevant surgical exposures, master technqiues in orthopaedic surgery.* Lippincott Williams & Wilkins, with permission.) **F:** The medullary canal is prepared by identifying the medullary canal of the host bone past the tip of the previous implant. Serial reaming with flexible reamers expands the canal. (Morrey BF, Morrey MC, eds. *Master Techniques in Orthopaedic Surgery: Relevant Surgical Exposures.* Lippincott Williams & Wilkins, with permission.) **G:** The soft tissue tension is demonstrated by the so-called "shuck test." With the elbow in 90 degrees of flexion and the provisional implants in place, a distal force is delivered through the forearm which places tension on the flexor and extensor musculature. The location of the humeral implant with this maneuver is the estimate of the best depth of insertion in order to avoid pistoning of the ulna and allow adequate flexion and extension. (By permission for Mayo Foundation for Medical Education and Research. All rights reserved.) **H:** Either 10 or 15 cm struts are commercially available and may be used. In some instances the graft is harvested from the humerus (smaller graft pictured) and the femoral (larger graft pictured).

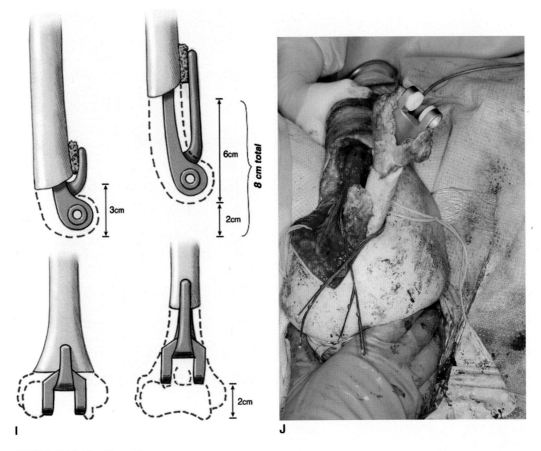

FIGURE 35.5 (*Continued*)

I: Up to 8 cm of distal humerus may be accommodated with simple strut reconstruction associated with the prosthesis. This implies up to 2 cm of shortening is allowed which has been demonstrated not to alter the kinematics of the elbow to any great extent. **J:** The struts are loosely applied to the distal humerus and secured as the cement cures.

Exposure of the Nerves

3. Dissection is started medially where the ulnar nerve is identified at the medial margin of the triceps. In this clinical setting the nerve has usually been translocated but it should be found in the proximal medial aspect of the triceps muscle. If an extensive exposure is necessary to place circumferential wires around the humerus, the nerve is isolated proximally and distally to the extent needed to assure that it is out of the field (Fig. 35.5C). For more proximal exposures of the humerus, the radial nerve is identified and found at the spiral groove. In some instances the radial nerve need not be dissected in detail but simply palpated. It may be retracted by mobilizing the lateral intermuscular septum from medial to lateral (Fig. 35.5D).

Triceps

4. The triceps muscle is left on the ulna if the reconstruction only involves the humerus. If the reconstruction is at the ulna, then the triceps is reflected from the ulna from medial to lateral. Great care is taken to leave the anconeus muscle in continuity (Fig. 35.5E).
5. The implant is removed and the distal aspect of the humerus is identified circumferentially.
6. The soft tissue is reflected from the anterior aspect of the humerus for a distance of at least 6 to 7 cm.
7. For joint replacement, the medullary canal of the humerus is identified and prepared (Fig. 35.5F). The trial implant is inserted at the proper depth. In instances where the joint has been resected, foreshortening the extremity can cause significant tensile stress on the bone cement interface, particularly at the ulna. Therefore, proper tensioning is required. We employ the so-called "shuck" test. This consists of placing the elbow at 90 degrees of flexion and observing the proper depth of insertion of the humeral component when the flexed forearm is displaced distally to the point resisted by the flexors and extensors (Fig. 35.5G).

Struts

8. An anterior strut reconstruction is predicated on the concept that the flange of the implant will be stabilized by the anterior strut and that the anterior strut will eventually heal to the host humerus. Allograft struts measuring 10 to 15 mm in width and 7 to 18 cm in length are applied to the anterior humerus (Fig. 35.5H). Depending on the length, the strut is stabilized with a No. 16 gauge wire. At least two circumferential wires are placed around

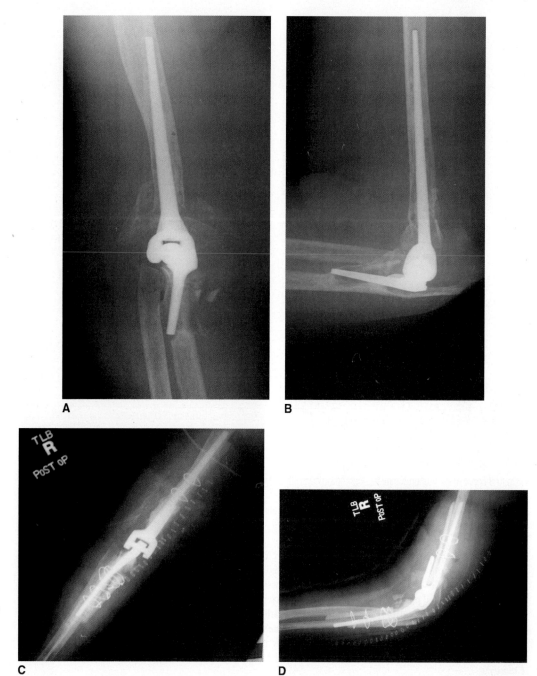

FIGURE 35.6

This 59-year-old female had an elbow replacement for rheumatoid arthritis and sustained a periprosthetic fracture **(A,B)** secondary to loosening. This was successfully managed with an anterior humeral strut and anterior/posterior ulnar strut **(C,D)**.

the graft proximal flange. If up to 8 cm of distal humerus has been lost, the long flanged humeral component is required. In instances in which less than 4 cm has been lost, then a standard flange is sufficient (Fig. 35.5I).

9. The medullary canal is irrigated and dried, a plug is inserted, and the cement is delivered with an injector system. The implant is then inserted to the previous defined depth. After the cement has hardened and excess has been removed, the ulnar component is cemented in place and the joint is articulated. Careful assessment of elbow flexion and extension and the tendency for pistoning of the ulnar implant with respect to the ulna is observed with the elbow in full flexion and full extension (Fig. 35.5J).

A clinical example is demonstrated (Fig. 35.6).

RESULTS

Former experience using struts for massive bone defects has not been documented. It is known, however, that struts used for periprosthetic fractures at the humerus heal in approximately 90% of instances (10). At the ulna, ulnar struts were reported in 22 instances for various ulnar pathologies. Once again the healing rate of the strut was reported as 91%. Overall, augmentation with allograft struts appears to be a viable option for the properly selected patient.

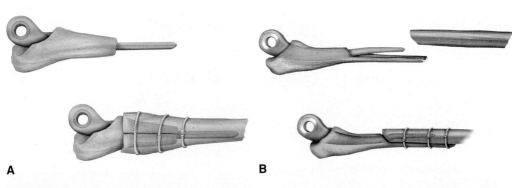

FIGURE 35.7

Three types of APC have been recognized. **A:** Circumferential graft is inserted within the expanded canal. The host bone may need to be split in order to be tightly collapsed with circumferential wires around the allograft. **B:** The implant is secured in the circumferential portion of the allograft. The distal or proximal portion is then slit creating a strut which is employed to secure the allograft to the host bone. Typically, the stem of the implant will bridge the allograft and be secured within the host bone as well. **C:** The side-to-side coaptation at the ulna. The triangular ulna is nicely matched with the triangular fibula which is the preferred graft for the ulna. For the humerus a section of circumferential allograft is removed in order to enhance the coaptation.

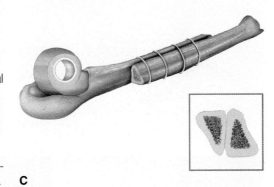

ALLOGRAFT PROSTHETIC COMPOSITE

Selection and Preparation

Three types of APC have been identified and employed in our practice (Fig. 35.7).

Type 1 is a circumferential graft into which the implant is inserted. A circumferential graft is then inserted into the expanded portion of host bone. The host bone is collapsed around the allograft with circumferential wires which, in turn, stabilizes implant (Fig. 35.7A).

Type 2 is a circumferential graft used proximally at the ulna or distally at the humerus. The distal portion of the graft is split, and the remaining portion of the cortical split is used as a strut in continuity. The implant is inserted through the circumferential portion of the APC and then into the canal of the host bone (Fig. 35.7B). The strut continues along the host bone and is secured with wire.

Type 3 is when the entire implant is cemented into a circumferential fibular or ulnar allograft, which is then grafted to the host ulna. A cadaver humerus is used to graft to the native humerus. The bones are opposed and stabilized with cerclage wires (Fig. 35.7C). In some instances, a narrow section may be removed from the humeral graft to provide better apposition and contact of the host bone.

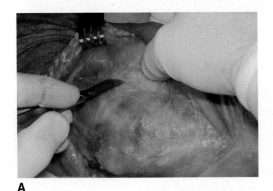

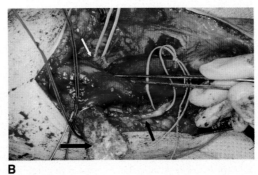

FIGURE 35.8

Humerus. **A:** The skin incision is extensive, following the previous incision. It usually has to be extended proximally or distally in order to address the bone deficiency. When necessary, the radial and ulnar nerves are identified and tagged. For the APC, the radial nerve is at greatest risk. **B:** When the defect is in the humerus, the triceps is left on the ulna and the humerus is "delivered" to the lateral or medial aspect of the extensor mechanism.

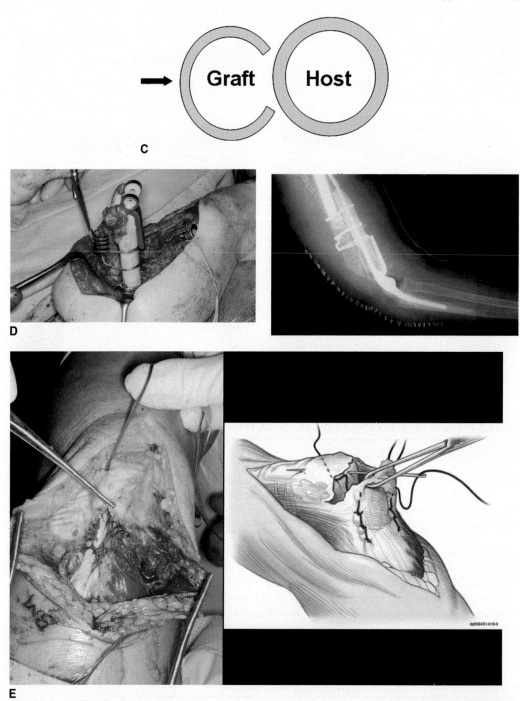

FIGURE 35.8 (*Continued*)

C: A section of bone may be removed from the humerus allograft in order for a better fit to the round humerus host bone.
D: The APC is secured to the host bone with circumferential wires. At least three wires are usually required for secure fixation.
E: If the triceps is deficient, a locking stitch is used in order to imbricate or otherwise stabilize the triceps mechanism. "By permission for Mayo Foundation for Medical Education and Research. All rights reserved."

Technique

1. *Patient Positioning*: The patient is positioned supine on the table. The arm is brought across the chest.
2. *Skin Incision*: A long skin incision is required to provide adequate exposure.
3. The nerves must be identified if the radial or ulnar nerve is symptomatic before the surgery. The nerves should be isolated with an effort to decrease the neurogenic symptoms. Identification of the nerves either by direct dissection or by palpation is absolutely necessary in this type of revision surgery (Fig. 35.8A).
4. *Triceps*. If the pathology involves the distal humerus, the triceps is left on the ulna or what remains of the ulna (Fig. 35.8B). If the pathology principally involves the ulna, elevate the soft tissue from medial to lateral

once the location of the ulnar nerve has been confirmed. In many instances, the triceps mechanism has been violated or is marginally competent; nonetheless, it is maintained in continuity for the ulnar reconstruction.

5. Allograft composite application (Humerus).

   Distal humerus. One of the three variations of APC reconstructions discussed above (see Fig. 35.7) is used to address deficiencies at the humerus.

   A. Intussusception

   The native host bone must be well secured to the APC. The key is for the host bone to heal to the APC. The surface between this composite and the host is critical. Hence, the canal of the host bone must be free of all membrane and fibrous material in order to enhance chance of incorporation. In some instances composite fixation may be used. This involves cementing a portion of the stem while osseous integration is anticipated through the remainder of the composite.

   B. Strut in Continuity with Circumferential Graft

   This is an effective means of bypassing deficient bone and reinforcing the native construct. The implant is securely cemented in the allograft and the strut provides a reliable fixation to the host bone. It is stabilized by monofilament wire.

   C. Side to Side

   If this construct is employed at the humerus, removal of a linear portion of the cortex of the graft enhances the likelihood of incorporation (Fig. 35.8C).

6. *Fixation*. For the humerus, 16- to 18- gauge monofilament wire is preferred. Cables are avoided: they are expensive, abrade soft tissue, are more prominent in a subcutaneous position and can harbor bacteria (Fig. 35.8D).

7. *Depth of Insertion*. The soft tissues are carefully assessed to determine the proper level of the axis of rotation. The tension of the tissues anteriorly and posteriorly is the first step in defining the depth of insertion (see Fig. 35.5G).

8. *Triceps*. If the triceps has been detached, it is securely repaired to the ulna or to the ulnar APC depending upon the nature of the pathology. A No. 5 nonabsorbable suture is employed for this purpose. Locking stitches are placed in the triceps mechanism in order to stabilize the tissue (Fig. 35.8E).

9. *Closure*. The closure is routine. The tourniquet is deflated prior to closure. A drain is not routinely used unless a hematoma is expected.

After Care

This is determined according to the expectation of osseous integration. A well fitted brace is sometimes prescribed in order to enhance the potential for osseous integration. Typically, fixation is considered adequate to allow passive assisted motion by 2 weeks, motion against gravity from 2 to 8 weeks, 1 to 2 lb of lifting from 8 to 12 weeks and then the typical restriction of 2 lb repetitive, 10 lb single event after 3 months if there has been radiographic confirmation of incorporation.

ULNA RECONSTRUCTION

The same three types of APC have been used for the ulna. In some instances, the ulnar stem may need to be bent in order to negotiate and enter the host bone from the APC.

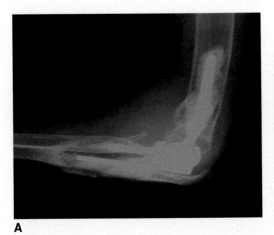

A

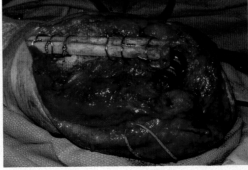

B

FIGURE 35.9

Ulna. At the ulna, osteolysis (**A**) is addressed with strut grafts that may be extended proximally in order to provide a lever arm for reconstruction of the sleeve of triceps mechanism (**B**).

FIGURE 35.10

The flat surface of the right fibula allograft nicely coapts to
the flat surface of the lateral aspect of the host ulna.

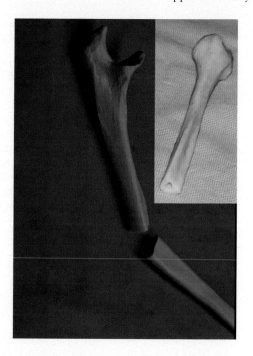

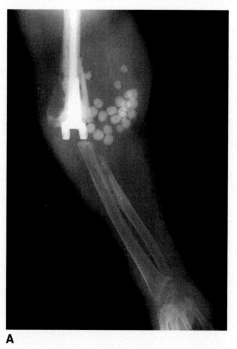

A

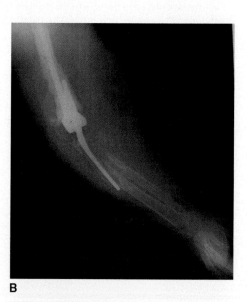

B

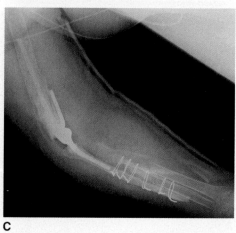

C

FIGURE 35.11

An allograft fibula used as a Type 3 ulnar graft. An infected revision (**A**) had failed a salvage revision implantation into the radius
(**B**). This was finally salvaged with a Type 3 APC fibula to ulna
side-to-side onlay graft (**C**).

Olecranon

In virtually all instances of APC at the ulna, the olecranon is deficient. The APC is carefully extended in order to restore the lever arm of the olecranon (Fig. 35.9). Side to side fixation is best accomplished at the ulna with a fibula allograft. Care is taken to prepare the surface of the allograft so as to broaden the contact with the host bone. The flat medial side of the right ulna nicely receives the flat surface of the left fibula (Fig. 35.10).

RESULTS

The outcome of 13 patients undergoing APC at Mayo was originally reviewed by Mansat et al. With an average of 42 months surveillance, the Mayo Elbow Performance Score revealed 4 excellent, 3 good, 1 fair, and 5 poor results. Nine of the thirteen patients had minimal pain. The mean arc of flexion was 97 degrees but five patients required a second procedure. The most common indication was infection which occurred in four patients. Since this report, a revised approach to the APC has been developed. The clinical results of the newer techniques shown here are under investigation. To date we have had one fracture of a healed Type 3 APC (Fig. 35.11). Preliminary assessment of 22 cases operated on from 2005 to 2009 reveal only one failure to date. This study is ongoing (11).

REFERENCES

1. Voloshin I, Schippert DW, Kakar S, et al. Complications of total elbow replacement: A systematic review. *J Shoulder Elbow Surg*. 2010. In press.
2. Dean GS, Holliger EH, Urbaniak JR. Elbow allograft for reconstruction of the elbow with massive bone loss. Long term results. *Clin Orthop*. 1997;341:12–22.
3. Figgie HE, Inglis AE, Mow C. Total elbow arthroplasty in the face of significant bone stock or soft tissue losses: Preliminary results of custom-fit arthroplasty. *J Arthroplasty*. 1986;1:71.
4. Mansat P, Adams RA, Morrey BF. Allograft-prosthesis composite for revision of catastrophic failure of total elbow arthroplasty. *J Bone Joint Surg*. 2004;86A(4):724–735.
5. Morrey BF, Sanchez-Sotelo J. Revision of failed total elbow arthroplasty with osseous deficiency. In: Morrey BF, Sanchez-Sotelo J, eds. *The elbow and its disorders*. 4th ed. Philadelphia, PA: Saunders/Elsevier, 2009:899–910.
6. Zakardas PC, Cass B, Throckmorton T, et al. Long-term outcome of resection arthroplasty for the failed total elbow arthroplasty. *J Bone Joint Surg Am*. 2010.
7. Loebenberg MI, Adams RA, O'Driscoll SW, et al. Impaction grafting in revision total elbow arthroplasty. *J Bone Joint Surg*. 2005;87A(1):99–106, 2005.
8. Blackley HR, Davis AM, Hutchison CR, et al. Proximal femoral allografts for reconstruction of bone stock in revision arthroplasty of the hip. A 9 to 15 year follow-up. *J Bone Joint Surg*. 2001;83A(3):346–354.
9. Kamineni S, Adams R, Morrey B. Strut graft for ulnar revision. *J Bone Joint Surg*. 2000.
10. Sanchez-Sotelo J, O'Driscoll S, Morrey BF. Periprosthetic humeral fractures after total elbow arthroplasty: treatment with implant revision and strut allograft augmentation. *J Bone Joint Surg*. 2002;84A(9):1642–1650.
11. Morrey M, Sanchez-Sotelo J, Morrey B. Allograft prosthetic composite: current concepts. In preparation, 2010.
12. Ullmark G, Sorensen J, Langstrom B, et al. Bone regeneration six years after impaction bone grafting: A PET analysis. *Acta Orthop*. 2007;78(2):201–205.

36 Distal Radius Osteoarticular Allograft

Miguel A. Ayerza, Luis A. Aponte-Tinao, and D. Luis Muscolo

Osteoarticular allografts of the distal part of the radius replace an articular surface for which prostheses are notreadily available. The reconstruction of distal radius after tumor resections, preserving wrist stability and function, is limited. Osteoarticular allografts are utilized for reconstruction of one side of the joint after tumor resection. Osteoarticular allografts do not sacrifice the side of the joint that is not compromised by the tumor, they can replace articular surfaces for which prostheses are not readily available, such as the distal radius, and can be attached to soft tissues.

INDICATIONS

- The procedure is appropriate for the treatment of a massive osteoarticular defect after tumor resection or massive traumatic bone losses of the distal radius (Figs. 36.1 and 36.2).
- At least one of the two major neurovascular bundles, the radial or the ulnar artery, must be free of tumor.
- The distal ulnar epiphysis must remain intact with its ligamentous insertions.
- Appropriate soft tissue coverage.

CONTRAINDICATIONS

- Patients with sarcomas in whom preoperative imaging studies demonstrate evidence of intra-articular compromise of the tumor.

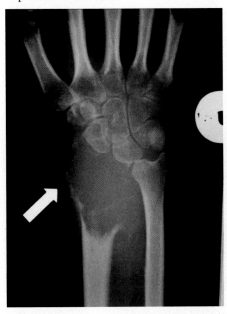

FIGURE 36.1

Anteroposterior radiograph of the distal forearm showing a giant cell tumor in the distal radius.

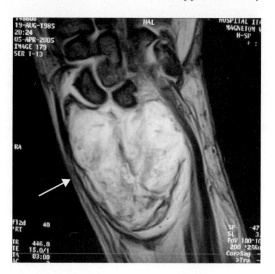

FIGURE 36.2

Coronal magnetic resonance image that illustrates the
extent of the tumor.

- Inadequate host soft tissue to reconstruct the defect.
- Patients with cartilage degenerative disease of the wrist.
- Absence of the distal ulna or ligament insertions.

PREOPERATIVE PREPARATION: ALLOGRAFT SELECTION

Fresh-frozen allografts are obtained and stored according to a technique that has been previously described (1).
Poor anatomical matching of both size and shape between the host defect and the graft can significantly alter joint
kinematics and load distribution, leading to bone resorption or joint degeneration. To improve accuracy in size
matching between the donor and the host, we developed measurable parameters based on CT scans of the distal
radius. In the axial view of the distal radius, we measure the maximum total width and anteroposterior width of
the radius. The allograft is selected on the basis of a comparison of these measures with those of the host.

TECHNIQUE

All operations are performed in a clean-air enclosure with vertical airflow and usually with regional anesthesia. The
patient is placed on the operating table in the supine position and an arm table is added with the upper limb placed
in position. A long dorsal incision is made following the third metacarpal, and the extensor tendons are exposed
(Fig. 36.3). Once these tendons are dissected, the wrist joint is identified and a dorsal carpal arthrotomy is performed
(Figs. 36.4 and 36.5). The biopsy track is left in continuity with the specimen. The distal radioulnar joint is identified and sectioned near the radius insertion to ensure that there is enough host tissue to reconstruct these ligaments
to the allograft. Palmar radio scaphoid ligaments are sectioned in the same fashion in order to preserve enough
host tissue for reconstruction. If there is an extraosseous tumor component, a cuff of normal muscle (i.e., pronator
quadrates) must be included in the resection. An osteotomy of the radius proximal to the tumor is performed at the
appropriate location as determined on the basis of the preoperative imaging studies. All remaining soft tissues at the
level of the transection are cleared. After the posterior and medial structures have been protected and retracted, the
osteotomy is performed perpendicular to the long axis of the radius (Fig. 36.6). Following the osteotomy, the distal
radius is pulled dorsally in order to expose the soft tissue attachments of the palmar space (Fig. 36.7). These palmar
soft tissue structures are transected and the distal radius is then passed off the operative field (Fig. 36.8).

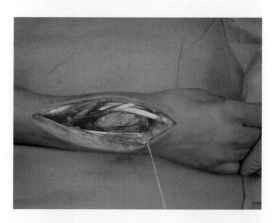

FIGURE 36.3

Intraoperative photograph that shows the extended
dorsal approach that is employed.

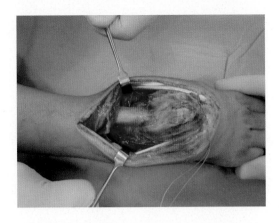

FIGURE 36.4

Intraoperative photograph showing wide exposure of the distal radius before the arthrotomy is performed.

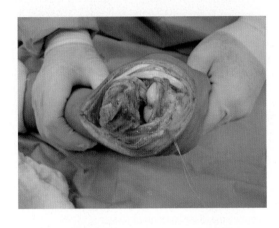

FIGURE 36.5

Intraoperative photograph obtained when the dorsal carpal arthrotomy is performed.

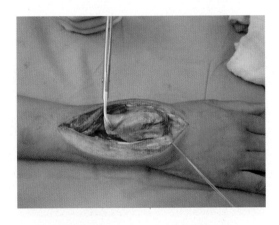

FIGURE 36.6

Intraoperative photograph made after the radius osteotomy is done.

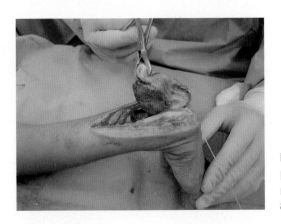

FIGURE 36.7

Intraoperative radiograph illustrating how the distal radius is pulled dorsally to expose anterior soft tissue attachments following the diaphyseal osteotomy.

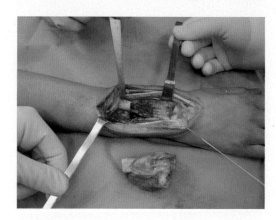

FIGURE 36.8

Intraoperative radiograph made after the distal radius is resected, showing the osteoarticular defect.

Simultaneous with the tumor resection, the allograft specimen is prepared on the back table. The graft is taken out of the plastic packaging and placed directly in a warm normal saline solution without antibiotics. After being thawed, the allograft is cut to the proper length and soft tissue structures such as the volar and dorsal capsule (Fig. 36.9) and the radioulnar ligaments are prepared for implantation (Fig. 36.10). It is crucial for joint reconstruction to have adequate soft tissue structures in order to repair them to the corresponding host tissues.

After resection of the tumor, the allograft is inspected to confirm that the size is appropriate and no degenerative changes are present (Fig. 36.11). Then the insertion of the allograft segment tailored to fit the bone defect is performed. In order to restore the anatomic relationship of the distal radioulnar joint, we repair the volar and dorsal ligaments by suturing corresponding tissues between the allograft and the host (Figs. 36.12 and 36.13).

We repair the palmar capsule suturing autologous capsular tissues to the capsular tissues provided by the allograft with two number-1 nonabsorbable sutures (Fig. 36.14). After the palmar capsular tissues are secured, the dorsal capsule is repaired suturing autologous tissues to those tissues provided by the allograft (Fig. 36.15).

Fitting the osteotomy between the host and donor in close apposition is a crucial step (Fig. 36.16), but the anatomic relationship of distal radioulnar joint should also be established. For that purpose, the radius allograft osteotomy should be performed considering proper alignment of the distal radioulnar joint.

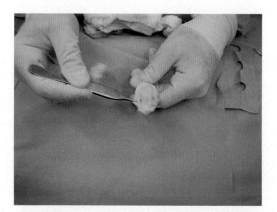

FIGURE 36.9

Intraoperative photograph after the donor graft has been thawed showing volar and dorsal capsule retained on the allograft for the joint reconstruction.

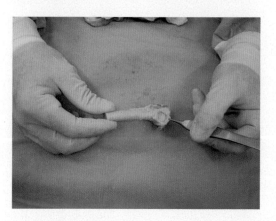

FIGURE 36.10

Intraoperative photograph of the graft showing adequate radioulnar ligaments that are prepared for implantation.

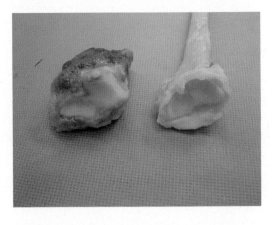

FIGURE 36.11

Intraoperative photograph after resection of the tumor that shows how the distal radius transplant is inspected to confirm that the size is appropriate and that no degenerative changes are present in the allograft.

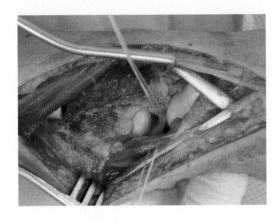

FIGURE 36.12

Intraoperative photograph that illustrates how host radioulnar ligaments are prepared for implantation.

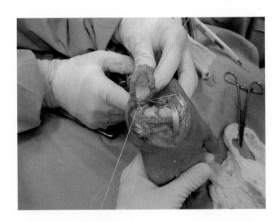

FIGURE 36.13

Intraoperative photograph made when the radioulnar joint is repaired suturing remnant ligaments from the host with the ligaments provided on the allograft.

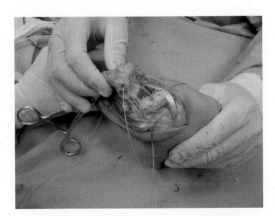

FIGURE 36.14

Intraoperative photograph made when the anterior and posterior capsule and ligaments of the host are repaired with the corresponding allograft tissues.

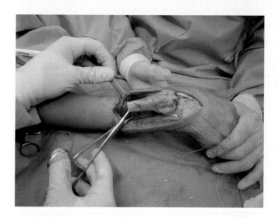

FIGURE 36.15

Intraoperative photograph after joint reconstruction of the wrist is completed.

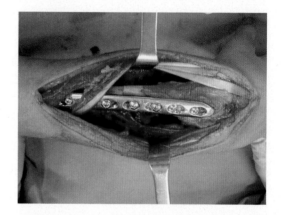

FIGURE 36.16

Intraoperative photograph showing the osteotomy junction between the host and allograft in close apposition, with adequate compression after internal fixation when the posterior plate is applied.

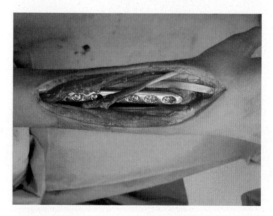

FIGURE 36.17

Intraoperative photograph showing that the plate is placed in order to cover as much length of the allograft as possible.

When the cortical bone is avascular, as on the allograft side, absolute stability offers the best conditions and chance for healing. The diaphyseal osteotomy is stabilized by internal fixation with a dorsal plate (Fig. 36.17) and, in order to minimize the risk of fracture, this buttress plate fixation should cover as much length of the allograft as possible.

One suction drain is inserted after lavage of the wound with saline solution, and a meticulous suture repair of the tendon sheds (peritenon) is performed. A layered closure of the subcutaneous tissues and skin is then completed.

POSTOPERATIVE MANAGEMENT

After reconstruction, the wrist is placed in neutral position and secured with a splint. After 2 days, the drain is removed and the wound is inspected. Ice or a cryotherapy device is used to help minimize postoperative swelling and discomfort. The goals during the first postoperative week are to minimize swelling. Passive flexion-extension exercises are started 2 weeks postoperatively with the goal of obtaining at least 30 degrees of flexion and 30 degrees of extension. After 3 weeks, gentle active pronation and supination exercises are initiated. At 4 weeks postoperatively, active-assisted wrist motion is initiated until full active extension and flexion are obtained.

PEARLS AND PITFALLS

- The procedure is best performed by an orthopedic oncologic surgeon with experience in hand/wrist surgery.
- All previous biopsy sites and all potentially contaminated tissues, including any needle biopsy tracks, should be removed en bloc.
- Poor anatomic matching of the size and shape of the allograft to the host defect significantly alters joint kinematics and load distribution, potentially leading to bone resorption or joint instability and degeneration.
- Reconstruction of the ligaments and joint capsule must be meticulous and precise since the longevity of these grafts is related, in part, to the stability of the reconstructed joint.
- Care must be taken to avoid malalignment that will put greater stress on the allograft cartilage.
- Uniform cortical contact, compression of the osteotomy gap, and rotational stability were noted to be better when internal fixation with plates and screws were used.
- To obtain a solid allograft construct, the internal fixation should span the entire length of the allograft.
- A locking compression plate is now used for the majority of our patients since greater mechanical stability of the reconstruction is obtained.

COMPLICATIONS

Osteoarticular allografts in the upper limb are used less frequently than other types of osteoarticular allografts. Although there are few reports of distal radius osteoarticular allografts, the orthopedic surgeon should expect similar complications as with other osteoarticular allografts such as allograft fractures and resorption, cartilage degeneration, joint instability, and delayed bone union or nonunion (Fig. 36.18) (1,2).

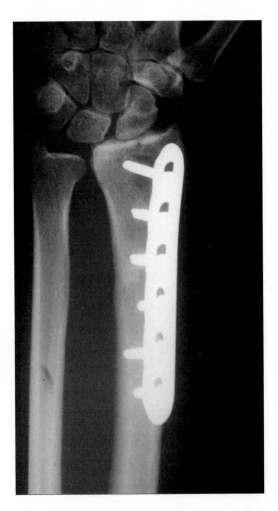

FIGURE 36.18

Anteroposterior radiograph 3 years after distal radius osteoarticular allograft reconstruction.

RESULTS

Osteoarticular allografts of the distal part of the radius replace an articular surface for which prostheses are not readily available. Kocher et al. (3) reported on 24 patients who had a reconstruction of the distal aspect of the radius with an osteoarticular allograft, done mostly after resection of a giant cell tumor. Eight eventually needed a revision, most frequently due to a fracture (four patients) or wrist pain (two patients). There were 14 other complications necessitating additional operative management. Of the 16 patients in whom the graft survived, 3 had no functional limitations, 9 reported limitations only with strenuous activities, and 4 had limitations in the ability to perform moderate activities. Bianchi et al. (4) retrospectively analyzed 12 patients with osteoarticular allografts of the distal radius. They reported one nonunion and eight distal radioulnar joint instabilities. Although they found subchondral bone alterations and joint narrowing in all cases, a painful reconstruction occurred in only one patient. They found a mean range of motion of 51 degrees of flexion and 37 degrees of extension. Szabo et al. (5) reported nine osteoarticular allograft reconstructions combined with a Sauve-Kapandji procedure after distal radius resection. Examination showed an average of 51 degrees of extension and 19 degrees of flexion of the wrist and 63 degrees of supination and 79 degrees of pronation of the forearm. Grip strength measured an average of 23 kg in five patients.

REFERENCES

1. Muscolo DL, Ayerza M, Aponte-Tinao LA. Massive allograft used in orthopaedics oncology. *Orthop Clin North Am.* 2006;37:65–74.
2. Mankin HJ, Gebhardt MC, Jennings LC, et al. Long-term results of allograft replacement in the management of bone tumors. *Clin Orthop.* 1996;324:86–97.
3. Kocher MS, Gebhardt MC, Manhin HJ. Reconstruction of the distal aspect of the radius with use of an osteoarticular allograft after excision of a skeletal tumor. *J Bone Joint Surg.* 1998;80A:407–419.
4. Bianchi G, Donati D, Staals EL, et al. Osteoarticular allograft reconstruction of the distal radius after bone tumor resection. *J Hand Surg [Br].* 2005;30:369–73.
5. Szabo RM, Anderson KA, Chen JL. Functional outcome of en bloc excision and osteoarticular allograft replacement with the Sauve-Kapandji procedure for Campanacci grade 3 giant-cell tumor of the distal radius. *J Hand Surg [Am].* 2006;31:1340–1348.

Index

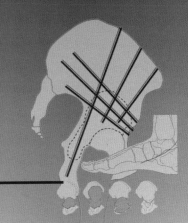

Note: Page numbers in *italics* indicate figures. Page numbers followed by t denote tables.